Backpacking Idaho

D0149739

From the book...

St. Joe River-Bacon Peak Loop (Trip 3)

A bonus of taking this trip in late August or early September is the chance to feast on the acres of huckleberries that carpet the ridges around Bacon Peak.

White Cap Creek (Trip 6)

Very rugged cross-country side trips provide access to several more lakes, meadows, and forests, so you can enjoy the solitude here for as long as your food and vacation time hold out.

Snake River Trail (Trip 7)

Your efforts are rewarded by the superb scenery, which features a continuous series of amazing views of the raging river, the ruggedly contorted canyon walls, and even occasional glimpses of the high Summit Ridge in Oregon.

Chamberlain Basin Loop (Trip 10)

One night I lay in my sleeping bag for almost an hour listening to wolves howl—a classic wilderness experience that I will not soon forget.

Middle Fork Salmon River (Trip 13)

Like all of the hot springs in this canyon, this is a great place to spend some time soaking sore muscles and enjoying the scenery.

Loon Creek Loop (Trip 14)

The jagged peaks here rise above 10,000 feet and are made up of a stunningly beautiful collage of gray, white, and reddish rocks. When you add this colorful geology to the area's cirque lakes, clear streams, and flower-covered meadows, you have a great place to go for a backpacking vacation.

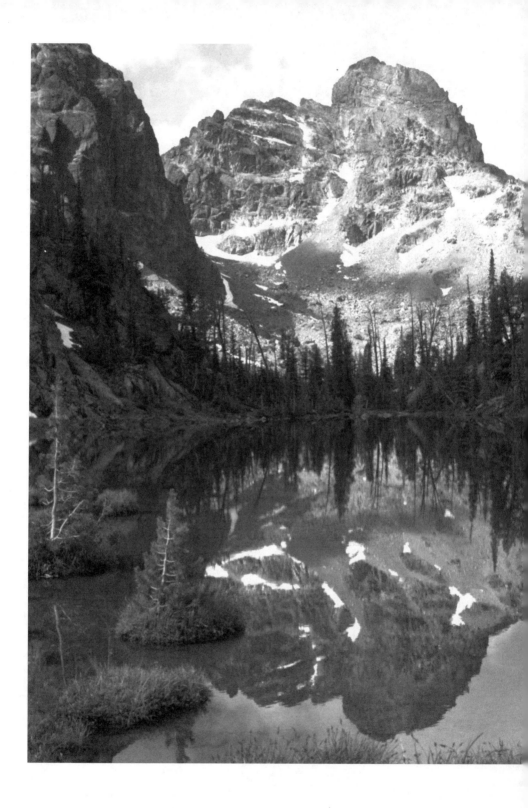

Backpacking
IDAHO

From
Alpine Peaks
to Desert Canyons

Douglas Lorain

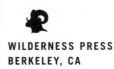

WILDERNESS PRESS
BERKELEY, CA

Backpacking Idaho

1st EDITION March 2004

Copyright © 2004 by Douglas Lorain

Front & back cover photos copyright © 2004 by Douglas Lorain
Interior photos by Douglas Lorain
Maps: Douglas Lorain
Cover design: Andreas Schueller
Book design: Andreas Schueller and Jaan Hitt

ISBN 0-89997-346-9
UPC 7-19609-97346-1

Manufactured in the United States of America

Published by: **Wilderness Press**
1200 5th Street
Berkeley, CA 94710
(800) 443-7227; FAX (510) 558-1696
info@wildernesspress.com
www.wildernesspress.com

Visit our website for a complete listing of our books and for ordering information.

Cover photos: Castle and Merriam peaks, White Cloud Peaks *(front)*;
Buffalo Hump over Hump Lake, Gospel Hump Wilderness *(back)*
Frontispiece: He Devil over tarn near Sheep lake, Seven Devils Mountains

SAFETY NOTICE: Although Wilderness Press and the author have made every attempt to ensure that the information in this book is accurate at press time, they are not responsible for any loss, damage, injury, or inconvenience that may occur to anyone while using this book. You are responsible for your own safety and health while in the wilderness. The fact that a trail is described in this book does not mean that it will be safe for you. Be aware that trail conditions can change from day to day. Always check local conditions and know your own limitations.

Acknowledgments

The help of many people made this book possible. First of all, I would like to thank the many wilderness rangers and fellow hikers who provided trip companionship and recommendations.

Special thanks go to the following persons:

My occasional hiking partner – Dave Elsbernd.

My friends – Bob, Barbara, and Natalie Fink, who graciously provided this dirty, bedraggled author with a place to shower, do laundry, and resupply on one of my long trips while doing research for this book.

My family – my parents Bob and Nancy Lorain, and my sister, Christine Ebrahimi, for putting up with the worry over my solo months-long backpacking sojourns into the remote Idaho back-country, for which I could provide no itinerary or date for my return.

As usual, my sister was invaluable in providing answers for all questions botanical.

Garth Barrow and the friendly young men of Boy Scout Troop 152 in Rigby, Idaho (Travis Ihler, Aaron Nelson, Matt Anderson, Tyson Aeschbacher, Brad Butikofer, and Dustin Berry) who kindly provided this tired hiker with much needed transport that saved me many miles of arduous road walking during a spell of record 100-degree weather.

Forest Service and Park Service personnel, who provided information, read drafts, or otherwise shared their considerable expertise – Duane Annis, Stacy Baker, Earl Baumgarten, Paul Christensen, Cathy Conover, Dennis Duehren, Carol Eckert, Kearstin Edwards, Jason Fisher, Michael Foster, Melissa Fowler, Tracy Gravelle, Pat Hart, Sheri Hughes, Donald L. Kole, Ivan Kowski, Gary Loomis, Laurie Matthews, Joni Packard, and Ann Schwaller.

While the contributions and assistance of the persons listed above were invaluable, all of the text, maps, and photos herein are my own work and sole responsibility. Any and all omissions, errors, and just plain stupid mistakes are strictly mine.

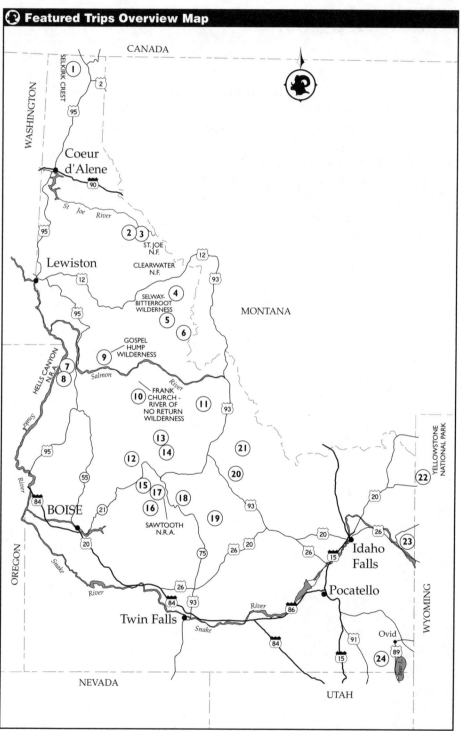

Contents

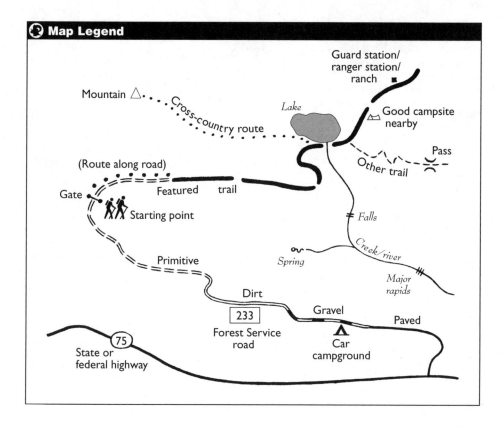

Map Legend

Mountain △

Cross-country route

Lake

Guard station/
ranger station/
ranch

Good campsite
nearby

(Route along road)

Pass

Other trail

Gate

Featured   trail

Starting point

Falls

Creek/river

Primitive

Spring

Major
rapids

Dirt

233

Forest Service
road

Gravel

Paved

75

State or
federal highway

Car
campground

Featured Trips Summary Chart

TRIP	RATINGS (1-10) SCENERY	SOLITUDE	DIFFICULTY	DAYS	MILES	ELEVATION GAIN
Best In -						
April and May:						
7 Snake River Trail	10	6	6	4-7	54	5300
June:						
5 Selway River Trail	7	5	5	4-6	50	4200
21 Central Lemhi Range Loop	8	9	8	4-6	45	10,300
20 Lost River Range Traverse	10	9	8	3-5	24	7300
8 Seven Devils Loop	8	6	5	2-4	28	4400
July:						
24 Bear River Range Highline Trail	8	7	5	3-4	25	2800
4 Warm Springs Creek Loop	6	7	7	3-4	32	5000
10 Chamberlain Basin Loop	5	7	7	4-7	50	10,300
12 Soldier Lakes Loop	7	6	7	3-5	40	7300
11 Bighorn Crags	9	4	6	3-6	46	9000
1 Long Canyon Loop	7	6	6	3-4	34	7500
16 Queens River Loop	9	7	5	3-4	31	5800
19 Pioneer Mountains Traverse	9	8	6	3-4	26	8200
15 Grand Sawtooths Loop	9	3	6	5-9	63	12,200
14 Loon Creek Loop	8	8	7	3-4	27	6100
August:						
17 Pettit Lake-Hell Roaring Loop	9	3	5	3-4	30	6000
6 White Cap Creek	6	8	5	5-7	52	5500
18 White Cloud Peaks Loop	10	5	8	3-5	28	5900
3 St. Joe River - Bacon Peak Loop	6	7	6	3-4	31	5000
22 Bechler River Trails	7	3	3	3-5	41	1700
September and October:						
2 Snow Peak - Mallard Larkins Loop	7	5	9	3-5	34	10,100
9 Gospel Hump Loop	7	8	10	5-8	68	12,600
13 Middle Fork Salmon River	7	6	6	6-8	67	4200
23 Snake River Range Traverse	8	6	8	3-6	45	9800

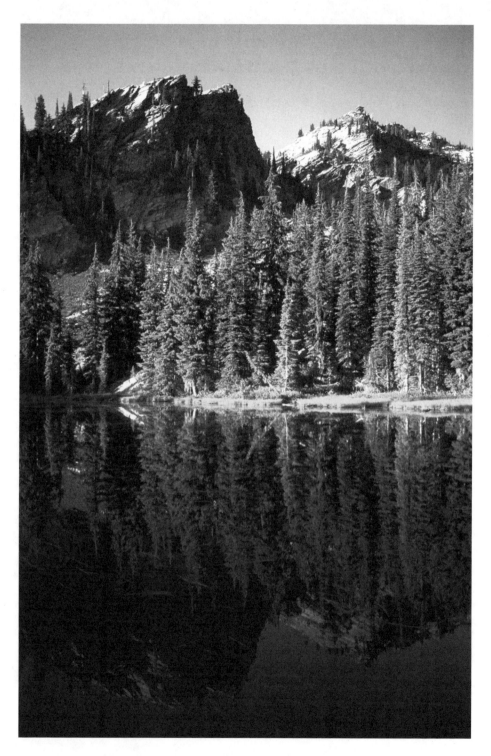

Snow Peak over Snow Peak Pond, Trip 2

Introduction

Idaho is a virtually undiscovered backpacker's paradise. Although the state has millions of acres of wilderness, it has no national parks and few well-known destinations to draw the crowds. As a result, Idaho remains a great place to "get away from it all."

What all those crowds heading for more famous hiking areas don't realize is that Idaho hides some of North America's most beautiful scenery. The mountains of Idaho are at least as scenic as anything found elsewhere in the American West and, in fact, they are far better than most. The canyon country is great too and is, if possible, even more spectacular than the mountains. These great gashes in the earth are incomparable in their depth, their scenic grandeur, and the abundance of their wildlife.

Idaho's nearly ideal climate helps to make exploring the state's natural wonders a joy. The weather here is consistently better than in bordering geographic regions, with fewer thunderstorms than in the Rocky Mountain states to the south and east, and much less rain than in soggy Oregon and Washington to the west. So Idaho boasts the ideal combination of solitude, outstanding scenery, and good weather — in other words, Shangri-La for backpackers.

There are many ways to see and appreciate the beauty of Idaho. Many parts of the state can be seen just as easily on dayhikes, rafting trips, bicycle tours, or even from your car. The focus of *this* book, however, is on the best ways for *backpackers* to see the state. Most of Idaho's best scenery is far from roads and can be truly appreciated only by those willing to hit the trails. After many years and thousands of trail miles, I have selected what I believe to be Idaho's very best backpacking trips. The focus is on *longer* trips — from 3 days to 2 weeks. These are beyond a simple weekend outing, but they make *terrific* vacations, and give you enough time to fully appreciate the scenery. Best of all, you'll have the chance to really get to know and love the state.

HOW TO USE THIS GUIDE

Each featured trip begins with an information box that provides a quick overview of the hike's vital statistics and important features.

This lets you rapidly narrow down your options based on your preferences, your abilities, how many days you have available, and the time of year.

Scenery

This is a subjective opinion of the trip's overall scenic quality, on a 1 (an eyesore) to 10 (absolutely gorgeous) scale. This rating reflects my personal biases in favor of flowers, photogenic views, and clear

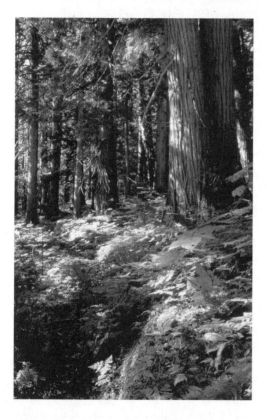

streams. If your tastes run more toward lush forests or rolling grasslands, then your own rating may be quite different. Also keep in mind that the rating is a *relative* one. **All** the featured trips are beautiful, and if they were located almost anywhere else in North America would justifiably draw crowds of admirers.

Solitude

Since solitude is one of the things that backpackers are seeking, it helps to know roughly how much company you can expect. This rating is also on a 1 (bring stilts to see over the crowds) to 10 (just you and the mountain goats) scale. It is worth noting, however, that by comparison to almost any other state, the Idaho backcountry is remarkably free of crowds. With few exceptions, it is rare to see more than one or two other

Along Long Canyon Trail, Selkirk Mountains, Trip 1

parties during a full day of hiking. In the years of research for this book, I spent hundreds of memorable nights camped near scenic lakes, fish-filled streams, or other idyllic locations throughout

Idaho, and more than 75% of the time I had these choice spots all to myself. Hikers who are accustomed to the relatively crowded trails of other states should, therefore, take this rating with a grain of salt.

Difficulty

This is yet another subjective judgment. The rating is intended to warn you away from the most difficult outings if you're not in shape to try them. The scale is *relative only to other backpacking trips*. Most Americans would find even the easiest backpacking trip to be a very strenuous undertaking. So this scale of 1 (barely leave the La-Z-Boy) to 10 (the Ironman Triathlon) is only for people already accustomed to backpacking.

Mileage

This is the total mileage of the recommended trip in its *most basic form* (with no side trips). I have never, however, seen the point of a "bare bones," Point-A-to-Point-B kind of trip. After all, if you're going to go, you may as well explore a bit. Thus, for many trips, there is a *second* mileage number (in parentheses below) that includes distances for recommended side trips. These side trips are also shown on the maps and included in the "Possible Itinerary" section.

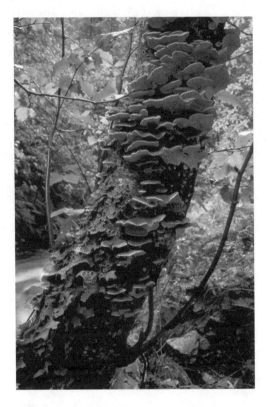

Mushrooms along lower Selway River Trail, Trip 5

I have made every reasonable effort (and some *unreasonable* ones) to ensure that the mileages shown are accurate. Users should *not*, however, assume that the numbers are exact. Idaho hiking guidebooks are notoriously lax about including mileages.

Wilderness maps for the state rarely, if ever, include mileages. Even the distances indicated on trail signs (when they are given at all) are often contradictory and usually unreliable.

Mileages for this book are shown to the nearest 1 mile (0.5 mile for short distances) and are based on a combination of map extrapolation and my own pedometer readings. These numbers can be considered accurate to within a margin of error of perhaps +/- 10%. To attempt to give mileages with any more precision would give the reader a false sense of accuracy. Hikers accustomed to tracking their progress with a higher degree of precision will need to adjust their mindset. Such exactness is not possible when traveling in the vast backcountry of Idaho.

Elevation Gain

For many hikers, how far *up* they go is even more important than the distance. This box shows all of the trip's ups and downs in a *total* elevation gain, not merely the *net* gain. As with the mileage section, a second number (in parentheses below) includes the elevation gain in recommended side trips.

Days

This is a *rough* figure for how long it will take the average backpacker to do the trip. In general, it is based on my preference for traveling about 10 miles per day. Also considered were the spacing of available campsites and the trip's difficulty. Hard-core hikers may cover as many as 25 miles a day, while others saunter along at 4 or 5 miles per day, a good pace for hikers with children. Most trips can be done in more or fewer days, depending on your preferences and abilities.

Shuttle Mileage

This is the shortest driving distance between the beginning and the ending trailheads. Since most trips in this book are loop trips, a shuttle mileage is usually not applicable.

Map(s)

Every trip includes a sketch map that is as up-to-date and accurate as possible. These sketch maps use bold lines to indicate the

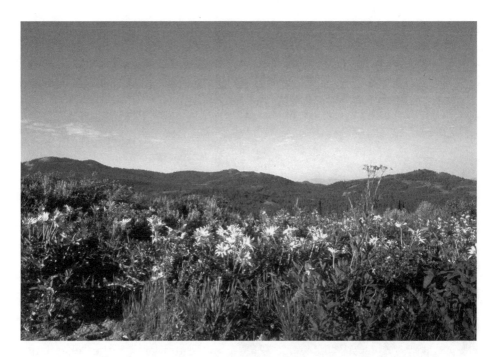

Along Highline Trail, Bear River Range, Trip 24

main route and all recommended side trips, so you can get an instant overview of the hike. As every hiker knows, however, you'll also need a good contour map of the area. This entry identifies the best available map(s) for the described trip. If you need USGS maps, they are now available free over the Internet from *www.topozone.com* or *www.maptech.com*. Simply center your search on a particular location, then print out a map on a scale from 1:24,000 to 1:200,000.

Season

There are *two* seasonal entries shown for each trip. The first tells you when a trip is usually snow-free enough for hiking (which can vary considerably from year to year). The second lists the *particular* time(s) of year when the trip is at its very best — when the flowers peak, or the fall colors are at their best, or the mosquitoes have died down, etc.

Permits and Rules

Compared to more crowded states in the American West, Idaho has very few restrictions on backcountry visitors. Except for

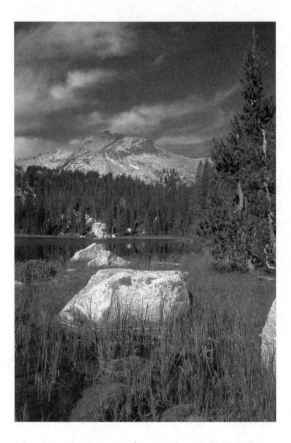

Plummer Peak over Three Island Lake, Sawtooth Mountains, Trip 15

Yellowstone National Park, most of which is in Wyoming, there are no trail quotas anywhere in the state, and hikers don't need to worry about making reservations. Very few areas even require that you fill out a free permit. Some places do have regulations that restrict the use of fires or the number of people in each party. These and other rules are noted in this section.

Contact

This is the telephone number for the local land agency responsible for the area. You can contact it to check on road and trail conditions before your trip.

Unfortunately, you should not expect to get much useful or reliable information from these local land managers. In researching this book, I asked dozens of Forest Service personnel hundreds of questions about trail lengths, when trail maintenance was last done (which can range from last week to not since the trail was built over 50 years ago), if a trail was snow-free enough for travel, and if a trail shown on the map even exists (they often don't). The answer was almost always "I don't know, we don't keep track of that information." Only *once* did I receive accurate and reliable information.

Special Attractions

This section focuses on attributes of a particular trip that are rare or outstanding. For example, almost every trip has views, but some have views that are *especially* noteworthy. The same is true of areas where you have a better than average chance of seeing wildlife, excellent fall colors, and so on.

Problems

This is the flip side to the "Special Attractions" section. It lists the trip's special or especially troublesome problems. Expect to read warnings about areas with particularly abundant mosquitoes, poor road access, grizzly bears, or limited water.

Tips and Warnings

Throughout the text are numerous helpful hints and ideas that come from my personal experience. Hopefully, these prominently labeled *Tips* and *Warnings* will make your trips safer and more enjoyable.

Possible Itinerary

This is given at the *end* of each trip. To be used as a planning tool, it includes daily mileages and total elevation gains, as well as recommended side trips. Although I have hiked every mile of every trip, many were not done exactly as written here. If I were to re-hike a trip, I would follow the improved itinerary shown here.

Variations

Not included with every trip, this self-explanatory section suggests the best ways to lengthen, shorten, or otherwise alter the recommended trip.

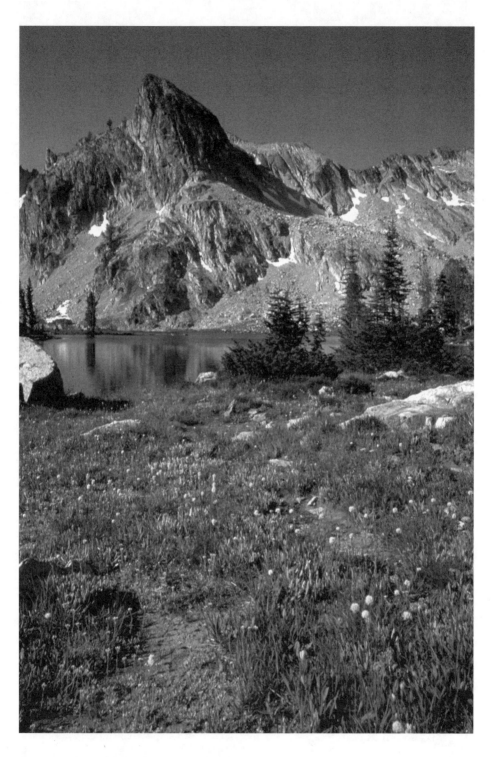

Lower Twin Lake, Sawtooth Mountains, Trip 17

Backpacking in Idaho

Authors of hiking guidebooks face a paradox. Without dedicated supporters the wilderness would never be protected in the first place. The best and most enthusiastic advocates are those who have actually visited the land, often with the help of a guidebook. On the other hand, too many boots can also be destructive. It is the responsibility of every visitor to tread lightly on the land and to speak out strongly for its preservation.

Although Idaho has over 4 million acres of officially designated wilderness, the job of protecting Idaho's precious wildlands is far from complete. You are strongly encouraged to join in the efforts to set aside more of the state's millions of acres of unprotected roadless terrain. But even land that is officially protected as wilderness needs continued citizen involvement. Issues like use restrictions, grazing rights, mining claims, horse damage, and entry fees all continue to present challenges. Remember: *you own this land*. Treat it with respect and get involved in its management.

To their credit, almost every agency official who reviewed this material stressed the need for hikers to leave no trace of their visit. But the time has come for us to go beyond the well-known "no trace" principles and leave behind a landscape that not only shows no trace of our presence, but is actually in *better* shape than before we visited it.

GENERAL BACKPACKING GUIDELINES

This book is not a "how to" guide for backpackers. Anyone contemplating an extended backpacking vacation will (or at least *should*) already know about equipment, the "no-trace" ethic, conditioning, how to select a campsite, food, first aid, and all the other aspects of this sport. There are many excellent books covering these subjects. It *is* appropriate, however, to review a few general backpacking guidelines and discuss some tips and ideas that are specific to Idaho:

Obviously, be scrupulous to leave no litter of your own. Even better, remove any litter left by others (blessedly little these days).

Do some minor trail maintenance as you hike. Kick rocks off the trail, remove limbs and debris, and drain water from the path to reduce mud and erosion. Report major trail-maintenance problems,

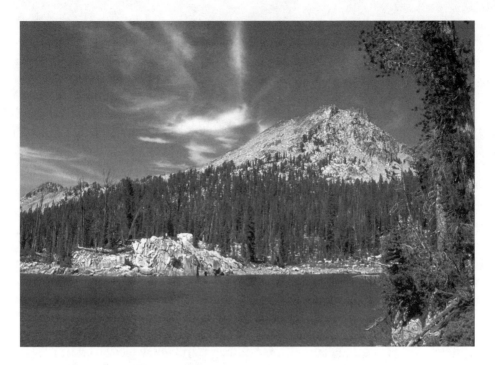

Peak 9918 over Lake Ingeborg, Sawtooth Mountains, Trip 15

such as large blowdowns or washouts, to the land managers so they can concentrate their limited dollars where those are most needed.

If you are a plant expert, **remove any introduced noxious weeds that you see**. Musk thistle, spotted knapweed, leafy spurge, and purple loosestrife are just some of the invasive species that land managers need help in eliminating.

Always camp in a place that either is compacted from years of previous use or can easily accommodate a tent without being damaged — sand, rocks, or a densely wooded area is best.

Never camp on fragile meadow vegetation or immediately beside a lake or stream. If you see a campsite "growing" in an inappropriate place, be proactive: place a few limbs or rocks over the area to discourage further use, scatter "horse apples," and remove fire-scarred rocks. Report those who ignore the rules to rangers (or offer to help the offenders move to a better location).

Never feed wildlife, and encourage others to refrain.

Do not build campfires. I have backpacked several thousand miles in the last 15 years and built just one fire (and that was only in an emergency). While there are still places in the forests of Idaho where you may be able to build a small campfire with a clear conscience, you simply don't need a fire to have a good time, and it damages the land. When you discover a fire ring in an otherwise pristine area, scatter the rocks and cover the fire pit to discourage its further use.

Leave all of the following at home: soap — even biodegradable soap pollutes; pets — even well-mannered pets are instinctively seen as predators by wildlife; anything loud; any outdated attitudes you may have about going out to "conquer" the wilderness.

IDAHO-SPECIFIC GUIDELINES

A parking pass is now required at all trailheads in the popular Sawtooth National Recreation Area and at some trailheads in the Ketchum Ranger District of the Sawtooth National Forest. In general, cars parked within 0.25 mile of any trailhead must display a pass. As of this writing, a three-day permit cost $5, and an annual pass was $15.

The winter's snowpack has a significant effect not only on when a trail opens, but also on peak wildflower times, stream flows, and how long seasonal water sources will be available. The best plan is to check the snowpack on about April 1, and make a note of how it compares to normal. This information is available through the local media, by contacting the Snow Survey Office in Boise at (208) 378-5740, or by checking the snow survey website at *www.idsnow.id.nrcs.usda.gov*. If the snowpack is significantly above or below average, then adjust a trip's seasonal recommendation accordingly.

Except on popular trails in places like the Sawtooth Mountains, trail maintenance in Idaho is not as regular as in most other western states. Most trails are cleared only once every few years, and many trails get no maintenance at all. You should expect to encounter downed logs or other obstacles as you hike. You should also expect that many minor trail junctions will not be signed, so watch the map and the surrounding terrain closely to locate obscure junctions.

A bit of advice for urbanites visiting the Idaho backcountry: in rural Idaho (and, for that matter, in much of the rural American West) the *correct* pronunciation of the word "creek" is *crik*, with a short "i" sound rather than a long "e" sound. Keep this in mind so you don't end up sounding like "ignorant city folk." Also, when you are passing an oncoming car on rarely used rural roads it is considered good etiquette to acknowledge the other driver with a small wave, whether you know the person or not. Failing to do so identifies you as a rude city visitor.

When driving on rural roads, beware of free-ranging livestock, which typically show little fear of cars and have a habit of loitering in the middle of the road. It may take considerable patience, honking, and/or swearing to get the animals to move off the road. Calves are particularly notorious for darting in front of cars when you least expect them to. In addition, ranchers regularly use the roadways to push their herds of sheep and cattle between pastures. Be prepared to occasionally get stuck behind (or in the middle of) slow-moving masses of smelly livestock.

General deer-hunting season in Idaho runs from early October to sometime in November. For safety, anyone traveling in the forest during this period (particularly those doing any cross-country travel) should carry *and wear* a bright red or orange cap, vest, pack, or other conspicuous article of clothing.

For most of Idaho, the general elk-hunting season begins in early-to-mid October and runs to mid-November, but in many backcountry game units the season begins on September 15. The exact season varies in different parts of the state. The seasons for hunting moose, mountain goat, bighorn sheep, and black bear usually do not attract enough hunters to cause a problem for backpackers.

Although Idaho's black bears are generally quite shy, they are common throughout the state's mountains and forests. You should hang all food and garbage at least 10 feet off the ground and 4 feet from the nearest tree trunk, so the bruins cannot reach it. This will also protect your food supply from an even more common and destructive group of thieves – chipmunks.

Grizzly bears are a subject of interest (and sometimes nightmares) for many hikers. In Idaho, there is a reasonable chance of encountering these impressive, but potentially dangerous, animals only in the mountains of the northern panhandle (Trip 1) and in or near Yellowstone National Park (Trip 22). When hiking in these areas, the following precautions are in order: never hike alone or at night; avoid areas with recent signs of bears; take special care to avoid spilling food or garbage near your camp; make plenty of noise while you hike; and hang all food and garbage at least 15 feet from the ground and 500 feet away from your camp. Since most of the trees along the ridgetops are rather small, it is sometimes difficult to

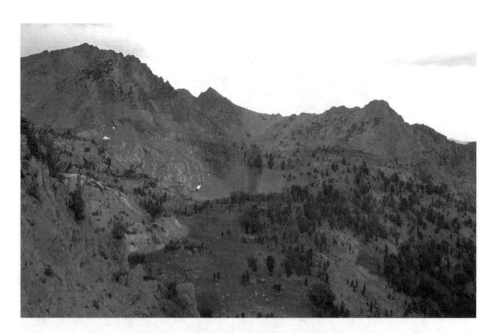

View East from Johnstone Pass, Pioneer Mountains, Trip 19

properly hang your food. You may want to bring a bear canister instead. Finally, remember that bears and dogs do *not* get along. Accordingly, the Park Service prohibits dogs, and the Forest Service *strongly* discourages bringing your dog. If you *must* bring your pet, be sure that the animal is on leash at all times. If you see a grizzly bear, consider yourself fortunate that you saw one of these rare and magnificent creatures in the wild, and report the sighting to the land managers — they like to keep track of such things.

Hikers frequently have to ford streams (large and small) on the trips described in this book and in Idaho in general. Early in the season, rivers and creeks run high with meltwater, which makes fording them a cold and potentially dangerous undertaking. The typical depth of the stream for the recommended season of the hike is noted in the text, but this can vary considerably from year to year. If a ford looks too deep, swift, or dangerous when you get there, don't risk it! Turn around and head back the way you came. The best and safest way to make a ford is to wear light-weight wading shoes or sandals, which will give you better traction, protect your feet from cuts and scrapes, and allow you to keep your boots and socks dry. Trekking poles to provide a third and fourth leg of support are also highly recommended.

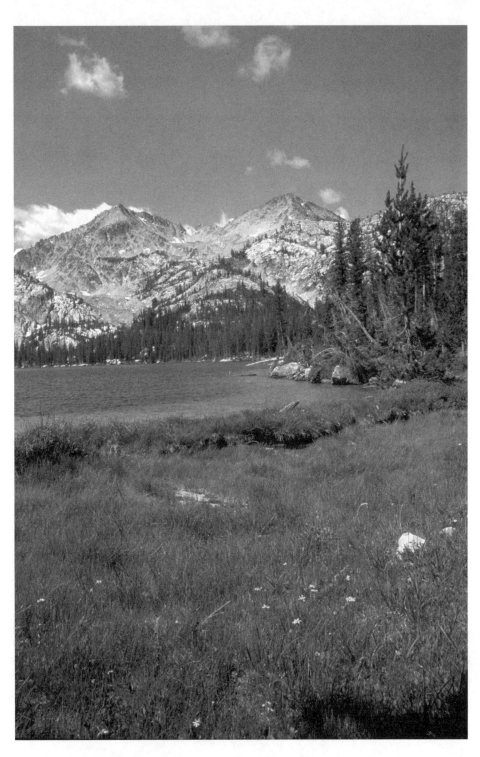

Toxaway Lake, Sawtooth Mountains, Trip 17

Wild Areas of Idaho

What follows is a general overview of the principal remaining wild areas in Idaho. All but one of these areas has at least one backpacking trip described in this book. Thus, whether you prefer deep river canyons, virgin forests, high mountains, or lonesome ridges, there's a choice of outstanding trips for you.

SELKIRK MOUNTAINS

Tucked in the far northern panhandle of Idaho, the craggy Selkirk Mountains are a long way from the state's main population centers. From Boise, for example, it's a 9-hour drive to the nearest Selkirk trailheads. As a result, most visitors to these mountains come from the much nearer metropolis of Spokane, Washington, to the west.

Pacific storms, also coming from the west, dump a lot more snow and rain in the Selkirk Mountains than they do in mountains to the south, making this the wettest part of Idaho. All this precipitation, along with the more northerly latitude, results in a relatively low timberline, so even though the peaks here are all below 8000 feet, there is plenty of alpine scenery to enjoy.

The precipitation also leads to incredibly lush forests, featuring species like western hemlock and western red cedar which are rare or absent from the rest of the state. These dense forests have suffered from two recurring catastrophes over the last 125 years: first, the insatiable desire of human beings for big trees to cut down; and second, a series of enormous fires that have repeatedly blackened the area. The rampant logging has left behind a landscape riddled with clearcuts that despoil most distant views. Evidence of the fires comes in the form of silvery snags along the ridgetops.

These mountains are the southern tip of a 250-mile-long range of peaks that stretch down from the interior of British Columbia, Canada. As a result, this range hosts an unusual assortment of northern animals not found in other parts of the state. Hikers may be fortunate enough to see mountain caribou – the most endangered large mammal in the United States – moose, lynx, gray wolf, or grizzly bear. Even though they are rarely seen, just knowing that these impressive animals inhabit the Selkirk Mountains adds a thrilling sense of possibility to your adventure.

These mountains provide many joys in addition to the wildlife. The biggest attraction is impressive scenery, mostly in the form of lovely cirque lakes and jagged granite peaks. A less obvious advantage this area has over the mountains in southern Idaho is that the lower elevations here don't require extra time for lowlanders to get accustomed to thin air.

One of the few disadvantages of hiking in the Selkirk Mountains is that this area has a higher percentage of cloudy and rainy days than the rest of the state (although it's still nowhere near as soggy as the mountains of Oregon and Washington to the west). Another disadvantage is the thick undergrowth, which makes cross-country travel much more difficult than in drier ranges to the south. But even with these problems, it is the rare pedestrian who, after a hike in these mountains, doesn't believe that the Selkirk's scenery, solitude, and wildlife far outweigh any downsides on their trip.

UPPER ST. JOE AND CLEARWATER RIVERS

Most of Idaho's mountains feature skyscraping peaks and towering cliffs that can accurately be described as *spectacular*. That word, however, would *not* be appropriate for the millions of acres of rolling, forested hills of north-central Idaho. The relatively gentle and picturesque hills and valleys of this region probably won't take a visitor's breath away, but that is only by comparison to other mountains in this scenery-rich state. Were these mountains located in almost any other state, they would be visited by thousands of hikers every year. In Idaho, however, this area is generally overlooked, except by anglers who enjoy the region's excellent fishing streams.

For decades, loggers and miners have eaten away at the wild character of this region, so there are few areas left where backpackers can get a meaningful distance from the nearest road. The wildest country, and the best scenery, is in the south near the watershed divide between the St. Joe and Clearwater rivers. Hikers here can enjoy good, if not great, mountain scenery, lots of wildlife (especially elk and mountain goats), and hundreds of miles of pleasant trails. These trails typically either follow the area's famous streams or climb to small lakes and huckleberry-covered ridges.

This entire region was at the center of one of the largest forest fires in recorded history. In August, 1910, a fire of almost unbelievable size and ferocity swept across northern Idaho, northwest Montana, and parts of northeast Washington. In the process it killed 85 people, most of them firefighters, and burned approximately 3 million acres. Incredibly, the firestorm consumed most of that vast acreage in just two days! This catastrophe was the catalyst for an aggressive fire-suppression policy in the United States Forest Service, which continued until recent times, when foresters realized that periodic natural fires are needed for forest health. In response to the 1910 disaster, the Forest Service built numerous fire lookouts and an extensive system of trails to service these remote facilities. Most of the lookouts are gone now, made obsolete by modern fire-detection techniques, but those that remain are among the area's most popular hiking destinations. This is understandable, because the lookouts provide not only a colorful history but also great views, which is, after all, why these locations were selected in the first place.

SELWAY-BITTERROOT WILDERNESS

Were it not for the adjoining, and even larger, Frank Church-River of No Return Wilderness, Selway-Bitterroot Wilderness would be considered huge. At approximately 1.8 million acres it certainly covers a lot of territory. In fact, the mind-boggling size of this wilderness is one of its main attractions, because visitors here have the opportunity to find the kind of complete solitude that is rarely possible in other wild areas of the United States.

Most of the wilderness' vast acreage is a seemingly endless sea of forested ridges, stream canyons, and relatively low peaks. Only a few places feature truly dramatic scenery with high, jagged peaks and cirque lakes. The most impressive of these areas are the relatively small Selway Crags, in the west-central part of the wilderness, and the Bitterroot Divide along the border with Montana. These are the only places in the wilderness where the dense forest cover is broken by exposed portions of the Idaho Batholith, the huge, uplifted dome of granite that underlies almost all the mountains of central Idaho.

Cutting through the heart of the wilderness is the scenic canyon of the Selway River, a beautiful stream that runs clear and cold, due in no small part to the roadless nature of its watershed. Wilderness

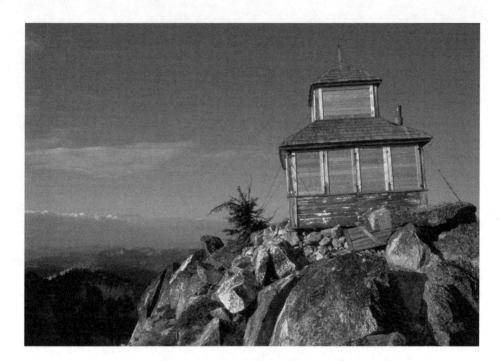

Grave Peak Lookout, Selway-Bitterroot Wilderness, Trip 4

rafters and kayakers vie for coveted limited-use permits to run this river, but hikers can backpack along the trail that parallels this scenic stream without any restrictions.

The wilderness' size makes it ideal habitat for wildlife that requires large territories to survive. Although you probably won't see one, the wilderness is home to wolverine, black bear, gray wolf, and mountain lion. It has even been proposed that grizzly bears be reintroduced to the area. This unusual wildlife adds an extra level of excitement to a trip in the Selway-Bitterroot Wilderness.

The greatest problems of hiking in this wilderness are the difficulty of walking such long distances and the poor road access to some trailheads.

HELLS CANYON NATIONAL RECREATION AREA

From the lofty, 9393-foot summit of He Devil, the highest point in the Seven Devils Mountains, you can see all the way down to the Snake River at the bottom of Hells Canyon, fully 8000 feet below. All that elevation change leads to a great variety of life zones. In just 4 or 5 miles as the golden eagle flies, the environment changes from a treeless alpine tundra of rocks, ice, and tiny wildflowers to a treeless desert complete with prickly-pear cactus. In recognition of this great geographic diversity, along with a similar diversity in scenery, wildlife, and cultural history, Congress set aside the Hells Canyon National Recreation Area in 1975, a 652,500-acre preserve that Idaho shares with the neighboring state of Oregon.

There are hundreds of miles of trails in the recreation area, nearly all of which provide the visitor with eye-popping scenery. In the craggy heights of the Seven Devils Mountains, the trails visit snow-streaked cliffs of dark basalt towering above cirque lakes of stunning beauty. In addition to the nearby mountain scenery, these high trails frequently allow hikers to look down to the bottom of the canyon and, with binoculars, spot other hikers walking on paths that provide a radically different experience. Snow almost never falls down there, and July wildflowers, which bloom so profusely in the mountains, are replaced by grasses that are dried brown by the desert sun as soon as early May.

Hikers looking up from those river-level trails are awed by equally impressive scenery and neck-craning vistas. The view extends up a seemingly endless series of basalt cliffs and grassy terraces where elk and bighorn sheep often roam. Those hikers would be well advised to spend some time looking *down* as well, to avoid an unexpected encounter with a rattlesnake, an abundant resident in this area. Other hazards lurking near your boots include poison ivy, especially near watercourses, and ticks, which are at their blood-sucking worst in the spring.

Finding water is another problem in the lower canyon, because the river is not always accessible from the trail and, by late in the season, only major tributary creeks are still flowing. Carry at least two quarts of water and refill them at every opportunity. The final, and perhaps the most oppressive, problem faced by canyon hikers is the heat. While midsummer temperatures top out in the comfortable 70s in the mountains, highs are typically over 100 degrees near the Snake River. And there is almost no shade. Spring and fall provide the most comfortable travel in the canyon. On the other hand, late June to early August is the best time to hike the trails in the Seven Devils Mountains. Thus, this remarkably diverse region provides great hiking for most of the year.

GOSPEL HUMP WILDERNESS

Covering some 206,000 acres of rugged topography, Gospel Hump Wilderness protects a remarkably diverse territory along the lower Salmon River in west-central Idaho. The scenic terrain here ranges from the contorted, low-elevation landscape of the Salmon River Breaks in the south to the rolling, high-elevation mountains, meadows, and plateaus in the north. As you would expect, the changes in altitude and terrain create a wide range of climates and vegetation types. The wilderness includes everything from steep, sun-baked hillsides covered with bunchgrass and scattered ponderosa pines to flower-covered mountain meadows surrounded by dense forests of lodgepole pines and subalpine firs.

What you will *not* encounter, anywhere in this wilderness, are crowds. As one of the least visited parts of the state, Gospel Hump Wilderness remains an excellent option for those looking to "get away from it all." Believe me, when you are in Gospel Hump Wilderness, "it all" is *really* a long way away. Only in October, when hunters arrive hoping to bag a trophy deer or elk, do very many people visit the backcountry. Of course, spring and summer hikers can also appreciate the wildlife, and they can expect to see more than just deer and elk. Bighorn sheep, for example, are common amid the rugged Salmon River Breaks, and you stand a good chance of seeing moose or mountain goats in the high country.

With all these crowd-pleasing attributes, you may be wondering why there aren't any crowds. The answer lies in access problems. The wilderness is a *long* way from the nearest population center, requiring several hours of driving from either Boise or Spokane to Grangeville, the small farming and lumber town nearest to the wilderness. And the drive isn't over there, because it's at least another hour-and-one-half from Grangeville to the nearest wilderness trailhead.

Once you get out of the car, you soon discover another price hikers must pay to enjoy the solitude of Gospel Hump Wilderness. Many of the trails here are rarely, if ever, maintained. Every trail shown on the map exists, at least in a *theoretical* sense, but it takes experience, and a bit of luck, to navigate the lesser-used routes.

FRANK CHURCH-RIVER OF NO RETURN WILDERNESS

The Frank Church-River of No Return Wilderness isn't just big, it's positively enormous. At more than 2.3 million acres, this is the second largest designated wilderness area in the contiguous United States. Amazingly, this seemingly endless expanse of rugged canyons, rolling mountains, and high plateaus feels even larger than it is, because the protected land is flanked by hundreds of thousands of acres of wild country that is not officially designated as wilderness (but should be). In addition, this wilderness is separated from the almost equally large Selway-Bitterroot Wilderness only by a primitive dirt road.

The average backpacker cannot reach the vast interior of this wilderness by ordinary means. It takes several days to hike into the center of this preserve from one of the outer trailheads. Access is made easier by methods that are very unusual in a designated wilderness. Much as in the wilds of Alaska, small bush planes provide regular service to several dirt airstrips scattered around the wilderness. These planes bring mail and supplies to remote wilderness ranches and guard stations, and provide convenient if rather expensive access for hunters, anglers, hikers, and other outdoor lovers.

Another common way of accessing the interior of this wilderness is to float its streams. Rafters joyfully descend some of North America's most exciting whitewater on the Middle Fork and the main stem of the Salmon River. A great way to see this wilderness is to pay a river operator to take you down the river, then offload and enjoy a long hike back to your car. Thus, if you can afford the price of a plane ride or a raft trip, almost every part of the wilderness is accessible, even for the average backpacker.

Regardless of how you choose to make your way into this wilderness, your efforts will be richly rewarded. Although the scenery is generally more subdued than in the higher mountains to the south and east, the area's lakes, forested plateaus, and ridges are still very attractive, and the river canyons are both deep and spectacular.

Perhaps more impressive than the scenery is the abundance of wildlife. Big-game animals like deer, elk, black bear, and bighorn sheep seem to be everywhere. The wilderness is especially appealing to species like mountain lion, gray wolf, and wolverine, which require large territories without the intrusion of human beings.

Probably the greatest attribute of Frank Church-River of No Return Wilderness is the simple thrill of knowing that you are hiking through the wildest land remaining in the lower 48 states. To the true wilderness lover, just knowing that the nearest road is over 30 miles away adds an indefinable sense of adventure and satisfaction to your trip.

The Forest Service sells two four-color contour maps that separately cover the north and south halves of the wilderness. Hikers, however, should not rely on these maps. To display all of this enormous wilderness requires that the maps be huge, two-sided, fold-out sheets, which are ungainly and awkward to use in the field. In addition, because the area is so big, even after breaking down the wilderness into these four large sections, the maps are still at a scale of 1:100,000, which is too small to be useful for hikers. So carry the Forest Service map for updated information about roads and trails, but bring USGS maps for greater detail.

SAWTOOTH NATIONAL RECREATION AREA AND VICINITY

Smack in the middle of Idaho – if such an irregularly shaped state can be said to have a "middle" – sits the 754,000-acre Sawtooth National Recreation Area, justifiably the most popular outdoor playground in the state. Within the borders of this compact area are many of Idaho's most outstanding outdoor attractions. Here you will discover part or all of four major mountain ranges — the Boulder, Sawtooth, Smoky, and White Cloud mountains. Another important range, the Pioneer Mountains, sits just outside the southeast side of the preserve. The recreation area also includes the headwaters of the world-famous Salmon River and the spectacular Sawtooth Valley, one of the most stunning mountain valleys in North America. Best of all, there are enough trails and hiking destinations to keep you happily exploring for decades.

In 1972, Congress set aside the Sawtooth Valley region as a national recreation area, with the stated purpose of assuring "the preservation and protection of the natural, scenic, historic, pastoral, and fish and wildlife values and provide for the enhancement of the recreation values." While this far-sighted act did not provide the full protection of a national park, which many conservationists would have preferred, it did put a check on the impending development of subdivisions, indiscriminate logging, and rampant road building that would have destroyed the unique qualities of this area.

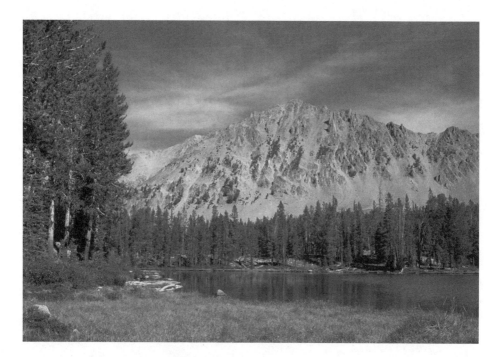

Lower Born Lake, White Cloud Peaks, Trip 18

Only 217,000 acres of the national recreation area are protected as wilderness, and all of that is in the Sawtooth Mountains. Therefore, hikers traveling in other areas must be prepared to encounter jeep and mining roads, motorbikes on the trails, and mining activity. The mining is allowed because thousands of claims existed before the national recreation area was established, and these were grandfathered in by the enabling legislation.

The mountain scenery here ranks with the best in North America, in no small part because of the unique geology. The most noteworthy rock is the beautiful pinkish granite of the Sawtooth Mountains. This unusual intrusion of granite formed during volcanic activity that took place only 50 million years ago and is distinct from the massive, 350-million-year-old Idaho Batholith, which underlies most of the mountains of central Idaho. In addition to being a different age and color, this rock fractures more easily, which made it especially susceptible to erosion by Ice Age glaciers. The ice left behind sharply serrated ridges and over 400 stunningly beautiful cirque lakes, which are often the destinations of hikers today.

Although the Sawtooths draw the crowds, the lesser-known mountain ranges in the Sawtooth National Recreation Area also offer outstanding scenery. The White Cloud Peaks are particularly spectacular, with dozens of stunning lakes, lots of multicolored rock, countless high peaks, and some of the most scenic trails in Idaho. The adjacent Pioneer Mountains contain scenery that is quite similar to the Sawtooths, but without the crowds. To the south, the Smoky and Boulder mountains are made up of porous rock, where water does not usually collect into lakes. Instead, you'll find view-packed ridges and plenty of wildflowers.

As is true in almost all the mountains of Idaho, the Sawtooths and their neighboring ranges have plenty of biting insects. Flies are an annoying problem, especially on sunny afternoons, but these pests can only survive below about 8000 feet. Mosquitoes are abundant at *all* elevations, but these invertebrate vampires generally disappear by about mid-August. So, if you plan a trip to the high lakes from late August through October, you should enjoy blissful, bug-free evenings.

LOST RIVER AND LEMHI RANGES

The highest mountains in the state of Idaho are in the east-central part of the state, about as far from major population centers as you can get in the lower 48 United States. The Lost River and Lemhi ranges run parallel to each other, rising from the canyon country along the Salmon River near Challis and petering out in the sagebrush plains near Arco about 100 miles southeast. The ranges are so little traveled that most of the highest peaks remain unnamed and are simply identified by their elevations.

The isolation ensures a high degree of solitude, even on holiday weekends. That solitude is enhanced by generally miserable road access and a scarcity of trails. A typical visit involves several miles of bouncing along at 5 miles per hour, preferably in a car you don't like very much, before you finally give up, pull off the "road," and walk the rest of the way to an unsigned trailhead. From there, you do your best to follow a sketchy path, but often give up on that as well, and continue your hike guided only by landmarks. Fortunately, the terrain is generally open, so navigation is easy.

Wildlife appreciates the isolation of these mountains, reveling in the quiet of a people-free landscape. So, if you make the effort to

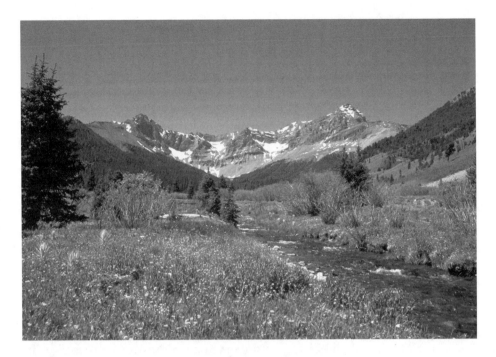

Upper basin of Dry Creek, Lost River Range, Trip 20

visit, you stand a good chance of seeing mountain goats, black bears, elk, moose, and even such relatively elusive animals as mountain lions.

Although tall, these mountains hide in the rainshadow of several mountain ranges to the west, so less snow falls here than on most Idaho mountains. The drier climate has some important consequences for hikers. First, trails open sooner in the year, with excellent hiking beginning in early-to-mid June. Second, the open forests have relatively little ground cover, which makes cross-country travel a reasonable option for getting around in these mountains. Third, surface water is at a premium. Lakes are rare, and the smaller streams typically dry up by late in the season. Hikers should plan to visit early in the summer and take advantage of every available water source. Water problems are most severe in the southern parts of these ranges, due to slightly lower snowfall and an abundance of limestone rock, which allows water to percolate down from the surface. A big advantage of the water shortage is a relative lack of mosquitoes, at least in comparison to the wetter ranges in other parts of the state.

OWYHEE AND BRUNEAU CANYONLANDS

The vast deserts of southwest Idaho hide a rarely visited landscape of rolling sagebrush plains that are spectacularly broken by the deep, narrow canyons of two desert streams, the Owyhee and Bruneau rivers. Extreme isolation and difficult access combine to ensure almost complete solitude for human visitors.

Hikers who do come here discover a harsh landscape that bears little resemblance to the scenery found in other parts of Idaho. First, unlike every other major hiking region in the state, there are no mountains here. Second, and most importantly, the weather is much drier.

The dry climate provides habitat for desert bighorn sheep, wild horses, badgers, sage grouse, and pronghorn antelope, which are absent from the forested environments in the rest of the state. Birds of prey are abundant, because they find good nesting sites on the canyon rims and plenty of prey in the form of jackrabbits and desert rodents. Look for golden eagles, prairie falcons, and several species of hawks, all in greater numbers than almost anywhere else in North America. Reptile enthusiasts will discover that this desert environment is home to the highest concentration of lizards in the state. In addition, rattlesnakes, a potentially dangerous reptile, are common enough that visitors must watch their step, especially when traveling in grassy areas near water.

Water is rare in this desert realm. The occasional springs, ponds, and small streams shown on maps usually dry up by early summer and cannot be relied upon by thirsty hikers. The lack of available water forces hikers to stay in the canyons, close to major rivers. These main streams have water all year, but even that flow is highly variable. Although kayakers and rafters drool at the exciting whitewater possibilities, the rivers are runnable only in the high water of spring, and in some years there is never enough water for rafting.

Rattlesnakes and water shortages aren't the only problems posed by the desert environment. Unless you enjoy heat stroke, this is no place to hike in midsummer. Temperatures stay in the 90- to 110-degree range from about mid-June to early September and, except for the occasional western juniper or streamside willow, trees are nonexistent. The dominant plant species is sagebrush, which isn't exactly famous as a shade tree. Spring and fall are the most comfortable seasons for a visit.

While the *absence* of trees creates one problem, it is the *presence* of a different plant that creates another. Poison ivy is common in the stream canyons and can be hard to avoid. Hikers should consider carrying one of those new soaps or creams designed to block the plant's rash-producing toxin. A final concern is that the canyons are prone to flash floods. Thunderstorms, especially in the summer, occasionally bring large volumes of water down these narrow defiles.

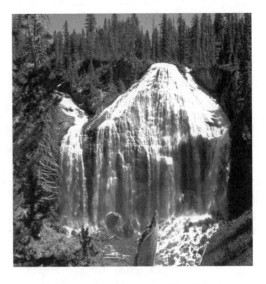

Union Falls, Yellowstone National Park, Trip 22

A brewing environmental controversy in these canyonlands centers around the impact of military training flights. Air Force pilots routinely use this remote area for low-altitude training, often roaring by less than 100 feet above the ground. Environmentalists are concerned that the flights cause stress to the wildlife and make two-legged visitors feel like they are hiking in a war zone. The Air Force claims to do its best to minimize the impact on particularly sensitive wildlife, such as bighorn sheep, and they point out that their pilots have to practice *somewhere*. For now, the debate, and the flights, continue.

Despite repeated attempts on the ground, and numerous calls to very knowledgeable BLM officials, I was unable to find a single extended backpacking trip in this area that I felt comfortable recommending in this book. Although the area features some outstanding dayhikes, there are no long hikes that are both accessible by car (or even by a decent, four-wheel-drive SUV) and can be enjoyably hiked, even by an athletic, experienced, and very determined backpacker.

YELLOWSTONE REGION

While most of world-famous Yellowstone National Park is in Wyoming, both Montana and Idaho proudly claim small parts of that magnificent preserve. Although the park's narrow western strip in Idaho has none of the geysers that made the park famous, in Yellowstone's southwest corner visitors will discover one of the highest concentrations of waterfalls in the Rocky Mountains. Trails along the Bechler River and its tributaries take visitors to waterfalls of every conceivable shape, size, and height.

This part of Yellowstone is accessible only by a gravel road from Idaho, so there are none of the crowds found in other parts of the park. And while wildlife may be less prevalent than it is in the more famous parts of Yellowstone, the animals here are less accustomed to people, so they are truly "wild" and therefore more natural.

Of course, one of the wildlife species for which Yellowstone is famous is the grizzly bear, and hikers may or may not be happy about the possibility of encountering this powerful denizen of the forest. The odds of seeing, much less being attacked by, a bear are extremely low, but backpackers are well advised to take extra precautions to avoid an encounter. Bear bells are not officially sanctioned, but they are not discouraged either. If you see a grizzly bear, give it a wide berth and consider turning around and staying out of its territory.

SOUTHEAST IDAHO MOUNTAIN RANGES

The southeast corner of Idaho is yet another scenic treasure in a state packed with glorious scenery. The landscape here is dominated by a series of relatively gentle mountain ranges separated by beautiful river valleys. The region has long been popular with vacationers, especially near Bear Lake, where people have built numerous summer homes and resorts. Despite this development, backpackers can still find solitude in the higher parts of the mountains, where the gentle, rolling hills become steeper and more rugged.

Winter snows are deep in these mountains and, when they melt, much of the water does something that is unique in Idaho. As part of the Great Basin, many of the streams here do not flow west toward the Columbia River and Pacific Ocean, as they do in the rest of the state, but travel *south* via the Bear River to Utah's Great Salt Lake, where the water simply evaporates and never reaches the ocean at all.

It's easy to get confused by the mountain ranges here, because their names bear little relationship to any sort of logical geography.

Often the name of what is clearly a single chain of mountains changes for no better reason than that a highway happens to cross the range. One continuous series of peaks, for example, goes by the name Big Hole Mountains in the north, is called the Snake River Range in the middle, and mysteriously changes again to become the Salt River Range in Wyoming.

Regardless of what you call them, these mountains are crucially important wildlife habitat, because they provide a corridor of wild land that connects the Greater Yellowstone Ecosystem to the north with the mountains of southern Wyoming and northern Utah. This corridor allows such species as moose and elk to extend their ranges and maintain the genetic diversity of their populations. In addition to these species, hikers stand a good chance of seeing mountain goats and black bears. There are even a few stray grizzly bears, although the species is so rare there is no need for hikers, even paranoid ones, to wear bear bells or lose sleep at night.

Autumn is a particularly fetching time to visit this area, because the mountains support an abundance of quaking aspens, narrowleaf cottonwoods, and Rocky Mountain maples. In late September and early October these species combine to create some of the best fall-color displays in the state. The mid-elevation hillsides, especially above Palisades Reservoir, come alive with colorful splashes of vivid yellows, oranges, and reds that will dazzle the eye and keep photographers happy for days. Just keep an eye on the weather, because the first hard freeze or strong wind will quickly end the year's foliage display.

These mountains are part of the Overthrust Belt, which is at the center of a long-standing controversy. Oil and gas companies believe that this area holds significant energy reserves, and they strongly advocate drilling and exploration. Conservationists, concerned about the impact of drilling on the region's wildlife, scenery, and recreational values, are fighting these plans. Before making up your mind on this controversy, visit this magnificent region and see what is at stake.

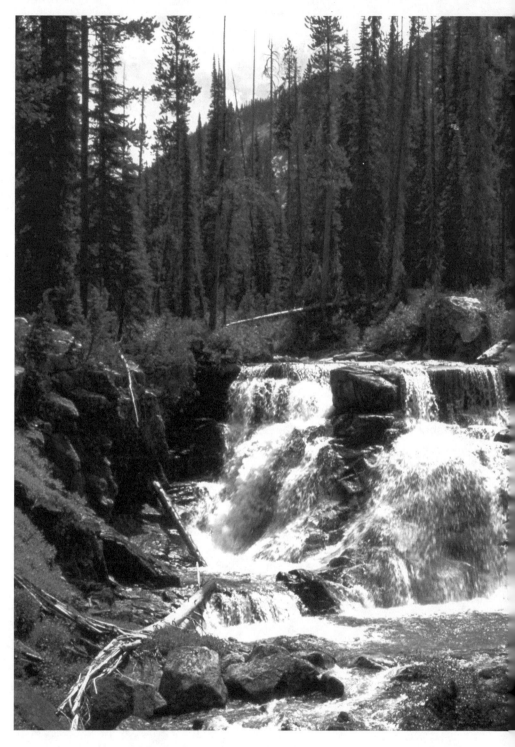

Smith Falls on South Payette River, Sawtooth Mountains, Trip 15

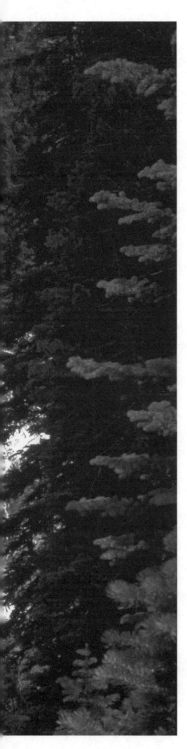

Featured Trips

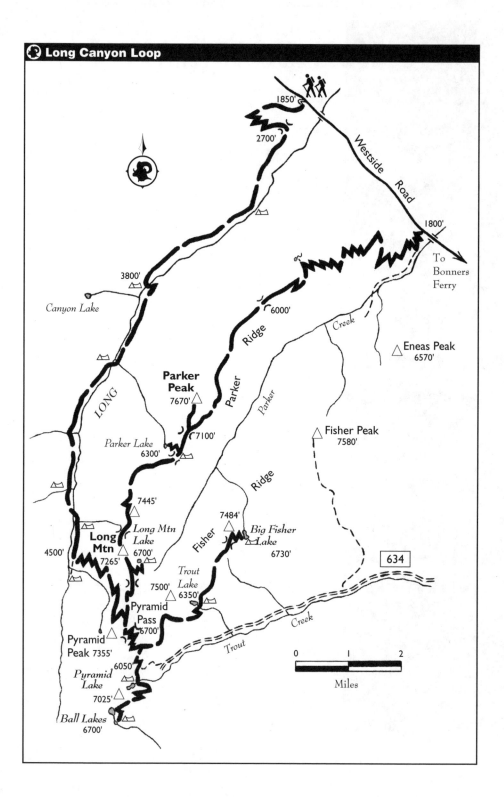

Long Canyon Loop

1850'

2700'

Westside Road

1800'

To Bonners Ferry

3800'

Canyon Lake

6000'

Creek

Eneas Peak 6570'

LONG

Parker Ridge

Parker

Parker Peak

7670'

7100'

Fisher Peak 7580'

Parker Lake 6300'

Ridge

7445'

7484'

Long Mtn

Long Mtn Lake

Fisher

Big Fisher Lake 6730'

4500'

7265'

6700'

Ridge

634

Trout Lake 6350'

7500'

Pyramid Pass 6700'

Creek

Pyramid Peak 7355'

6050'

Trout

Pyramid Lake

0   1   2

7025'

Miles

Ball Lakes 6700'

Long Canyon Loop

1

RATINGS (1–10)			MILES	ELEVATION GAIN	DAYS	SHUTTLE MILEAGE
Scenery	Solitude	Difficulty	34*	7500	3-4	4
7	6	6	(52)*	(13,000)	(4-6)	

* These numbers exclude the road walk back to the Canyon Creek trailhead.

MAPS USGS - Pyramid Peak, Smith Falls, Smith Peak.

USUALLY OPEN Mid-July to October.

BEST Late July to September.

PERMITS None.

RULES Maximum group size of 12 people, unless you specifically notify the Bonners Ferry Ranger District; fires are strongly discouraged; staying more than three nights at any given campsite is prohibited.

CONTACT Bonners Ferry Ranger District, (208) 267-5561.

SPECIAL ATTRACTIONS Unusual wildlife; lush rainforests.

PROBLEMS Grizzly bears; relatively wet weather; limited water and few campsites along Parker Ridge.

HOW TO GET THERE From the junction of U.S. Highways 2 and 95 about 2 miles north of Bonners Ferry, drive 12.6 miles north on Highway 95 to a junction. Go straight on State Highway 1 for 1.1 miles, then turn left (west) on a county road, following signs to Copeland Bridge and Westside Road. Stay on this paved road for 3.5 miles, taking a bridge over the Kootenai River, and come to a T-junction. Turn right on paved Westside Road and drive 3.5 miles to the Parker Creek trailhead, where there is room for only one or two cars to park. If you have two cars, leave one here.

To reach the recommended starting point, continue another 3.5 miles on Westside Road, then turn left (uphill) at a signed junction with a narrow, gravel, deadend road that goes 0.1 mile to the small parking lot for the Canyon Creek trailhead. **Note:** This trailhead is on private land. The public is allowed to park but not to camp here.

INTRODUCTION As the wettest range in the state of Idaho, the Selkirk Mountains support forests that are so lush they resemble the rainforests of the Pacific Northwest coast. The trees include such relatively unusual Idaho species as western red cedar, western hemlock, western yew, and Pacific dogwood, while the undergrowth is a mass of ferns, mosses, and lichens that assails the hiker with a stunning display of greenery. In a grand sampling of this wet environment, the first half of this hike takes you up Long Canyon, the last, major, unlogged valley in the Selkirk Mountains, where a magnificent shady forest provides a hiking experience unlike anything else in the state.

But there is more to admire here than dense forests. Along the ridges there are jagged peaks, hidden cirques filled with small, scenic lakes, and expansive views of the deep, green valleys below. In addition, wildflowers bloom in profusion, especially along the open ridgetops, where the forests have yet to recover from a series of large forest fires. This superior hike is the finest backpacking adventure in the Selkirk Mountains because it includes the best of the area's low-elevation forests as well as some of the range's most beautiful lakes and ridgetop views.

> **Warning:** *This is grizzly bear country. Please heed the guidelines given on page 12. Remember that bears and dogs do not get along. Accordingly, the Forest Service strongly discourages bringing your dog. If you must bring your pet, be sure that the animal is on leash at all times.*

DESCRIPTION The trail, which has been significantly rerouted from what is shown on the USGS maps, follows an overgrown road for the first 200 yards, then narrows to a foot trail and wanders gradually uphill through a nicely varied forest. The mix of evergreen trees here is more diverse than just about anywhere else in the state. Douglas-firs and western red cedars are the most common species, but there are also western larches and grand firs, as well as ponderosa pines, western white pines, and western hemlocks. The ground cover is kept in check by the deep shade of the canopy, but in places you will find pipsissewa, Oregon grape, lady fern, and thimbleberry, among other species.

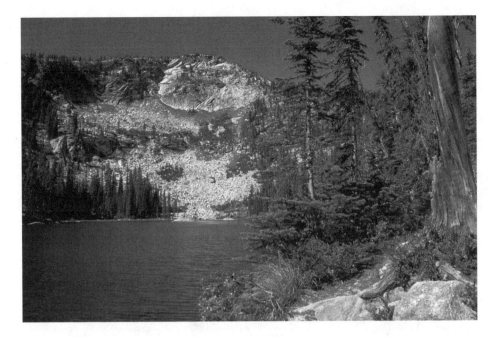

Peak 7500 over Trout Lake

The well-maintained trail climbs seven moderately long but well-graded switchbacks, then cuts through a woodsy gap in the ridge and emerges high on the slopes of Long Canyon. The trail then curves to the right and makes a rather steep and rocky uphill traverse well above cascading Long Canyon Creek, which can be heard, but not seen, deep in the canyon on your left. Although this traverse stays above the best forests, it has the advantage of going past some excellent viewpoints of Long Canyon and densely forested Parker Ridge to the south.

The trail levels briefly, then goes downhill at an irregular grade to a nice campsite beside rollicking Long Canyon Creek. Above this campsite, you travel across a forested hillside a little above the stream, maintaining a steady uphill grade that keeps pace with the cascading creek. About 3 miles from where it first met the creek, the trail drops to a pair of good campsites on either side of where you cross the stream on a log.

You make two quick switchbacks away from the creek and walk upstream for 1.5 miles through some of this area's best forests to a second creek crossing, which requires a knee-deep ford in early summer or a slippery rock-hop in late summer. There is a fair campsite immediately after the crossing hidden in the creek's dense riparian undergrowth of devils club, lady fern, horsetail, and Douglas maple. For the next few miles you make several steep little ups and downs through a dense forest that has no views, but which provides plenty of up-close green scenery. Although the trail generally stays well away from Long Canyon Creek, finding water is never a problem, since you hop over numerous tiny side creeks along the way. In fact, if anything, there is *too much* water, as frequent rains leave behind lots of mud and wet vegetation that overhangs the trail and soaks passing hikers. Fortunately, several wooden boardwalks have been installed over the worst muddy places to help keep you clean and dry.

About 2.5 miles from the second creek crossing, you pass a good campsite just before a rock-hop crossing of a fairly large, unnamed creek that flows down from Smith Lake. From there, it's another 0.5 mile to the third and final crossing of Long Canyon Creek, which is usually an easy ford, although by late summer it is possible to cross on slippery rocks. About 200 yards later, you pass a decent campsite beside a small tributary creek, then walk a little less than 1 mile to a signed junction. The unmaintained trail straight ahead goes a short distance to a good creekside campsite.

You turn left at the junction and begin the long, steady climb out of Long Canyon. The 2200-foot ascent starts with 30 mostly short and always gently graded switchbacks, followed by a half-mile-long traverse. Although there isn't much in the way of views, it's interesting to observe the changes in vegetation as you climb. The cedars and Douglas-firs in the lower canyon slowly give way to lodgepole pines, Engelmann spruces, and western white pines, while the understory makes a transition to huckleberries, alders, and beargrass. Once the traverse ends, 20 more switchbacks take you up to a nice viewpoint and a junction.

The return route of your loop goes sharply left on Parker Ridge Trail #221, but first you'll want to spend a day or two on a pair of extended side trips to the high lakes and scenic terrain at the head of Trout Creek Canyon. To do so, go straight and wind gradually uphill past the base of aptly named Pyramid Peak to the narrow, viewless defile of Pyramid Pass. The trail then descends several switchbacks on a hillside covered with huckleberries to a junction beside a small wooden bridge. Here you have a choice of side trips, both of which are highly recommended.

To do the shorter side trip, turn sharply right and wander down a few gentle switchbacks to a junction beside a visitor registration box. You turn right and make a circuitous, 0.5-mile ascent to irregularly shaped Pyramid Lake, a shallow pool with good campsites near its outlet and a superb view of an unnamed, craggy peak to the southwest. For more scenery and exercise, continue on the trail to the equally scenic Ball Lakes. To reach them, turn sharply left at the outlet of Pyramid Lake and climb a boulder-strewn slope on seven moderately steep switchbacks to the top of a ridge. You then wander up and down through lovely subalpine-fir forests for 0.5 mile to a signed fork. The trail to the left descends several hundred yards to Lower Ball Lake, while the path to the right goes just 50 yards to slightly larger Upper Ball Lake. Both lakes are set in very scenic granite basins and have good campsites.

To do the longer side trip, return to the junction below Pyramid Pass and go northeast, following signs to Trout and Big Fisher lakes. This trail goes gradually uphill across the partly forested southeast side of Fisher Ridge, where you'll have fine views ahead of Trout Creek Canyon and back to the peaks around Pyramid Lake. After about 1 mile the trail levels off, contours around a high point in the ridge, then descends 250 feet to Trout Lake. This gorgeous lake sits beneath a high granite mountain and has a couple of very good campsites above its east shore. Beyond Trout Lake the trail makes a moderately steep, 1-mile climb to the top of Fisher Ridge, then ascends the ridgeline to a 7400-foot pass with fine views down to Big Fisher Lake. From here, you steeply descend to the shores of this very scenic lake, where the trail ends. The best campsites are on the lake's southwest shore, but the best views are from the east shore back up to the high ridgeline you just descended.

To finish the loop trail, go back over Pyramid Pass and return to the junction with the Parker Ridge Trail. Go north (uphill) and steeply climb through an area that was swept by fire several decades ago and that still hides some silvery snags amid the new forest. After a little over 0.5 mile of steep uphill, you reach the ridgecrest at a rocky saddle, where you'll have exceptional views west to Smith Peak, north down Long Canyon, and northeast down the wooded canyon of Parker Creek and up to Fisher Peak. The trail then turns to follow the ridgecrest and slowly climbs for 400 yards to a junction

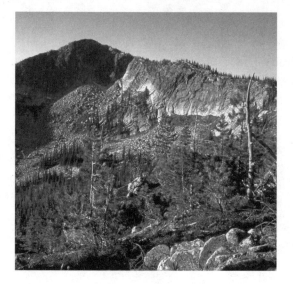

Along Parker Ridge Trail

with the 0.5-mile spur trail that switchbacks down to Long Mountain Lake. This side trip would be worthwhile if only to appreciate this small, deep lake's lovely setting surrounded by heather and perky subalpine firs in a basin of white granite rocks. But the best reasons to make the side trip are that this lake is one of the few permanent water sources on Parker Ridge and it has an excellent campsite.

The main trail continues straight from the Long Mountain Lake junction and ascends Parker Ridge to a point just below the rolling summit of 7265-foot Long Mountain. High-elevation wildflowers are abundant on this open ridge, especially pussy toes, lousewort, and white heather. Views are similarly grand, featuring outstanding vistas up and down the spine of the Selkirk Mountains, into the green depths of Long Canyon, and north to the vastness of Canada.

From Long Mountain, you go down to a saddle, then climb partway up a tall, rocky, pyramid-shaped summit. Before reaching the top, the trail cuts to the left, makes an up-and-down traverse across the west side of this peak, then drops again in steep switchbacks and follows the undulating ridgecrest as it curves east. There are plenty of possible campsites along this scenic ridge, but the only water is from snowfields that may, if you are lucky, linger into early August. At a saddle about 3.5 miles from Long Mountain is the junction with the 0.7-mile side trail to Parker Lake. This lake has excellent fishing, but it isn't as spectacular as most of the other lakes in this range, and camping near the shore is limited by brush and steep slopes. You'll still want to visit this lake, however, because it's the last reliable source of water until a small spring about 6 miles ahead. If you choose to camp here, the best sites are on the ridge near the main trail, although they force you to walk a long way to get water.

The main trail bears right at the Parker Lake junction and climbs fairly steeply to a long, ridgetop saddle where there is another junction. The trail that goes straight makes a steep, 0.5-mile climb to the former lookout site atop prominent Parker Peak, where you can take in many of the same views you had along the ridge, but from a higher and better grandstand. The Parker Ridge Trail bears right at the junction, goes steadily downhill across the rocky east face of Parker Peak, then regains about 250 feet and returns to the wide and heavily forested ridgetop.

It's all downhill from here, most of the time in dense woods, which reverse the previous pattern of a change in tree species that you noticed on the way up. The descent starts quite gently as it goes through a long, woodsy saddle, then makes a series of well-graded switchbacks. At the third switchback turn, a trail goes straight about 10 yards to a small spring with welcome water. Unfortunately, there is no flat ground nearby to accommodate a tent. The last part of the descent takes you across large, grassy areas with good views of the farmland and meandering river in the Kootenai River Valley. At the 43rd switchback, a little before the bottom of the long downhill, you meet Parker Creek Trail #14. Here you turn left and go down nine short switchbacks to the Parker Creek trailhead on Westside Road.

POSSIBLE ITINERARY			
	Camp	Miles	Elevation Gain
Day 1	First crossing of Long Canyon Creek	8	2300
Day 2	Pyramid Lake	11	3200
Day 3	Pyramid Lake (dayhike to Ball Lakes and Big Fisher Lake)	13	3700
Day 4	Ridge above Parker Lake (with side trip to Long Mountain Lake)	8	2700
Day 5	Out (with side trip to Parker Peak)	12*	1100*

* These numbers exclude the road walk back to the Canyon Creek trailhead.

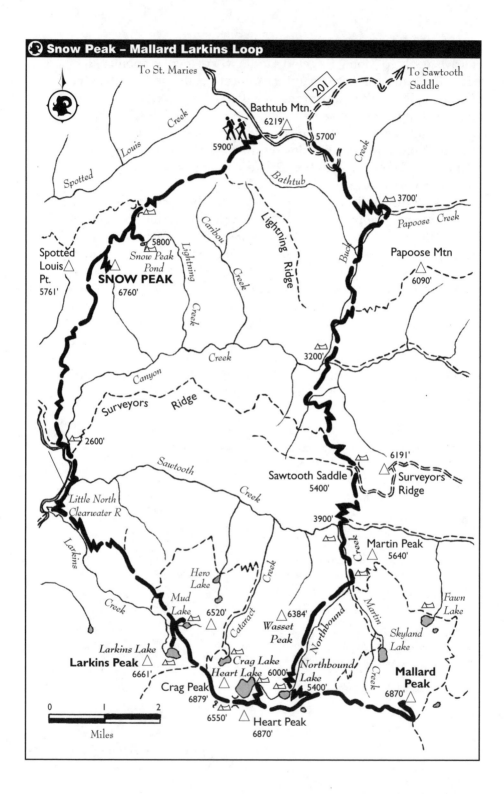

Snow Peak – Mallard Larkins Loop

To St. Maries

201

To Sawtooth Saddle

Louis Creek

Spotted Creek

Bathtub Mtn.
6219'

5900'

5700'

Bathtub

Creek

3700'

Papoose Creek

Caribou Creek

Lightning Creek

Lightning Ridge

Buck

Spotted Louis Pt.
5761'

5800'
Snow Peak Pond

SNOW PEAK
6760'

Papoose Mtn
6090'

Creek

3200'

Canyon

Surveyors Ridge

Creek

Sawtooth Saddle
5400'

6191'

Surveyors Ridge

2600'

Sawtooth

Creek

3900'

Little North Clearwater R

Larkins

Martin Peak
5640'

Creek

Hero Lake

Creek

Cataract Creek

Martin Creek

Fawn Lake

Mud Lake
6520'

Wasset Peak
6384'

Skyland Lake

Northbound

Larkins Lake

Larkins Peak
6661'

Crag Lake

Heart Lake
6000'

Northbound Lake
5400'

Mallard Peak
6870'

Crag Peak
6879'

6550'

Heart Peak
6870'

0   1   2
Miles

2 Snow Peak – Mallard Larkins Loop

RATINGS (1–10)			MILES	ELEVATION GAIN	DAYS	SHUTTLE MILEAGE
Scenery	Solitude	Difficulty	34	10,100	3-5	N/A
7	5	9	(42)	(12,400)	(4-6)	

MAPS USGS - Bathtub Mountain, Buzzard Roost, Mallard Peak, Montana Peak.

USUALLY OPEN July to early October.

BEST Mid-July (for flowers) or mid-August to mid-September (for huckleberries).

PERMITS None.

RULES The usual no-trace principles apply.

CONTACT St. Joe Ranger District, Avery Office, (208) 245-4517.

SPECIAL ATTRACTIONS Huckleberries; wildlife; great views from two fire lookouts.

PROBLEMS Long road access; rough, obscure, and very brushy trail from Snow Peak down to the Little North Fork Clearwater River.

HOW TO GET THERE From the small town of St. Maries, go 1 mile north on State Highway 3, then turn right (northeast) onto St. Joe River Road, following signs to Calder and Avery. Stay on this good paved road, which eventually becomes Forest Road 50, for 69 miles to a junction with Bluff Creek Road (Forest Road 509). Turn right, immediately cross a bridge over the St. Joe River, and climb 8.1 miles on this narrow gravel road to a fork. Bear left onto Forest Road 1250, following signs to Pineapple Saddle, and drive 3.4 miles to a four-way junction. Turn left, following signs to Beaver Creek, and proceed 3.9 miles to the Snow Peak trailhead in a saddle below the rounded summit of Bathtub Mountain. The trailhead comes complete with an outhouse, a horse feeding station, and a primitive car campground near a small spring just west of, and below, the parking lot.

INTRODUCTION This ruggedly difficult loop takes you into the heart of the very scenic Mallard Larkins Pioneer Area. The "pioneer area" designation is an administrative rather than a legislative classification, which is not the same permanent protection as wilderness status, but which provides for similar management of the area as roadless and machine-free. Regardless of what you call it, this lovely region features plenty of crowd-pleasing attributes, including scenic lakes, good fishing, and great views.

A special feature of this area is its unusual abundance of wildlife. Elk seem to be everywhere, and moose can sometimes be seen near the rivers and lakes. Mountain goats are found on all of the area's craggy mountains, and a particularly well-known herd lives on the cliffs of Snow Peak. In addition, black bears are common enough that hikers should hang their food to keep it safe from marauding bruins.

All this wildlife attracts hunters during the elk season in October. If you visit then, make yourself conspicuous by wearing bright red or orange clothing.

"Larkin" was the name of an early homesteader in this area, but the origin of the name "Mallard" is unknown, although it probably does *not* refer to the duck, since the only waterfowl found on the area's high lakes are a few goldeneyes.

> *Tip:* Do not do this loop clockwise, because going up the exposed, hard-to-find, and mostly dry trail between the Little North Clearwater River and Snow Peak would be *no fun at all*.

DESCRIPTION Snow Peak Trail #55, which is blessedly closed to motor vehicles to reduce the impact of noise on the mountain goats, begins in a dense ridgetop forest of firs and mountain hemlocks. Beneath these lichen-draped trees, the forest floor is covered with huckleberries, beargrass, and grouse whortleberries. The wide and well-maintained trail immediately gets your thigh muscles warmed up with a 450-foot ascent on a wide ridge. This climb is the first of many ups and downs along this rolling ridge, none of which is overly steep, but when taken together add up to a significant amount of elevation gain. At the 1-mile point you bear right at the junction with the Lightning Ridge Trail, then spend the next 2 miles

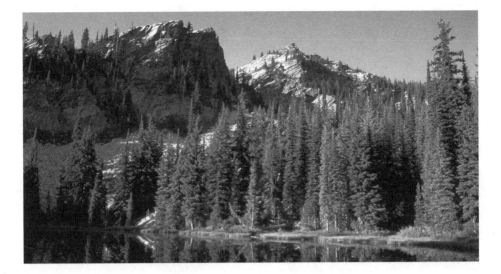

Snow Peak over Snow Peak Pond

going down, up, then down again to a saddle and a junction with the Spotted Louis Trail #104.

You bear slightly left at the junction and, 30 yards later, come to a pleasant campsite with water from a tiny spring to the east. Although there are no views here, a night at this camp is rewarded with the sounds of an unusually high concentration of owls, which hoot for hours from their perches in the trees. Expert birders will recognize the calls of great horned, barred, and screech owls, and they may pick out the distant sound of a great gray or a pygmy owl as well.

A little less than 1 mile of steady uphill from this campsite takes you to an unsigned junction at a forest opening with a first-rate view of rugged Snow Peak. The 0.5-mile deadend trail to the left winds downhill to shallow Snow Peak Pond, where there is an excellent campsite with a terrific view up to the nearby cliffs of Snow Peak. This pond is also a fine spot to watch mountain goats leaping from ledge to ledge in a display that would make a prima ballerina look clumsy.

The main trail goes straight at the unsigned junction and climbs around the back side of a rocky ridgeline to an unsigned fork. The trail to the left (uphill) is the not-to-be-missed side trip to the top of Snow Peak. This short, scenic path steeply ascends through open forests and sloping meadows with nice displays of colorful arnica, yarrow, paintbrush, lousewort, pink heather, and other wildflowers. From the wooden lookout building atop the rocky pinnacle of Snow

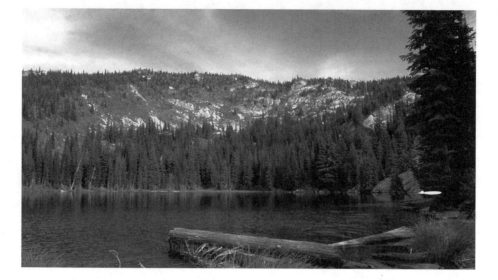

Mud Lake

Peak the views are breathtaking. No single landmark dominates the scene, but the view over a seemingly endless sea of wooded peaks, ridges, and river canyons is inspiring. In addition to the views, you stand a good chance of seeing mountain goats on the crags near the lookout. A sign tells the history of the prolific Snow Peak herd, which has been used since 1960 as a "mother herd" for transplanted goats throughout the American West.

Back on the main trail, you go south, make a gentle descent across a partly forested hillside, then contour around a sloping basin and go gradually down the spine of a ridge on the southwest side of Snow Peak. After this deceptively gentle start, you plunge very steeply downhill on a rarely, if ever, maintained trail that includes a fair amount of deadfall and is overgrown with miles of miserable brush. The builders of this trail were of the old school, shortest-distance-between-two-points mentality, so there are few switchbacks to ease the grade. The brush combines with numerous elk paths to make things very confusing. The proper trail generally stays close to the top of the ridge, although you need to watch carefully, because there are several confusing detours down the hillside on your left. If you get lost (and you will) just persevere in struggling along the ridgetop until you relocate the trail and, when you get back to civilization, write a letter to the Forest Service asking them to send a trail crew to maintain this important connecting trail at least once every 10 or 15 years. After descending 3700 feet, the seemingly endless downhill finally concludes at an unsigned junction just above the confluence of Canyon Creek and the Little North Fork Clearwater River.

Tip: A considerably longer but better maintained alternate route to reach this point follows the Spotted Louis Trail from the junction northeast of Snow Peak to Little North Fork Clearwater River. From there, you turn left and hike Trail # 50 to Canyon Creek.

Delighted to have that rough and miserable section completed, you turn left (downstream) on good Trail #50 and make a knee-deep ford of clear Canyon Creek. Immediately on the south side of the creek is a broken-down building called Trappers Cabin and a very good campsite, or rather it *would* be good if not for the almost constant presence of large horse parties that make the spot very aromatic and home to thousands of horse flies. Atop a little spur ridge just past this camp is a junction with the Surveyors Ridge Trail, where you go straight, sticking with the Little North Fork Clearwater River Trail. Less than 0.5 mile later, you make an easy ford of Sawtooth Creek, then gradually climb a heavily forested hillside to a junction just after you begin to switchback down the south side of a spur ridge.

You bear left (uphill), following signs to Larkins Lake, and start a long ascent of the steep-sided canyon that holds cascading Larkins Creek. The climb has an irregular grade, but it is often very steep as it works its way up the southwest-facing slope of the canyon. The first mile goes across mostly open, sun-exposed slopes, then the canyon walls become increasingly wooded, so the remainder of the climb is in the shade. The trail eventually pulls away from the creek, climbs six moderately steep switchbacks, then turns southeast and steadily climbs a wide, wooded ridge to an unsigned and unmapped junction with a trail that goes sharply left.

You go straight and keep slowly plugging away uphill, often under the shade of huge, old-growth western red cedars, to a signed junction with the very rough Hero Lake Trail. Bear right and soon reach a confusing junction with a very good horse trail that is not shown on any map. Your trail turns left (uphill) and ascends through a series of small, brushy meadows filled with aster, coneflower, groundsel, pearly everlasting, paintbrush, and other tall wildflowers. Eventually, the trail leaves these lush meadows and crosses an open, view-packed hillside carpeted with huckleberries.

Partway up this hillside is a signed junction with the 0.5-mile side trail, right, to Larkins Lake. Set directly beneath the cliffs of Larkins Peak, this scenic lake has plenty of fish and some good campsites. Just 10 yards beyond the Larkins Lake turnoff is an unsigned junction with the 150-yard side trail that goes left and uphill to Mud Lake. This beautiful, misnamed lake has an excellent campsite of its own and a fine view of the long ridge of Gnat Peak.

The main trail goes straight at both of these junctions and keeps climbing the open hillside for 0.5 mile to the top of the ridgeline east of Larkins Peak. The trail then curves left and traverses the south side of a knoll to an unsigned junction with Trail #240, which angles in from the right. Go straight and, just 200 yards later, reach a junction with the irregularly maintained Cataract Creek Trail.

Tip: For a nice side trip, turn left and go 1 mile down this trail to scenic Crag Lake, which has a couple of nice, secluded campsites.

Your route, now called Heart Pass Trail, goes straight and makes a gradual uphill traverse around the south side of Crag Peak. After a little over 0.5 mile, you pass a nice, view-packed campsite beside a (really) tiny spring, then reach a high saddle between Crag Peak and Heart Peak. Just north of this saddle is sparkling Heart Lake, the largest and arguably the most scenic lake in the Mallard Larkins area.

From the saddle, the trail goes downhill across the steep, rocky north face of Heart Peak to an unsigned junction. The trail to the left drops very steeply to the shores of gorgeous Heart Lake, which is well worth a visit. If you want to spend the night at this deep lake, you'll find a couple of excellent campsites above the northeast shore. Here you can happily while away several hours fishing or watching mountain goats on the sheer cliffs that drop into three sides of the lake.

Warning: Treacherous snowfields often remain on the north-facing slope of Heart Peak until late July or early August.

After returning to the main trail, you hike a little over 1 mile east, still going downhill across a north-facing slope, to the junction with Northbound Creek Trail #111. This is the best maintained of the several trails that go north from the Mallard Larkins area back toward your car.

Having completed the Mallard Peak side trip, head north (appropriately enough) on the Northbound Creek Trail and descend

Mallard Peak Fire Lookout

Before returning to the Snow Peak trailhead, take some time for a scenic side trip. This time your goal is the excellent view from the historic fire lookout atop Mallard Peak. To reach it, go straight at the Northbound Creek junction and follow a gentle trail for a little less than 1 mile to a junction with the little-used Martin Creek Trail. Bear right, make a steady uphill, then contour across the south side of a scenic ridge covered with brushy Douglas' knotweed to a four-way junction at the top of a spur ridge. Look for mountain goats on the crags just southeast of this junction.

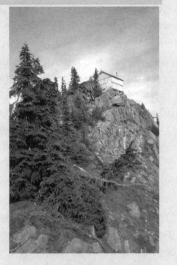

To reach Mallard Peak, you turn left and climb steeply for 0.5 mile to the cliff-edged mountain top. The wooden lookout building here was originally built in 1929 and is now on the National Register of Historic Places. It was restored in the 1980s through the volunteer efforts of Ray Kresek, an avid lookout buff from Spokane, Washington. From this site, you can enjoy views north and west over most of the area covered by this hike, as well as south to the rugged Clearwater River country.

nine gentle switchbacks to a couple of excellent campsites at the northeast end of beautiful Northbound Lake. The trail then crosses the lake's outlet, goes down several short switchbacks, and follows splashing Northbound Creek. Although this section has a fair amount of brush and frequent muddy areas, it also treats the hiker to a feast of unusually large and abundant huckleberries in late August and early September. About 2.5 miles beyond Northbound Lake, you rock-hop the creek and immediately come to a nice campsite beside a junction with the Martin Creek Trail.

You bear left and, in the next mile, make two more rock-hop crossings of Northbound Creek to a good campsite just before the shallow ford of Sawtooth Creek. By late summer the water is low enough to reveal a string of conveniently placed stepping stones, which will get you across with dry feet. Rest and fill your water bottles here, because you now face a long, tough uphill. It begins with three short switchbacks that take you to a junction with the Sawtooth Creek Trail. Go straight on the dusty and more-heavily-used trail, then climb at a relentless, moderately steep grade for nearly 2 miles on an open, south-facing slope that can be oppressively hot in midsummer. Eleven switchbacks keep the grade from becoming excessively steep, but it's still a tiring climb. At the top of Surveyors Ridge, you intersect a primitive road, where you turn left and walk 50 yards to the roadend trailhead at Sawtooth Saddle. This is an alternate starting point for this trip if you are willing to make the long, bumpy drive to this remote location.

To continue the loop, take Surveyors Ridge Trail #40, which angles down from the north side of the trailhead parking area. This gently graded trail slowly loses elevation for 1 mile on the heavily forested north side of Surveyors Ridge to a junction with Buck Creek Trail #100. You turn right (downhill) and steadily lose 1600 feet in a little less than 2 miles to a calf-deep ford of Canyon Creek. About 50 yards up the opposite bank is a junction with Upper Canyon Creek Trail #99.

You bear left, staying on the Buck Creek Trail, and, 100 yards later, come to a nice campsite beside Buck Creek. A short distance past the camp, the trail appears to cross the creek, but the correct route stays above the east bank and heads upstream through lush woods. Frequent crisscrossing elk paths and several muddy spots confuse things in this area, but numerous blazes make the proper route obvious. A little over 0.5 mile from Canyon Creek, you ford Buck Creek, then, just 100 yards later, get wet again as you recross the flow at a calf-deep ford.

A bit less than 0.5 mile past these two crossings, you hop over a tiny side creek, then make a short, steep climb to a junction with Papoose Mountain Trail #101. You go straight and descend to a third crossing of Buck Creek, this time on a log.

Warning: The section of trail above this crossing does not get maintained very often, so you are forced to struggle through dense riparian vegetation and to make frequent, frustrating detours around some huge blowdown. Fortunately, there is only about 0.5 mile of this tough hiking before the trail heads up onto the hillsides above the water, where the route is in much better shape.

Not quite 1 mile from the Papoose Mountain junction is the first of five more creek crossings, none of which is very deep, but nearly all of which require that you get your feet wet. Immediately after the fourth crossing, this time over Papoose Creek, you come to a junction with Papoose Creek Trail #627. Turn left and soon come to a nice campsite just before you cross Buck Creek for the last time.

The trail is now well-maintained as it makes a long, 2000-foot climb through forests back up to Bathtub Mountain. The climb begins with a dozen, moderately graded switchbacks to the top of a ridgeline, then the trail turns northwest and ascends along the top of the ridge. After 1.5 miles, you climb several short switchbacks, then come to a junction with an abandoned road. The trail resumes across the overgrown road, then goes uphill at a gentle grade, makes one switchback, and meets the road for a second time. This time you follow the road for 30 yards, then angle to the right on a foot trail that travels through open woods to a signed trailhead on a good gravel road. To return to your car, turn left and follow this gently ascending road for 1 mile back to the Snow Peak trailhead.

VARIATIONS You can shorten this hike to a 31-mile loop and avoid the trip's most difficult ups and down by starting from Sawtooth Saddle. This variation follows the Surveyors Ridge Trail to the Little North Clearwater River, then returns via the southern section past the lakes in the Mallard Larkins area. To reach Sawtooth Saddle, drive about 20 miles past the Snow Peak trailhead on a bumpy and rough road that requires a slow pace. Since this shorter loop misses Snow Peak, you will want to leave time for a dayhike to this major highlight on the way back from your backpacking trip.

POSSIBLE ITINERARY			
	Camp	**Miles**	**Elevation Gain**
Day 1	Snow Peak Pond	4	1000
Day 2	Mud Lake (with side trip to the top of Snow Peak)	12	4400
Day 3	Northbound Lake (with side trips to Larkins Lake, Heart Lake, and Mallard Peak)	10	2600
Day 4	Lower Buck Creek	8.5	1600
Day 5	Out	7.5	2800

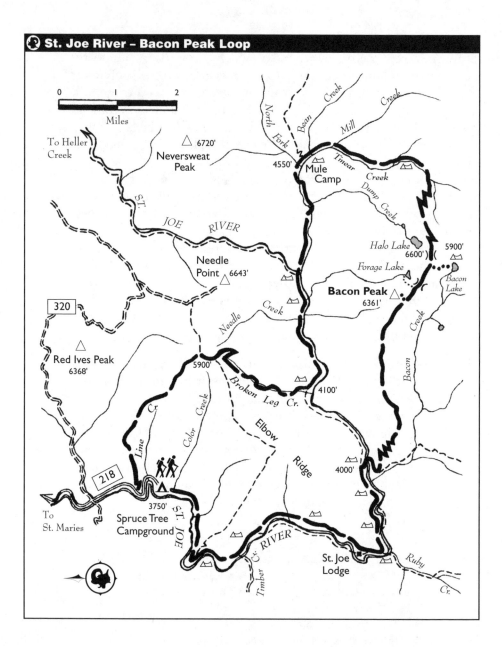

St. Joe River – Bacon Peak Loop

0   1   2
Miles

To Heller
Creek

△ 6720'
Neversweat
Peak

North Fork

Bean Creek

Mill Creek

4550'
Mule
Camp

Tmear Creek

Dump Creek

ST. JOE RIVER

Needle
Point △ 6643'

Halo Lake
6600')(

5900'

Forage Lake

Bacon Peak
6361'

Bacon Lake

320

Red Ives Peak
6368'

Needle Creek

5900'

4100'

Broken Leg Cr.

Color Creek

Lime Cr.

Elbow
Ridge

Bacon Creek

4000'

218

3750'
Spruce Tree
Campground

ST. JOE

To
St. Maries

Timber Cr.

ST. JOE RIVER

St. Joe
Lodge

Ruby
Cr.

50   Backpacking Idaho

3 St. Joe River – Bacon Peak Loop

RATINGS (1–10)			MILES	ELEVATION GAIN	DAYS	SHUTTLE MILEAGE
Scenery	Solitude	Difficulty	31	5000	3-4	N/A
6	7	6	(33)	(6200)	(3-5)	

MAPS USGS - Bacon Peak, Chamberlain Mountain, Red Ives Peak.

USUALLY OPEN July to early October.

BEST August and September.

PERMITS None.

RULES The usual no-trace principles apply.

CONTACT St. Joe Ranger District, Avery Office, (208) 245-4517.

SPECIAL ATTRACTIONS Huckleberries; excellent fishing.

PROBLEMS Two potentially difficult river fords, especially in early summer.

HOW TO GET THERE From the small town of St. Maries, go 1 mile north on State Highway 3, then turn right (northeast) onto St. Joe River Road, following signs to Calder and Avery. Stay on this good paved road, which eventually becomes Forest Road 50, for 76 miles to a prominent junction. Turn right onto Forest Road 218, and drive 9.8 miles on this single-lane road to a bridge just after the Red Ives Ranger Station, where the pavement ends. Immediately after the bridge, you bear right at a junction, staying on Road 218, and drive 2.0 miles on this pothole-filled gravel road to the trailhead parking area at the south end of the loop through Spruce Tree Campground.

INTRODUCTION The St. Joe River is unquestionably one of the most beautiful rivers in Idaho (or anywhere else, for that matter). Its crystal-clear waters flow through a densely forested canyon of lush vegetation that surrounds the hiker in a landscape of every conceivable shade of green. If the surrounding scenery weren't enough, the river's cool waters hide lots of large plump trout making the stream one of the country's best fly-fishing rivers. The St. Joe River is managed as a catch-and-release fishery; barbless hooks are required.

The trail along the upper reaches of the St. Joe River is a wonderful hike any time that it's open, but if you want to include a visit to the high lakes and viewpoints around Bacon Peak, then it's better to go in late summer or early fall, when the two fords of the St. Joe River that this side trip requires won't end up washing you all the way downstream to St. Maries. A bonus of taking this trip in late August or early September is the chance to feast on the acres of huckleberries that carpet the ridges around Bacon Peak.

DESCRIPTION The gently graded trail heads upstream following a long-abandoned road that stays on the woodsy hillside a little above the St. Joe River. Although the trail is (blessedly) closed to motor vehicles, it is very popular with equestrians, so you can expect plenty of horse apples and a fair amount of dust.

> **Tip:** After it rains (a frequent occurrence in this relatively wet part of the state) the dust is turned into messy mud, so bring a pair of gaiters to help your boots and legs stay clean and dry.

At the 1.5-mile point, you pass the junction with Elbow Ridge Trail #79 and follow the river in a sharp turn to the southeast. Just 0.5 mile later, you descend to a forest opening with a nice, grassy campsite, then walk a few hundred yards to the end of the old road.

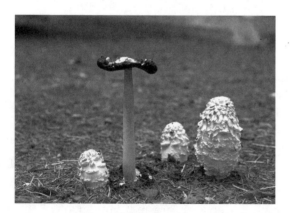

Inky cap mushrooms along St. Joe River

Now on a lovely trail, you closely follow the rippling waters of the clear St. Joe River through a lush forest of Engelmann spruce, Douglas-fir, western hemlock, and a mix of other conifers. All these trees combine with the dense riparian shrubbery to create a lovely green tapestry. The next junction is with Timber Creek Trail #54, where you go straight, soon pass a very inviting riverside campsite, and then come to a horse trail that angles off to the right on its way to St. Joe Lodge. You bear left, go up and down across the woodsy hillside above the river for 1 mile, then descend to a grassy flat with lots of wildflowers and a good campsite. Another mile of up-and-down hiking takes you past the buildings of St. Joe Lodge to a junction with a short spur trail that goes down to this guest facility. You go straight and soon reach a junction with Ruby Creek Trail #71.

Tip: *There is an excellent riverside campsite just 50 yards down the Ruby Creek Trail.*

The St. Joe River Trail bears left and follows the stream as it makes a sharp turn to the northeast. A little over 0.5 mile past the Ruby Creek junction the trail passes a campsite and then splits. A horse trail goes to the right and immediately fords the river, while the hiker's trail bears left and climbs the river's north bank to a fine viewpoint. After this, you descend to a reunion with the horse trail, then hike a few hundred yards to an excellent campsite that is the perfect place to relax by the river, fish, and enjoy the sights and sounds of running water.

About 0.5 mile past this campsite, you leave the St. Joe River Trail and veer right (downhill) on Pass Creek Trail #61, which soon comes to a good campsite just before a ford of the St. Joe River. In early summer this ford is a major obstacle, with the water typically running halfway up your backpack. By late summer the water remains cold enough to numb your toes, but the ford is only about calf-to-knee-deep and is not particularly dangerous. Leave your wading shoes on after you make this ford, because it turns out that this is only part of the river. Just 80 yards later, but unseen from the first ford, you have to cross a second, equally large but not as swift branch of the river.

The trail climbs steadily away from the river through viewless forests to a junction with Bacon Loop Trail #66. You turn left and make a 1-mile, switchbacking ascent to a ridgeline and a small, muddy elk wallow.

Warning: *Several confusing elk paths converge here. Look for the uphill trail on the left marked with blazes to identify the route meant for two-legged travelers.*

The trail now makes a long, dry climb along the top of the ridge. Although the ascent is tiring and often steep, it also has many benefits. In addition to the usual spruces and firs, the forests here have large numbers of western larch trees, which put on a nice display of gold and orange in October. Another welcome part of the local botany is huckleberries, which get more abundant as you gain elevation, and provide tasty treats for hungry hikers from mid-August to early September. Finally, the trail passes through several small, ridgetop meadows, which are filled with bracken fern, coneflower, and goldenrod, and allow you to enjoy excellent vistas to the south over the canyon of Bacon Creek and its surrounding ridges. Bacon Creek is the first of many features in this area that carry either the name "Bacon" or the name "Bean." The names were bestowed by early prospectors in honor of their rather monotonous diets.

About 1800 feet up from the St. Joe River, the trail passes through a small burn area, after which the grade becomes noticeably less steep on a traverse across the south side of Bacon Peak.

Tip: For an easy and rewarding side trip, make the short, cross-country scramble to the viewpoint atop the tilted pile of shale at the summit of Bacon Peak. The views over the St. Joe River Canyon are excellent.

The trail soon reaches a view-packed saddle above Forage Lake. If you want to visit this deep and very scenic lake (a perfectly reasonable desire, given its dramatic setting), then avoid the impressive cliffs directly above the water and scramble instead down the very steep, brushy slope west of Forage Lake. There are a couple of mediocre but very scenic campsites near Forage Lake's outlet.

The main trail goes down to a low point at the southeast end of the saddle, then turns uphill and traverses the side of a ridge. A short distance from the saddle, sparkling Bacon Lake becomes visible in a basin to the south. To reach this lake, leave the trail and descend steeply over mostly open slopes, then pick up a sketchy bootpath that contours through forests to a very good campsite on the lake's north shore.

The main trail climbs to the top of the view-packed ridge, then continues to an overlook, where you can peer down on Halo Lake in a deep cirque to the north. After this, you reach a high point just below the summit of a craggy peak, then make a lengthy descent over steep slopes covered with flowery meadows and open forests. Ten switchbacks are placed at strategic intervals along the way, so the trail is reasonably well graded. About 1.5 miles from the top,

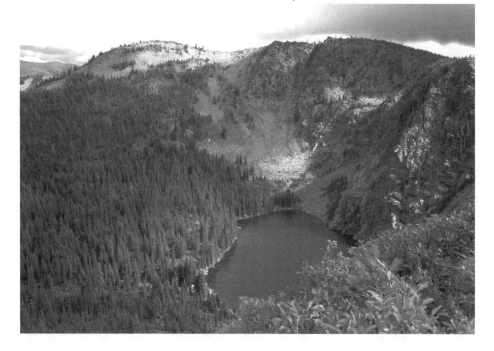

Forage Lake nestled below Bacon Peak

you rock-hop over small Tinear Creek, which, unless you made the side trip to either Forage or Bacon Lake, has the first water and campsites since the St. Joe River, 7 miles back.

For the next 2 miles you go gently downhill through dense forests beside cascading Tinear Creek, then make rock-hop crossings of both Mill Creek and Bean Creek. Immediately after the second of these crossings you come to a wooden corral and a hunter's camp. A few hundred yards later is the junction with Bean Divide Trail #610, where you go straight and make a rock-hop crossing of North Fork Bean Creek. About 100 yards after this crossing is a small sign identifying Mule Camp, which is a nice place to spend the night, whether you have any mules or not.

The trail turns west, following Bean Creek, soon makes two chilly fords of the creek, then makes a lengthy up-and-down traverse to a ford of the St. Joe River. Like the earlier ford of the St. Joe, this crossing can be a major challenge in early summer, but by late summer it is only knee-deep (although *very* cold). There is an excellent campsite immediately after this ford.

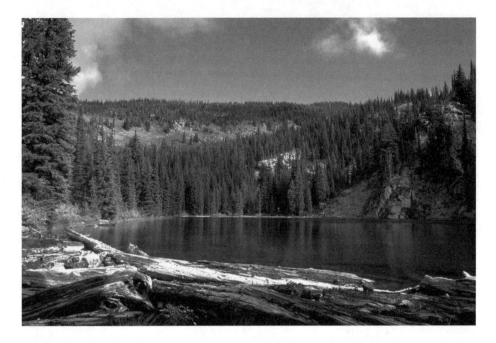

Bacon Lake

About 200 yards past the St. Joe River ford is a junction with the St. Joe River Trail, where you bear left and begin a lovely walk down the river's scenic canyon. You soon pass a good campsite, then go across a series of grassy meadows and rocky areas that alternate with forests to create a very pleasant mix of riverside scenery. About 2.5 miles from the Bean Creek junction is a spacious camp area and the junction with Broken Leg Trail #230.

Here you face a choice. If you go straight, you'll return to Spruce Tree Campground via the St. Joe River Trail, repeating much of the route you hiked on the way in. To enjoy some different scenery on a shorter return route, turn right on the Broken Leg Trail.

Warning: *Although 2.5 miles shorter, this rugged trail gains 1700 feet more elevation than the riverside route.*

The Broken Leg Trail starts by going gradually uphill for a few hundred yards to an easy hop over its small namesake creek. For the next mile the trail crosses and recrosses tiny Broken Leg Creek several times, then finally settles on the west side and makes a very steep, woodsy climb. The creek eventually disappears, but the trail keeps going uphill, making two long switchbacks near the top of the climb and coming to a junction with the Elbow Ridge Trail. You go straight, still heading uphill, and, less than 0.5 mile later, intersect the Line Creek Trail. You turn sharply left and make a short additional climb to a high point on the ridge, where you can rest and enjoy exceptional views east over a series of forested canyons and ridges to the distant mountains of Montana.

The trail then heads northwest in a long, unevenly graded descent that is sometimes very gentle and at other times quite steep, but rarely anything in between. The gentle sections eventually cease, so the last 1.5 miles take you steeply downhill until your jammed toes get relief at the Line Creek trailhead on Forest Road 218. To return to your car, turn left and walk 0.8 mile along this road back to Spruce Tree Campground.

VARIATIONS If you want to skip the difficult fords and just experience the river without the high lakes and views, then remain on the St. Joe River Trail all the way upstream to a remote trailhead near Heller Creek Campground. To leave a car at this trailhead, follow a rough dirt road that heads east from the Red Ives Ranger Station.

POSSIBLE ITINERARY			
	Camp	**Miles**	**Elevation Gain**
Day 1	St. Joe River (above Ruby Creek)	7	500
Day 2	Bacon Lake (with side trips to Bacon Peak and Forage Lake)	8.5	3500
Day 3	Broken Leg Creek	10.5	1000
Day 4	Out	7	2200

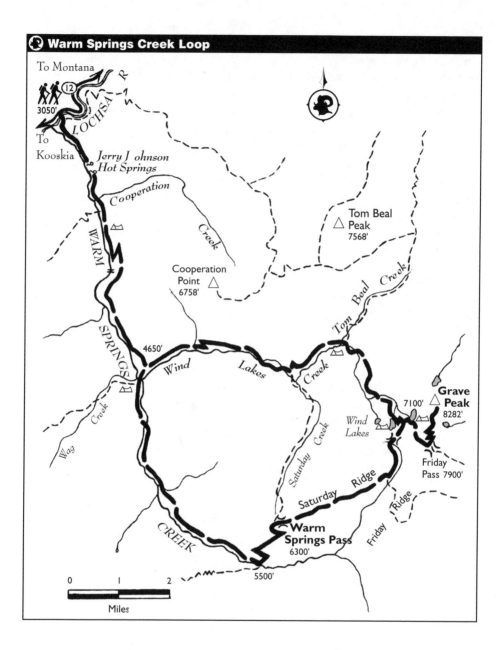

Warm Springs Creek Loop

To Montana

3050'

To Kooskia

LOCHSA R

12

Jerry Johnson Hot Springs

Cooperation Creek

WARM

SPRINGS

Wag Creek

Creek

4650'

Wind Lakes

CREEK

Cooperation Point 6758'

Tom Beal Peak 7568'

Tom Beal Creek

Creek

Wind Lakes

Saturday Creek

Saturday Ridge

Friday Ridge

Warm Springs Pass 6300'

7100'

Grave Peak 8282'

Friday Pass 7900'

5500'

0   1   2

Miles

4 Warm Springs Creek Loop

RATINGS (1–10)			MILES	ELEVATION GAIN	DAYS	SHUTTLE MILEAGE
Scenery	Solitude	Difficulty	32	5000	3-4	N/A
6	7	7	(36)	(6300)	(3-4)	

MAP USFS - Selway-Bitterroot Wilderness - North Half.

USUALLY OPEN July to October.

BEST Mid-July to August.

PERMITS None.

RULES Maximum group size of 20 people and 20 stock animals.

CONTACT Powell Ranger District, (208) 942-3113.

SPECIAL ATTRACTIONS Great views from Grave Peak; easy road access.

PROBLEMS Mosquitoes in July; rowdy visitors at the hot springs; some brushy and muddy sections of trail.

HOW TO GET THERE From Kooskia, drive 77.5 miles east on U.S. Highway 12 to the well-signed Warm Springs Creek trailhead near a prominent trail bridge over the Lochsa River. (Coming from the east, this trailhead is 23.3 miles west of Lolo Pass.) Parking is available about 50 yards east of the bridge on the north side of the highway. As often happens at trails to hot springs, break-ins often occur at this trailhead; leave nothing of value in your car.

INTRODUCTION This short and relatively easy introduction to the Selway-Bitterroot Wilderness includes just enough high viewpoints, shy wildlife, clear fishing creeks, scenic mountain lakes, and attractive forests to give you a taste of what this area has to offer. If you like this trip, then you'll be delighted to know that the wilderness has another 600 miles of similar trails – more than enough to keep your feet busy for years to come.

DESCRIPTION The trail crosses the foot-and-horse bridge over the Lochsa River and immediately comes to a junction. The wide and well-used hiker's trail turns right and travels through a dense forest of grand firs and drooping western red cedars beside the clear waters of Warm Springs Creek. Beneath this shady canopy, the lush ground cover includes lady, maiden-hair, and sword ferns, and a wide variety of early-summer wildfowers such as star-flowered smilacina, queens cup, twisted stalk, and trillium.

The trail follows the creek for a little over 1 mile to where you'll smell a hint of sulfur in the air and see steam rising from Jerry Johnson Hot Springs. The first spring, a little below the trail, drops as a small cascade directly into the creek. Just 100 yards past this spring is a popular day-use area and several more hot springs. (Jerry Johnson Hot Springs is managed as a day-use area; no overnight camping is allowed.) The springs all look very inviting, but they are usually crowded with noisy visitors, especially on weekends, so most backpackers will want to stay only long enough for a relaxing soak, then move on to a quieter location. The best bathing is at the south end of the springs area in several rock-rimmed pools, where the water is the perfect temperature for a comfortable soak.

> *Tip: Bathing here is clothing-optional, so leave your modesty at home. Try visiting on a weekday in September, when the springs are often deserted. On a crisp autumn morning I had the springs all to myself and sat soaking in a warm pool for almost an hour, quietly watching a moose browse just 40 yards away.*

About 1 mile past the last hot springs is an ankle-deep ford of Cooperation Creek. There is usually a convenient log a short distance downstream, if you want to keep your feet dry.

A few hundred yards after this crossing is a junction with Bear Mountain Trail #213. You go straight, pass a very good campsite, then make two switchbacks and slowly ascend a steep, brushy hillside well above Warm Springs Creek. The scenery here is highlighted by the boisterous stream, which tumbles over numerous cascades and small waterfalls in the rocky canyon on your right. About 2 miles past the campsite the trail briefly returns to the creek, then climbs away from the water through a lodgepole-pine forest to a junction and the start of the loop.

For a clockwise circuit, go left on Wind Lakes Creek Trail #24, which soon begins to climb beside its pretty namesake stream.

After 1 mile, you hop over a small side creek, then make four short, uphill switchbacks followed by a 0.5-mile contour that takes you back to Wind Lakes Creek. The often-brushy trail then wanders uphill through dense thickets of thimbleberries, which ripen in August, to a creek crossing. For most of the hiking season this crossing is a calf-to-knee-deep ford, although in late summer you can use slippery stepping stones to get across without getting wet. Less than 1 mile later is another ford, where there is no alternative to getting your feet wet.

About 500 yards after the second ford is a signed junc-

Grave Peak over Upper Wind Lake

tion with a rough and unmaintained trail up Saturday Creek to Warm Springs Pass. You turn left (uphill), following signs to Tom Beal Creek, and climb at an irregular grade for about 1.5 miles to a junction just after a rock-hop crossing of good-sized Tom Beal Creek. Bear right and immediately hop over what's left of Wind Lakes Creek to a decent campsite on the opposite bank.

The trail crosses the creek again just 100 yards after this campsite, then climbs steadily through numerous boggy areas with an assortment of tall, showy, water-loving wildflowers such as false hellebore, valerian, groundsel, and mountain boykinia. After about 1 mile the trail enters drier terrain and the forest changes to mostly subalpine firs with a few western white pines. The ground cover also switches to plants that prefer drier ground such as beargrass, heather, and thickets of brushy, head-high huckleberries.

You hop over the creek a final time, steeply climb another 400 feet, then level off just before the first Wind Lake. There are fine views across this scenic lake to the sharp pinnacle of Grave Peak to the east. The lake also has good fishing and several excellent (but buggy) campsites near the north shore.

The trail crosses the lake's trickling outlet creek, then makes a very steep, 300-foot ascent to a junction beside a beautiful, meadow-rimmed pond with a very photogenic view of Grave Peak. The main loop trail turns right at this junction, but first you'll want to make a fabulous side trip to Upper Wind Lake and the top of Grave Peak. To do so, go straight and walk 200 yards to large and very scenic Upper Wind Lake, which has a spectacular view of Grave Peak and a very good campsite above its southwest shore.

The trail to Grave Peak, which starts from the southwest end of Upper Wind Lake, goes through forest, then climbs the spine of a very steep, rather rocky ridge where only a few stunted subalpine firs, whitebark pines, and alpine larches survive the harsh conditions. Also struggling to survive in this high-elevation environment are several species of small wildflowers, including lousewort, phlox, partridgefoot, and pink heather. The trail reaches the top of the ridge at a grassy knoll, then descends a short distance to a junction just below Friday Pass. You turn left (north), go through a small notch in the ridge, then descend four quick switchbacks and make an up-and-down traverse across the west side of a jagged high point. The faint trail then switches to the east side of the ridge and steeply picks its way up through rocks to the lookout on the summit of Grave Peak.

The old wooden building, which is no longer staffed, would be worth a visit if only to admire its quaint cupola-style architecture. But it's the remarkable setting and great views that really grab your attention. The peak sits at the apex of three knife-edge ridges (one of which you just climbed) and looks down on sparkling lakes in each of the basins below the summit. The expansive views include the rugged Bitterroot Divide to the east, the Selway Crags to the southwest, the deep chasm of the Lochsa River Canyon to the north, and an infinity of forested hills, ridges, and basins in every direction. Give yourself plenty of time to fully enjoy the scene.

To complete the loop, return to Upper Wind Lake and walk back to the junction 200 yards west of the lake. Turn left (south), hike a few hundred yards to a low saddle in an old burn area, then drop to a delightful meadow at the head of Warm Springs Creek. The trail then descends a fairly steep and rocky hillside beside the burgeoning creek to an easily overlooked junction, where you bear right (slightly uphill) onto Saturday Ridge Trail #8.

Tip: If you miss the junction, you will soon come to a crossing of Warm Springs Creek and know that you have to backtrack a few hundred yards to relocate the proper trail.

The Saturday Ridge Trail goes across the southeast side of its namesake ridge in a long, rolling traverse that gradually gains more elevation than it loses. Along the way you pass through many sloping meadows, which feature July-blooming beargrass, August-ripening huckleberries, and all-season views of Friday Ridge to the east and Hungry Rock to the south. You eventually reach the wide, undulating top of the ridge, follow it for about 1 mile, then descend at a moderate grade to a junction at forested Warm Springs Pass. Turn left and continue the woodsy downhill, losing another 800 feet on a winding trail to a junction just above Warm Springs Creek.

You go straight and begin the long tour down Warm Springs Creek. The trail has no spectacular views or other highlights, but except for some steep little ups and downs and several boggy areas the walking is easy and pleasant. Not quite 5 relatively uneventful miles from the junction, you make an easy, calf-deep ford of Warm Springs Creek, and then, 1 mile later, come to a large and very good camp area just before a junction with Wag Creek Trail #917 to McConnell Mountain. Turn right and immediately make a knee-deep ford just below where Warm Springs Creek and Wind Lakes Creek converge. About 500 yards after this ford, you close the loop at the junction with the Wind Lakes Creek Trail. To return to your car, bear left and retrace your route past the hot springs to the trailhead.

POSSIBLE ITINERARY			
	Camp	Miles	Elevation Gain
Day 1	Tom Beal Creek Junction	11	2900
Day 2	Upper Wind Lake (with side trip to Grave Peak)	7	2800
Day 3	McConnell Mountain Junction	11	500
Day 4	Out	7	100

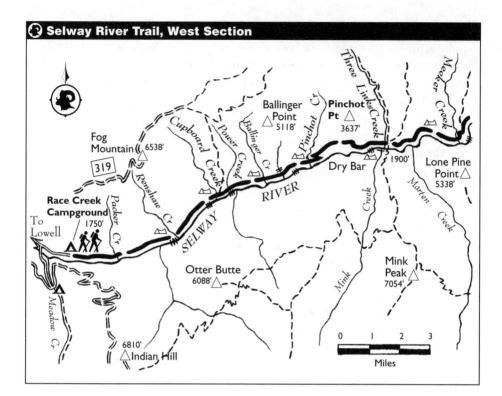

Fog
Mountain 6538'

319

Race Creek
Campground
1750'

To
Lowell

Meadow Cr

Packer Cr

Renshaw Cr

Cupboard Creek

Power Creek

Ballinger Cr

SELWAY

RIVER

Ballinger
Point
5118'

Pinchot Cr

Pinchot
Pt 3637'

Three Links Creek

Meeker Creek

Dry Bar

1900'

Lone Pine
Point 5338'

Mink Creek

Marten Creek

Otter Butte
6088'

Mink
Peak
7054'

6810'
Indian Hill

0   1   2   3

Miles

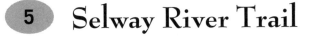

5 Selway River Trail

RATINGS (1–10)			MILES	ELEVATION GAIN	DAYS	SHUTTLE MILEAGE
Scenery	Solitude	Difficulty	50	4200	4-6	252
7	5	5				

MAPS USFS - Selway-Bitterroot Wilderness - North & South Halves.

USUALLY OPEN May to early November.

BEST July to October (for fishing).

PERMITS None.

RULES Maximum group size of 20 people and 20 stock animals.

CONTACT Moose Creek Ranger District, (208) 926-4258.

SPECIAL ATTRACTIONS Good stream fishing; whitewater rafters to watch; canyon scenery.

PROBLEMS Very long car shuttle; rattlesnakes.

HOW TO GET THERE To reach the recommended starting point at the lower trailhead at Race Creek, drive 22 miles east from Kooskia on U.S. Highway 12 to a junction at the tiny resort town of Lowell. Turn right (southeast) onto the Selway River Road, following signs to the Selway Wild and Scenic River, and immediately cross a bridge over the Lochsa River. Drive 18.8 miles on this winding road, which turns from pavement to pothole-filled dirt and gravel after 6.8 miles, to a junction just past the Selway Falls Guard Station. Go straight and drive a final 1.1 miles to the signed trailhead at Race Creek Campground. The trail leaves from the east end of the large parking area.

To reach the upper Selway River trailhead, return to Highway 12, turn east, and drive 113 miles on this scenic road over Lolo Pass and into Montana to a junction with U.S. Highway 93 at Lolo. Turn right (south) on Highway 93 and drive 58 miles to a junction just

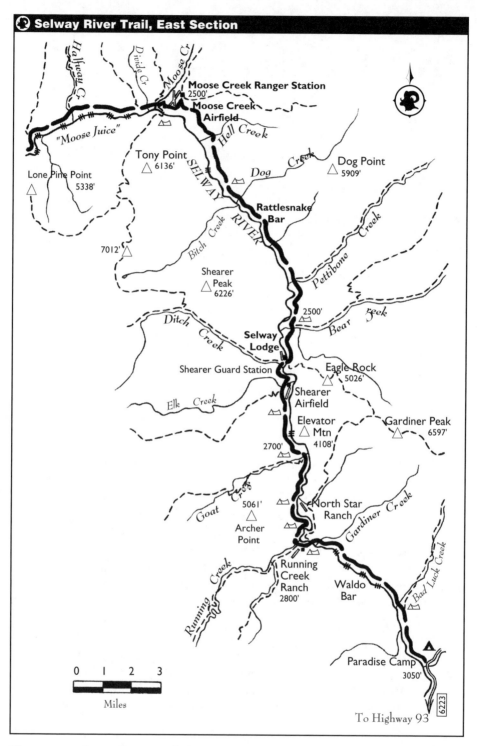

Halfway Cr.

Divide Cr

Moose Cr.

Moose Creek Ranger Station
2500'

Moose Creek Airfield

Hell Creek

"Moose Juice"

Tony Point
△ 6136'

Dog   Creek

Dog Point
△ 5909'

Lone Pine Point
△ 5338'

SELWAY

Bitch Creek

RIVER

Rattlesnake Bar

Pettibone   Creek

7012' △

Shearer Peak
△ 6226'

2500'

Bear   Creek

Ditch   Creek

Selway Lodge

Shearer Guard Station

Eagle Rock
△ 5026'

Elk   Creek

Shearer Airfield

Elevator Mtn
△ 4108'

Gardiner Peak
△ 6597'

2700'

Goat   Creek

5061'
△

North Star Ranch

Gardiner   Creek

Archer Point

Running   Creek

Running Creek Ranch
2800'

Waldo Bar

Bad Luck Creek

Paradise Camp
3050'

6223

To Highway 93

before a bridge over the Bitterroot River. Turn right (southwest) on State Highway 473 (also called West Fork Road), following signs to Trapper Creek Jobs Corps Center, and proceed 14.4 miles to a junction 0.5 mile past the West Fork Ranger Station and immediately before a bridge over West Fork Bitterroot River. Bear right on Nez Perce Road and drive 16.5 miles on this alternating paved and gravel road to Nez Perce Pass, where you reenter Idaho. The pavement continues for another 8.4 miles as the road winds downhill beside the rushing waters of Deep Creek. Once the pavement ends, you follow a bumpy, gravel road for 10.5 miles to a junction with the Magruder Road to Elk City. Go straight, following signs to Paradise Campground, and drive 11.4 miles on narrow and bumpy Forest Road 6223 to a bridge over White Cap Creek and the well-signed Selway River trailhead on the left. It takes a full day to complete this very long car shuttle.

In the summer months you may be tempted to try a shorter car shuttle that follows the very rough dirt road through the Magruder Corridor. Unfortunately, this route usually requires four-wheel drive, especially when the road is wet, and it is so slow it actually takes longer to drive than the recommended road described above.

INTRODUCTION Snaking through the heart of its namesake wilderness, the swift-flowing Selway River is a recreational Mecca for rafters and kayakers who love challenging whitewater and pristine canyon scenery. To preserve the wilderness character of the canyon, the Forest Service strictly limits the number of rafting permits to just one launch per day – a policy which forces floaters to apply for one of the coveted permits months in advance of their trip and makes this one of the country's toughest rivers to get permission to run. But hikers can enjoy the same scenery on the Selway River Trail with no permits required and no restrictions on the number of pedestrians.

The Selway River is managed as a catch-and-release fishery, with the season running from late May to November; barbless hooks are required. On tributary streams you can catch and keep two fish, and the season runs from July through November.

If you are doing the trip as a one-way hike, you'll want to walk downstream from the Selway River trailhead. But since the access road over Nez Perce Pass does not open until sometime in June, early-season hikers must use the Race Creek trailhead. In addition, hikers who want to do a shorter, up-and-back trip, usually begin from the Race Creek trailhead, because it has easier road access. To accommodate these hikers, I have described this trip from the Race Creek trailhead.

Warning: Rattlesnakes are common along this trail, so watch your step, and check the area carefully before you sit down to rest.

DESCRIPTION The first thing you notice as you start hiking upstream from Race Creek Campground is that in this relatively wet part of Idaho the vegetation is unusually lush. Droopy western red cedars hang over the riverbank, while grand firs, Douglas-firs, and ponderosa pines dominate elsewhere. Typical species in the thick undergrowth include thimbleberry, bracken fern, sword fern, wild rose, and honeysuckle, which displays showy clusters of orange, tubular-shaped flowers in June.

Warning: Much of this thick vegetation hangs over the trail, so, after it rains, you will get soaked without gaiters and rain pants.

For variety, the trail also passes through a few open, rocky areas with lots of May and June wildflowers like harebells, clarkia, yarrow, stonecrop, and skyrocket gilia.

The trail's early miles are easy, because there are almost no noticeable ups and downs and you stay under the shady canopy of large trees. You also never stray far from the lovely, green-tinted river, which has frequent gravel bars and sandy beaches that are great for lazy rest stops beside the water. After about 1.5 miles, you take a log across small Packer Creek and pass a sign marking where you enter the Selway-Bitterroot Wilderness. The first good riverside campsite comes a mile later where the river bends around a large gravel bar, but if this doesn't suit you there are even better camps at Renshaw Creek just 0.5 mile later. Shortly after Renshaw Creek, the trail leaves the big trees and crosses a relatively open, brushy slope, where a few blackened snags provide evidence that this is an old burn area. The sun can beat down rather mercilessly on this south-facing hillside, but the grade remains gentle, so the hiking is still comfortable.

Not quite 6 miles from the trailhead is a very good campsite just before you cross the bridge the over rushing Cupboard Creek. A few feet past the bridge is a junction with the Cupboard Creek Trail, which appears to be well used even though the sign indicates that the trail is not maintained.

Camp Critters

The popularity of the riverside camps with both boaters and hikers has attracted a few animal pests. The most common thieves are black bears and chipmunks, which are easily foiled by hanging your food. You might also see a porcupine, which gives you the chance to get a good look at one of these common, slow-footed forest residents. On close inspection you soon realize that despite their prickly appearance, porcupines might even be described as "cute" if not exactly cuddly. On the other hand, although porcupines are generally inoffensive, they have a destructive habit of chewing on sweaty pack straps, boots, and fly-rod handles for the salt. So you'll need to hang these items with the food to keep them safe from the quilled pests. A final noteworthy resident of this area is the spotted sandpiper, several of which often fly up and down the shore here, piping out their distinctive alarm calls whenever a hiker temporarily intrudes on their territory.

Tip: *The next 2 miles of the canyon are a good area to watch for ospreys, a large hawk that builds a bulky, tree top nest and dives for fish in the river. Ospreys compete with river otters, belted kingfishers, and human anglers for their share of the Selway's famous trout.*

From Cupboard Creek it's 0.5 mile to Power Creek, whose title greatly overstates both the stream's size and significance, then another mile across view-packed slopes to the sturdy bridge over Ballinger Creek, where a grassy, river-level flat provides a choice of excellent campsites.

A short distance past Ballinger Creek the trail crosses the trickling flow of Cascade Creek, which would hardly be worth mentioning except that its water drops over a scenic, wispy waterfall just above the trail. You then hike across grassy, wildflower-filled slopes with good views of a series of noisy river rapids to a sandy beach with a good boater's campsite. Just past this campsite you take a log across the clear flow of Pinchot Creek, then gradually pull away from the water in two lazy switchbacks followed by an extended uphill traverse. For the next 1.5 miles the trail goes up and down across a steep, grassy slope dotted with picturesque ponderosa pines, where the views 200 feet down to the river's rapids and across to the forest-covered walls on the opposite side of the canyon are excellent. The trail then gradually works its way downhill across the slopes of Pinchot Point, returns to the river near Dry Bar, and continues another mile to a wooden bridge over loudly cascading Three Links Creek.

About 100 feet past this bridge is a major trail junction. Although the signs here are small and hard to find, it would be impossible to miss this junction, because the Mink Peak Trail that goes to the south (right) immediately crosses an elaborately large cable suspension bridge over the rampaging Selway River.

Tip: If you want to camp in this area, the best sites are on the south side of the river. To find them, cross the bridge, then bear right on an unsigned bootpath. This route takes a log over Mink Creek and, 100 yards later, deadends at a nice campsite.

Two other important trails converge at the junction on the north side of the river. The Three Links Trail goes sharply left (north) to follow the creek of the same name, and an unsigned path angles slightly left (northeast) on its way up to Sixty-two Ridge.

Your trail goes straight and closely follows the north bank of the Selway River. The canyon scenery here is always pleasant and often spectacular, as the river alternates between loud rapids and quiet riffles, while the mostly forested canyon walls stretch skyward thousands of feet on either side. The river's many twists and turns give you the chance to enjoy this scenery from different angles.

About 1.5 miles from Three Links Creek, you pass an inviting riverside campsite and, 100 yards later, splash across tiny Tango Creek, whose meager flow is just enough to provide water if you camp nearby. Another 1.5 miles takes you through a small burn area and across partly forested canyon slopes to the bridge over good-sized Meeker Creek, after which you make a quick, 150-foot ascent to a junction with the Meeker Ridge Trail. You go straight and for the next mile make a series of gentle ups and downs through a fairly large burn area. The fire that left behind this charred landscape must have been quite intense, because fire scars on the other side of the canyon indicate that the flames managed to jump the river. As often happens in a wildfire, many of the trees survived the blaze, giving the forest a patchwork appearance. The undergrowth was burned as well, leaving the ground crowded with bracken ferns, which thrive in the open sunlight.

You reenter the shady forest canopy shortly before a grove of impressive western red cedars, where you might camp, although the trickle of water here dries up by midsummer. From here, it's another 0.5 mile to the bridge over clear-flowing Halfway Creek and a junction with the Halfway Creek Trail. The sign says that this trail is not maintained, which may explain why it is so overgrown and appears to be virtually unused.

You go straight and for the next 3.5 miles hike through a narrow section of the canyon where the river dances along in what is essentially one continuous, churning rapid. Rafters refer to this exciting section below Moose Creek as the "Moose Juice," and it's a good place to watch for boaters. You

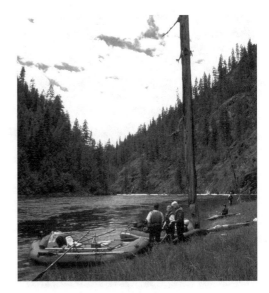

Rafters near Pinchot Creek

may even see one or two boats flip over in the maelstrom of class 4 whitewater.

Tip: If you're a photographer, it's a good idea to have your camera immediately available to catch action shots of the boaters.

The trail makes its way through this ruggedly scenic section via a series of little ups and downs that take you over the top of several small cliffs and rock outcroppings. In general, you never get very far from the river, although at one point you climb to an overlook that is 200 feet above the water. Eventually, you pass a signed junction with the unmaintained Goat Mountain Trail, then cross small Divide Creek on a log and come to a junction with the Big Rock Trail. You turn right and immediately cross a long suspension bridge over the boisterous flow of Moose Creek, which almost anywhere else would deserve to be called a "river."

Once across the bridge, the trail ascends two short switchbacks to another junction, this time with the Moose Ridge Trail, which drops to some excellent, but very popular, boater's camps on either side of a prominent bridge over the Selway River. The main trail bears left and climbs the spine of a minor ridge to the large flat that holds the Moose Creek Airfield. This remote airfield gets a surprising amount of use and has two long runways that cross in the middle of the field.

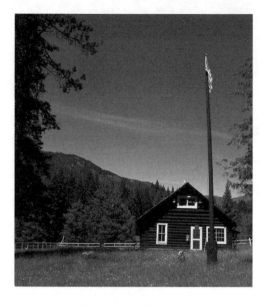

Moose Creek Ranger Station

You bear right at a signed junction with a spur trail to the airfield and loop around and below the south end of the two landing strips. The trail then curves to the left and makes its way through woods to a junction about 200 yards from the Moose Creek Ranger Station. Although the Selway River Trail turns sharply to the right here, it's worth your time to first go left and make a short side trip to visit the historic log buildings at the ranger station. It's particularly interesting because this facility is a throwback to the early twentieth century, when most ranger stations were so isolated they had no road access and were staffed by just one or two hardy rangers who rarely saw many visitors.

Tip: *The station has piped water, which gives you the chance to refill your water bottles.*

The main Selway River Trail follows the canyon in a prominent turn to the southeast making a long, sun-exposed traverse on the canyon walls several hundred feet above the river. The trail stays high for about 1 mile, crossing several small gullies and side ridges along the way, then gradually descends to a crossing of Hell Creek, a pretty little stream whose uninviting name is difficult to explain. The trail then remains above the river for another mile before it finally returns to the water's edge not far from a good boater's campsite.

For the rest of the trip the Selway River Trail rarely rises more than 100 feet above the water, and even though there are many ups and downs along the way, none of them are sustained for very long, so the hiking is relatively gentle and easy. In addition, the scenery remains excellent throughout and helps to pull you along as the trail goes through open forests and across dry slopes of rocks, grasses, and shrubs where you can enjoy frequent views up and down the canyon.

The next major tributary stream is clear-flowing Dog Creek, which you cross on a bridge. You then walk about 1 mile to Rattlesnake Bar, whose name serves as a useful reminder that these reptiles are common in the Selway River canyon. Still staying fairly close to the beautiful river, you travel upstream to a junction, where you go straight and almost immediately cross a bridge over the narrow gorge that holds swift-flowing Pettibone Creek.

Your trail keeps going south, following the twisting river through two short but particularly attractive sections where the Selway flows in deep, green pools through narrow chasms below the trail. You then make a short, woodsy climb over a small side ridge and descend through open, parklike stands of ponderosa pines to a junction with the Bear Creek Trail. There is a good campsite at the edge of a small, grassy flat near this junction.

You veer right, almost immediately cross a bridge over wide Bear Creek, one of the Selway River's largest tributaries, then walk 1 mile through the lush understory of a shady forest to a junction just before a bridge over the river. Turn right and cross the bridge to reach private and cozy Selway Lodge, which has several scattered buildings and a dirt airstrip.

The public trail curves to the left past the main lodge buildings, then goes through a gate and ascends a bit to the south end of the landing strip. You go through another gate and almost immediately reach a junction with the Ditch Creek Trail. Here you go straight and walk past a wooden storage building to a bridge over rushing Ditch Creek. Now the wide trail climbs a bit through relatively dense forests to a fork. To visit the Shearer Guard Station and Airfield, bear left and soon walk past the station's two log cabins to the airfield's grassy landing strip. This public landing strip is often used as an access for backcountry fishing and hunting trips.

The main trail goes right at the fork, takes a log over Elk Creek, then comes to a junction with the Goat Ridge Trail. You go straight and skirt the west side of the Shearer Airfield to the south end of the landing strip and a reunion with the trail that went past the guard station. About 0.5 mile beyond the airfield, you pass just above a superb campsite on a sandy, riverside beach beneath a grove of towering, old-growth pines, firs, and cedars. From here, it's an easy 2-mile walk past the impressive ramparts of Elevator Mountain to a

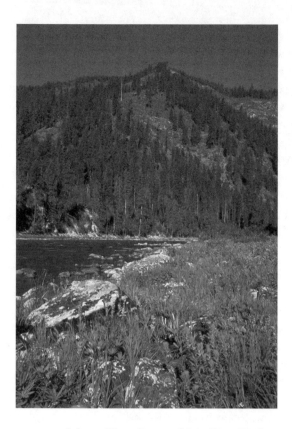
Selway River Canyon Near Bear Creek

sturdy wooden bridge over good-sized Goat Creek. There are some nice campsites below the bridge just before you cross the creek.

Immediately after the Goat Creek bridge is an unsigned junction with a trail that angles right. You go straight, hike through some brushy areas near the river, then break out onto relatively barren canyon slopes and come to a good (but horsy) campsite directly below some impressive rock pinnacles. On the other side of the river you can see the scattered buildings and private airstrip of isolated North Star Ranch. About 1 mile south of this campsite you'll pass above two even better ones before and after where the trail has been blasted into the rock about 30 feet above the water.

Soon after these campsites, the trail crosses a bridge over wide and shallow Running Creek, then comes to a junction. The Selway River Trail goes left, follows the fence around private and comfortable-looking Running Creek Ranch, then comes to the last of the large, curving, wood-and-cable bridges over the Selway River. There are some good campsites in a sandy area on the right just before you cross the bridge.

Immediately on the other side of the bridge is a junction, where you turn right and soon cross small Gardiner Creek on stepping stones.

> **Tip:** *Fill your water bottles here, because this is the last reliable and easily accessible source for about 5 miles.*

South of Gardiner Creek the trail goes up and down across open slopes that support lots of bracken fern and, in early summer, a colorful assortment of wildflowers. Unfortunately, by August, the only thing still blooming is spotted knapweed, a noxious, introduced species that has become the bane of the northern Rocky Mountains.

About 2 miles past Gardiner Creek you come to a good viewpoint above Waldo Bar, then hike another 3 miles over generally open and rather barren terrain to a rock-hop crossing of small Bad Luck Creek. There is a fair campsite on the left just beyond the creek crossing. About 400 yards after this campsite is an unsigned junction with a trail that goes sharply left on its way up the canyon of Bad Luck Creek. You go straight and complete the last 2 miles of the hike in a relatively dense forest of mixed ponderosa pines, Douglas-firs, and grand firs, with lots of western red cedars on the river-banks. The lush understory is filled with elderberry, sword fern, Oregon grape, twisted stalk, Douglas maple, and mountain ash, all of which are rare or absent from the drier slopes to the north. The trail ends at the small parking lot for the upstream trailhead.

POSSIBLE ITINERARY

	Camp	Miles	Elevation Gain
Day 1	Ballinger Creek	7.5	300
Day 2	Moose Creek	14	1200
Day 3	Bear Creek	11	1500
Day 4	Running Creek	9.5	600
Day 5	Out	8	600

VARIATIONS If you are hiking from mid-July through early October, when the surrounding high country is free of snow, you can make a long, rugged, semi-loop out of this trip by returning along high, ridgetop trails south and west of the Selway River corridor. One particularly scenic route goes west from Shearer Guard Station, climbs Goat Ridge, then passes Grave Meadow Peak on its way to Indian Hill Lookout, just a short car shuttle from the Race Creek trailhead.

Another option is to do this trip as a scenic, up-and-back hike from Race Creek to Moose Creek. This lovely route passes many of the best river rapids and is often open as early as late April or early May.

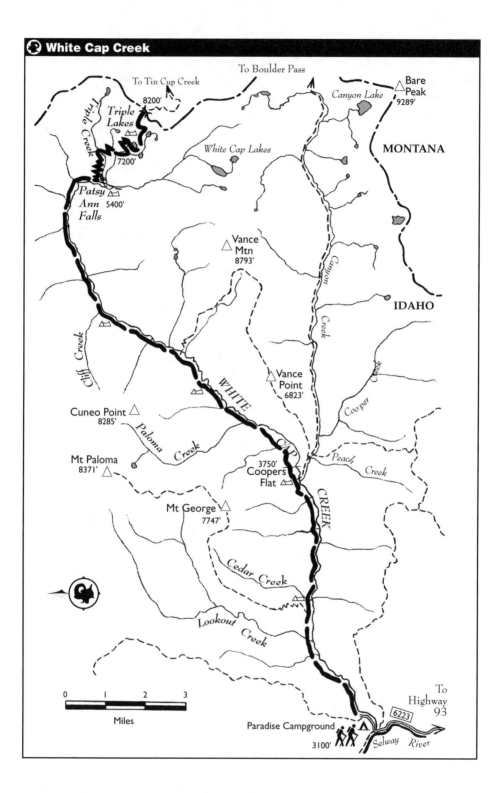

White Cap Creek

To Boulder Pass

To Tin Cup Creek

Bare Peak
9289'

Canyon Lake

8200'

Triple Lakes

7200'

White Cap Lakes

MONTANA

Little Creek

Patsy Ann Falls
5400'

Vance Mtn
8793'

IDAHO

Cliff Creek

WHITE

Vance Point
6823'

Canyon Creek

Cooper Creek

Cuneo Point
8285'

Paloma Creek

CAP

Peach Creek

Mt Paloma
8371'

3750'
Coopers Flat

Mt George
7747'

CREEK

Cedar Creek

Lookout Creek

0 1 2 3
Miles

To Highway 93

6223

Paradise Campground

3100'

Selway River

6   White Cap Creek

RATINGS (1–10)			MILES	ELEVATION GAIN	DAYS	SHUTTLE MILEAGE
Scenery	Solitude	Difficulty	52	5500	5-7	N/A
6	8	5	(55)	(6500)	(5-7)	

MAP USFS - Selway-Bitterroot Wilderness - South Half.

USUALLY OPEN July to October.

BEST Mid-July to mid-August.

PERMITS None.

RULES Maximum group size of 20 people and 20 stock animals.

CONTACT West Fork Ranger District, (406) 821-3269.

SPECIAL ATTRACTIONS Solitude; wildlife.

PROBLEMS A few rattlesnakes in the lower canyon of White Cap Creek; long drive from almost anywhere in Idaho.

HOW TO GET THERE From Salmon, drive 69.5 miles north on U.S. Highway 93 – over Lost Trail Pass and into Montana – to a junction where you turn left, following signs to Painted Rocks State Park. Drive 1.2 miles to a T-junction with State Highway 473, then turn left and stay on this paved road for 11.4 miles to a junction 0.5 mile past the West Fork Ranger Station and immediately before a bridge over West Fork Bitterroot River. Bear right here on Nez Perce Road and drive 16.5 miles on this alternating paved and gravel road to Nez Perce Pass, where you reenter Idaho. The pavement continues for another 8.4 miles as the road winds downhill beside the rushing waters of Deep Creek. Once the pavement ends, you drive a bumpy, gravel road for 10.5 miles to a junction with the Magruder Road to Elk City. Go straight, following signs to Paradise Campground, and drive 11.4 miles on narrow and bumpy Forest Road 6223 to a bridge over White Cap Creek and the Selway River trailhead. Turn right

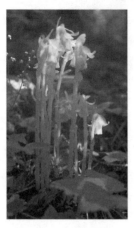

Indian Pipe

and drive another 0.6 mile to the trailhead parking area just past Paradise Campground, which caters to outfitters and equestrians. **Note:** Parking is not allowed at the Paradise Guard Station or along the road that continues beyond the trailhead.

INTRODUCTION Most of the trips in this book head for outstanding scenic attractions where tall peaks scratch the sky or great canyons dig deep into the crust of the earth. The majority of central Idaho's vast wilderness, however, is an endless sea of relatively unspectacular forested terrain, where the top attraction isn't the scenery but the chance to immerse yourself in the kind of solitude that hasn't been possible in the rest of the United States for over 100 years.

No book about backpacking in the Gem State would be complete without at least a few hikes where scenery takes a back seat to the simpler joy of tasting what the early explorers experienced. The trail up White Cap Creek, a major tributary of the Selway River, provides only modest scenery but plenty of solitude, and eventually gives you access to a group of isolated lakes perched high on the sides of the granite summits of the Bitterroot Range. Very rugged cross-country side trips provide access to several more lakes, meadows, and forests, so you can enjoy the solitude here for as long as your food and vacation time hold out.

DESCRIPTION This trip's long, respectful approach to the high country begins with a short walk past the Paradise Guard Station to the signed trailhead on a turnaround loop at the end of the road. The well-maintained trail then heads upstream beside the clear waters of large White Cap Creek, where anglers will find good sport casting for cutthroat trout and non-anglers can simply enjoy the attractive forests.

The trail spends the first 1.5 miles traversing partly forested slopes about 100 feet above the creek, where there are pleasant views across the canyon of a vigorous young forest that is growing back after an old fire. The trail then follows the creek more closely through a dense forest with a lush understory that reminds some hikers of the rainforests in western Oregon and Washington. Wildlife is abundant in this intensely green environment, with deer, elk, black bears, and an occasional moose all making their homes here. Even more common are feisty red squirrels, which use their loud, raspy calls to angrily scold any and all intruders. One brazen little fellow even spent 5 minutes deliberately dropping pine cones on my head while I rested against a tree in "his" territory.

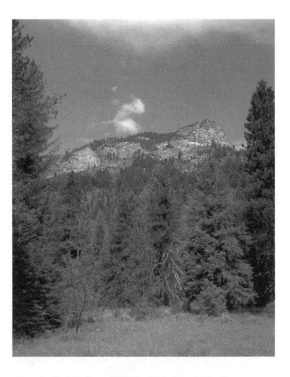

Cuneo Point from White Cap Creek Trail

At a little past the 2-mile point, you take a bridge over Lookout Creek, then wander through dense forests and small, fire-scarred areas to an unsigned junction with a trail that angles uphill to the left. You go straight, pass a decent campsite next to small Cedar Creek, then continue with the gentle, woodsy, creekside ascent. At about the 5-mile point, the trail climbs to the drier and more open slopes about 200 feet above the creek and comes to an unsigned fork. Either trail will work, because the two routes rejoin after just 150 yards.

The trail remains well above the stream for the next 2.5 miles, then descends and crosses a densely forested flat near the water to a major junction. The Canyon Creek Trail goes right and crosses a large, wooden bridge over White Cap Creek to the small meadow, excellent camps, and old log cabin at Coopers Flat.

Warning: From late August to mid-November a hunting outfitter monopolizes almost all the available space at Coopers Flat, so you may have to find someplace else to spend the night.

The White Cap Creek Trail goes left at the junction and soon resumes its gradual, forested climb. In July, the forests here come alive with tall, showy beargrass blossoms, while on the forest floor the smaller, perky, white blooms of bunchberry and queens cup struggle for recognition. Later in the season these roles are reversed, as the beargrass is left with nothing but a dead stalk, while the bunchberry shows off clusters of bright orange berries and the queens cup displays a large blue berry at its center.

For the first few miles after Coopers Flat, the trail goes through viewless but attractive forests, staying well away from the sight, or even the sound, of White Cap Creek. The only significant landmark along the way is Paloma Creek, which in the high runoff of early July can be a tricky ford, but by late summer is an easy rock-hop. More gentle hiking then takes you to some nice campsites in a small meadow at an unsigned junction with a faint trail that crosses the creek and heads southeast toward Vance Mountain. The hiking remains pleasant, but the scenery uninteresting, for the next 2 miles, until you cross a bouldery slope where you'll gather the first good views of the high, granite peaks and spires of the Bitterroot Range that hem in this wilderness canyon. This forest opening soon closes, however, as you return to the trees and walk another mile to a very good campsite near White Cap Creek. Approximately 500 yards past this campsite is a ford of Cliff Creek, which can be difficult in early summer, but is no challenge at all by August.

Beyond Cliff Creek the trail goes through two large, brush-covered avalanche chutes, where you can take a moment to admire both the views of the surrounding peaks and the monumental efforts of the trail crews who had to cut a swath through hundreds of downed trees. The pace of the climb gradually increases as you reenter forests and follow the canyon in a slow curve to the east and then south. To compensate for the extra effort, this part of the canyon has more openings in the tree cover, which improve the views and scenery. Less than 1 mile after completing its turn to the south, the trail makes two short switchbacks and ascends to an unsigned fork.

The trail to the right goes 100 yards to a crossing of Triple Creek just below the tall, sliding cascade of Patsy Ann Falls. After that, the trail continues another 300 yards to a very good campsite on the opposite side of a rock-hop crossing of White Cap Creek. Old maps show the trail continuing beyond this campsite all the way up to the remote White Cap Lakes. I spent nearly a full, miserable day in the rain and fog attempting to follow faint traces of this old trail, which has not been maintained in decades. I came back surly, soaked to the

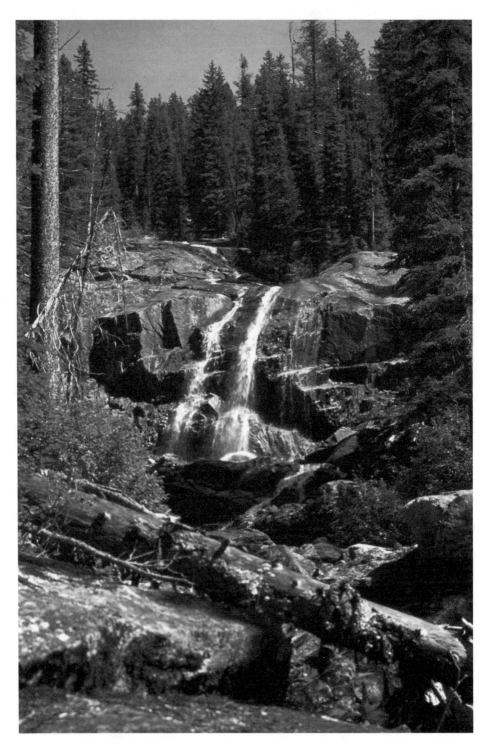

Patsy Ann Falls

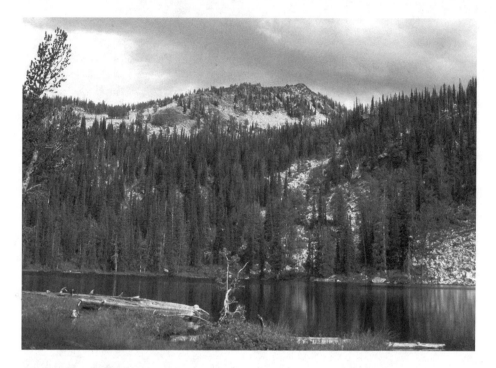

Middle Triple Lake

bone from miles of tough bushwhacking through rain-soaked, 10-foot-high brush, and completely confused by misleading elk trails that merely led up the wrong side canyons. I finally determined that it just wasn't worth it, especially since I wouldn't be able to see anything in the rain anyway. I recommend this route only for hardy souls who enjoy the challenge of tough, cross-country travel and who are willing to endure the considerable hardships of bushwhacking in order to gain nearly guaranteed solitude, excellent fishing opportunities, and the chance to see lots of elk.

For a much easier destination, bear left (uphill) on the maintained trail as it makes 10 short switchbacks up the hillside beside Patsy Ann Falls. The climb is tiring, but it provides continuously improving views down the impressive canyon of White Cap Creek. At the top of the switchbacks, the trail levels off and follows Triple Creek into a forested basin that comes alive in July with the blossoms of beargrass, spiraea, and wild carrot, while tall mountain boykinia crowds the banks of the creek.

You splash across Triple Creek, then make two uphill switchbacks, followed by a long, southerly traverse to a small creek. You cross the creek on rocks, follow it upstream for about 0.5 mile, then cross it again and make five switchbacks up an open, rocky hillside to Middle Triple Lake. This scenic lake has views of several rocky summits to the east, is surrounded by forests of subalpine firs and whitebark pines, and has good campsites along its west shore.

Beyond this lake, the trail climbs past Upper Triple Lake, arguably the most scenic of the trio, then keeps going up to an 8200-foot pass on the border with Montana. The views east down to Tin Cup Lake and the canyon of Tin Cup Creek make the long climb worthwhile. Unless you plan to do any of several tough, cross-country side trips, this is the place to turn around and head back the way you came.

VARIATIONS Consider turning this into a long, one-way hike by going over the pass above the Triple Lakes and exiting through Montana along the Tin Cup Creek Trail. Allow an extra day on this traverse for a very scenic side trip past Kerlee Lake to the top of El Capitan, one of the highest summits in the Bitterroot Range.

An alternate destination for this hike is Boulder Pass. To reach it, hike 14 miles up the Canyon Creek Trail from Coopers Flat through a canyon with similar scenery to that along White Cap Creek. From Boulder Pass, it's well worth continuing east 0.5 mile into Montana, then turning right (south) and climbing to scenic Boulder Lake, which has good campsites and a view of 9289-foot Bare Peak.

POSSIBLE ITINERARY

	Camp	Miles	Elevation Gain
Day 1	Coopers Flat	9	1100
Day 2	Cliff Creek	9	1000
Day 3	Middle Triple Lake (with side trip to the pass east of the Triple Lakes)	11	3700
Day 4	Meadow at Vance Mountain Trail junction	13	100
Day 5	Out	13	600

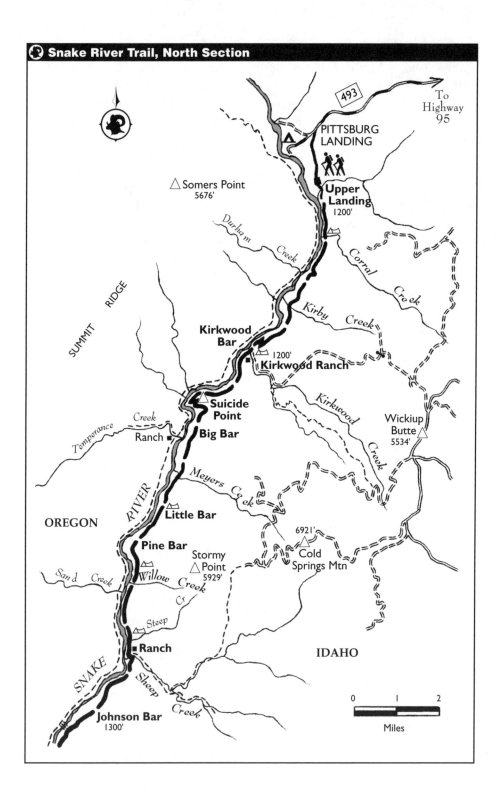

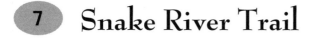

7 Snake River Trail

RATINGS (1–10)			MILES	ELEVATION GAIN	DAYS	SHUTTLE MILEAGE
Scenery	Solitude	Difficulty	54	5300	4-7	N/A
10	6	6				

MAP USFS - *Hells Canyon National Recreation Area.*

USUALLY OPEN Year round (except during winter storms).

BEST Mid-April to mid-May / October.

PERMITS None.

RULES All fires within 0.25 mile of the Snake River must be in a fire pan and ashes must be packed out.

CONTACT Hells Canyon National Recreation Area, Riggins Office, (208) 628-3916.

SPECIAL ATTRACTIONS Jaw-dropping canyon scenery; whitewater rafters to watch; historic sites; wildlife.

PROBLEMS Rattlesnakes; ticks; extreme summer heat; poison ivy.

HOW TO GET THERE From Grangeville, drive 18.0 miles south on U.S. Highway 95 to the bottom of the Salmon River Canyon, where you turn right (northwest) at a junction, following signs to Hammer Creek Recreation Area. (Coming from the south, this turnoff is about 28 miles north of Riggins.) After 0.9 mile, turn left, cross a bridge, and immediately turn left again onto Deer Creek Road. This road is initially paved, then turns to good gravel and climbs 10.9 miles to the Hells Canyon National Recreation Area boundary at Pittsburg Saddle. The narrow road then goes steeply downhill for 6.0 miles to a major junction. Turn left, following signs to Upper Landing, and drive 1.3 miles on a single-lane paved road to the signed trailhead parking lot.

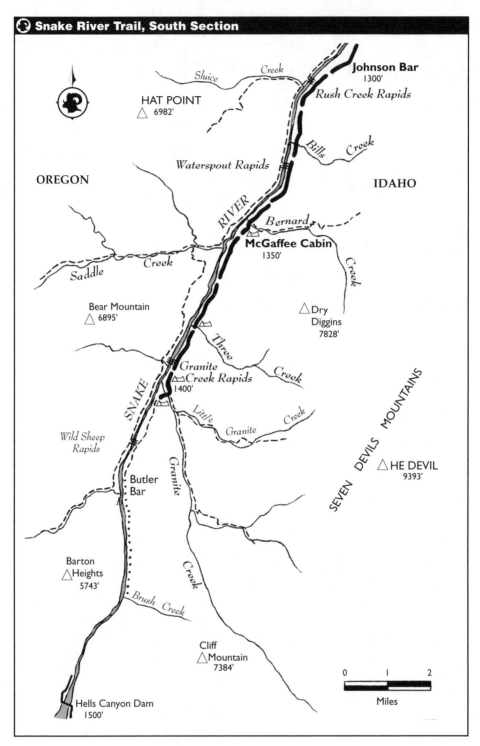

INTRODUCTION No matter how much you've heard about it before you go, nothing can really prepare you for the awesome depth and breath-taking scenery of Hells Canyon. From river level, the view extends up a mind-boggling 8000 feet to the craggy heights of Idaho's Seven Devils Mountains. Across the river, the Summit Ridge is not as high, but it's still over a vertical mile up from the Snake River to Hat Point, the highest point on the Oregon side.

Spectacular views are only one of the area's attractions, although those alone would be more than enough reason to visit. If your schedule precludes taking a vacation during the summer months, Hells Canyon is an excellent alternative, because when most trails in Idaho are buried under several feet of snow, the low-elevation path along the Snake River provides excellent early- or late-season hiking. Spring is probably the best time to visit, because that is when the canyon is green and the wildlife is most abundant.

Wildlife isn't the only reason that spring is the best time for a visit. From mid-April to mid-May temperatures in Hells Canyon are relatively cool, the canyon is green, the flowers are blooming, and the seasonal tributary creeks provide reliable sources of water. Spring hikers, however, must also contend with a greater number of rattlesnakes and ticks, so watch your step and check yourself from time to time to remove any blood-sucking hangers-on.

The most important reason that spring and fall are the best times to visit is that from late May to about mid-September temperatures in Hells Canyon would make the Devil himself feel appropriately at home. In addition, since the only trees at the bottom of the canyon are thorny hackberries and a few isolated ponderosa pines, shade is at a premium. The best plan is to get an early start and do most of your hiking in the morning, when the trail is shaded by the canyon walls.

The fragile Snake River corridor sees a fair amount of use, especially by boaters. To minimize the impact, the Forest Service stresses the need for all visitors to practice no-trace techniques. Jet boaters and rafters are required to pack out all human waste from the river corridor. Although this is unrealistic for backpackers, it is important that you properly bury your deposits as far away from the river as possible, and otherwise minimize your impact on the land.

DESCRIPTION From the large trailhead parking lot, walk the remaining 0.3 mile of road to the picnic area at Upper Landing, where the official footpath begins.

Any thoughts you may have had about a gentle riverside hike are soon dashed as the trail almost immediately begins a series of short, rugged ups and downs. This roller-coaster pattern, which will continue for most of the hike, is necessary because the trail must negotiate countless little rock outcroppings. Sometimes the trail is simply blasted into the rock, but usually it is forced to go over or around these obstacles. Only on occasional riverside benches or at the outwash areas near the mouths of tributary creeks is the terrain gentle and the trail relatively flat.

Your efforts are rewarded by the superb scenery, which features a continuous series of amazing views of the raging river, the ruggedly contorted canyon walls, and even occasional glimpses of the high Summit Ridge in Oregon. Closer at hand are the rocks, nearly all of which are covered with strange patterns of colorful lichens. Even the canyon's sounds are impressive, as when the honking calls of a pair of Canada geese or the loud rattle of a belted kingfisher reverberate off the canyon walls and create an echoing stereo effect. Unfortunately, the less pleasant roar of jet boats does the same thing, but these interruptions are fairly brief. After 1 mile, you pass a possible campsite about 200 yards before you hop over Corral Creek.

Warning: *Watch where you step and especially where you sit down to rest here, because rattlesnakes, black-widow spiders, poison ivy, and prickly pear cactus are all common.*

Shortly after the creek, the trail goes up a side gulch, then out to a clifftop overlook about 250 feet above the water, where you'll get your last good look back to the Pittsburg Landing area.

The trail generally stays well above the river for the next few miles, crossing steep slopes and descending to river level only once, at about the 3.5-mile point. During the canyon's beautiful, but all-too-brief green season, these bunchgrass-covered slopes are tinged with green and sprinkled with colorful wildflowers. Look for the blues of brodiaea and larkspur, the yellows of balsamroot and lomatium, the cream color of death camas, the white of prairie star, and the pink of phlox, among many others. Unfortunately, the only water along the way comes where you cross the meager flow of Kirby Creek.

At about the 6-mile point, you descend six short, fairly steep switchbacks to Kirkwood Bar, a large, grassy, river-level flat. On the

Hellishly Wild

From late winter through mid-spring, animals seem to be everywhere in Hells Canyon and they come in a wide variety of forms. The river teems with fish including sturgeon, rainbow trout, catfish, bass, salmon, and steelhead. Canada geese and merganser ducks float on the water, and you are likely to see elk, mountain goats, and bighorn sheep grazing on ledges that overlook the canyon. More secretive creatures include western fence lizards, which scurry away from you in rocky areas, furtive cottontail rabbits that seem to be afraid of anything that moves, and elusive mountain lions, which prowl throughout the canyon and keep the deer, elk, and bighorn sheep constantly on guard. You need to be alert as well, because at least once during your trip you can expect to be startled by the heart-stopping sound of a rattlesnake, warning you to keep your distance.

Not nearly as dangerous, but equally nerve-rattling, is the sudden squawk and furious flapping of chukars, an introduced member of the partridge family that has a habit of remaining out of sight until the last possible second, then frightening unprepared hikers with a sudden flurry of activity. Other common birds in the canyon include swooping white-throated swifts, perky canyon wrens, majestic golden eagles, and showy black-billed magpies.

north end of Kirkwood Bar are several developed campsites complete with picnic tables, fire pits, and flush toilets. There is no potable water, however, so you will have to treat or filter the water from Kirkwood Creek, a boisterous little stream that crosses the flat through an oasis of dense riparian vegetation dominated by black hawthorns, red birches, chokecherries, and syringas.

Kirkwood Bar also holds historic Kirkwood Ranch, which the Forest Service now runs as a museum. Even if you aren't camping here, try to schedule a minimum of half an hour to tour the ranch, look at old photos, read the interpretive signs, and examine the many outbuildings and scattered farm equipment. If you have any questions, these can be answered by the friendly Forest Service volunteers, who are stationed here year round. Hidden just a short walk up the jeep track along Kirkwood Creek are several more historic sites, including a prehistoric Indian pit house and the old Carter homestead. Kirkwood Ranch is the usual turnaround point for this trail's relatively few dayhikers, so from here on the already uncrowded trail gets even more lonesome.

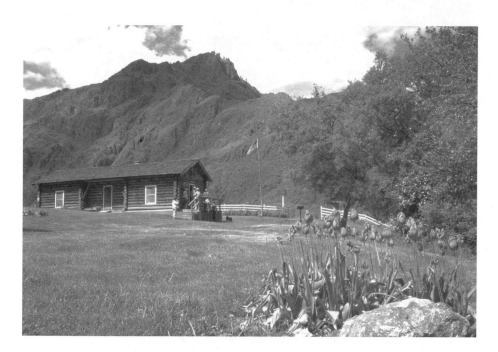

Kirkwood Ranch National Historic Site

For the next mile past Kirkwood Bar, you make several small ups and downs to a bend in the river that opens up views of Oregon's Summit Ridge, which remains blanketed with snow into late May. The next major highlight is Suicide Point, a high overlook which you reach after a short, stiff ascent. The view from Suicide Point is dramatic, including not only the river and the canyon walls, but also the distant ramparts of Summit Ridge and a spur of Idaho's lofty Seven Devils Mountains. Suicide Point supposedly got its name from a Native American *Romeo and Juliet* legend about a pair of young lovers who were members of two feuding tribes, the Nez Perce and the Shoshone. Lamenting their forbidden love, the couple leaped to their deaths from this point above the river.

From Suicide Point, you work your way down to Big Bar, a large, sloping, grassy bench that the trail crosses. On the Oregon side, you can see the fences, barns, and ranch house of Temperance Creek Ranch, an isolated but friendly place that is now leased to a hunting and fishing outfitter.

Tip: The grassy areas south of Temperance Creek Ranch are a particularly good place to see elk in the morning and evening.

At the south end of Big Bar, you make a brief climb, then go into the twisting canyon of Meyers Creek, where you can rest beside the splashing stream and refill your water bottles. The trail then crosses a small grassy area above Little Bar, which is visible below the trail and has some very good campsites, although the only nearby water is from the river (a questionable source, due to farm runoff in southern Idaho). Just past Little Bar, you come to the gully holding usually dry Caribou Creek, where you will see a small stone cabin about 75 yards above where you cross the gully.

The trail descends from Caribou Creek, travels close to the river for a little less than 1 mile, then climbs to another grassy, table-like bench where the river makes a sweeping turn to the south. After crossing this bench, you drop a bit and come to Pine Bar, where a patch of ponderosa pines provides a welcome area of shade. There is a good campsite below the trail here, while above the trail is a steep, exposed area of alum beds that are distinguished by colorful yellow and orange soils.

The trail then climbs over a rock outcropping, where there are fine views up and down the river, then drops to tiny Willow Creek, which usually has water, at least in the spring. History buffs might want to spend a little time exploring the rocks in this area for some ancient petroglyphs. They can be hard to find, but are very interesting and provide graphic evidence that people have lived in Hells Canyon for thousands of years. As always, never touch or otherwise deface this important archeological site.

Continuing south, the trail goes through a particularly dramatic section of the canyon, where the trail makes a series of ups and downs to avoid the very steep walls. You go past the Sand Creek game warden cabin, which is on the Oregon side, then drop back to the river and come to a possible campsite on a small, sandy beach near tiny, but usually flowing, Steep Creek. A few more ups and downs take you through a wooden gate and past an incongruous mail box (serviced by a weekly mail boat) to Sheep Creek Ranch, a pleasant oasis that features poplar trees, a surprisingly green lawn, and lilac bushes that bloom in April and May. Just past the ranch house is a junction.

You turn right, cross Sheep Creek on a wooden bridge, then travel less than 0.5 mile to Johnson Bar, where the canyon opens up. There are large, grassy benches on both sides of the river here, from

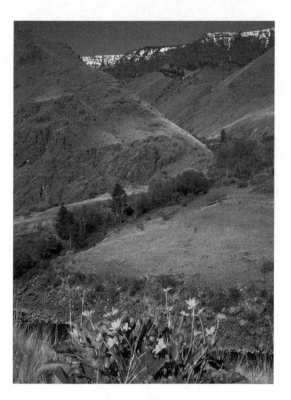

Above Rush Creek Rapids

which you can look downstream into the narrow section of the canyon you just came through and crane your neck to gaze upward more than 5700 vertical feet to the high, sometimes snowy ridgeline around Hat Point in Oregon. A sharp eye can even pick out the 90-foot-tall metal fire lookout tower atop Hat Point.

A little less than 2 miles of nearly level hiking take you across waterless Johnson Bar to the roaring maelstrom of Rush Creek Rapids, where it's fun to watch rafters struggling to negotiate this class-4 whitewater. The canyon then gets narrower and turns south, to where intervening ridges block the view of Hat Point. As compensation, you can now see the even higher peak in Idaho that has Dry Diggins Lookout on the top.

Another mile of easy, mostly level walking leads to the remains of a collapsed stone hut just before you reach tiny Bills Creek.

The trail gets more rugged now as it takes you past Waterspout Rapids, makes a long ascent to a high overlook, then goes back down to river level at a junction with the very faint trail up Bernard Creek.

> **Warning:** *Beware of poison ivy, which seems to be everywhere in this area. Fortunately, the sumac, which also grows abundantly here and throughout the canyon, is not the poisonous variety.*

You go straight, take a bridge over the clear, rushing waters of Bernard Creek, and soon come to the nicely restored McGaffee cabin, where a sign on the door says WELCOME STRANGERS – COME ON IN. It's worthwhile to accept this invitation and spend some time poking

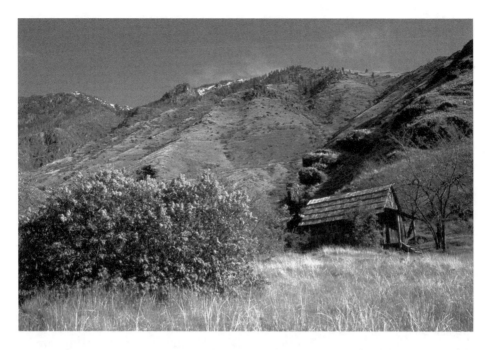

Historic McGaffee cabin near Bernard Creek

around this old homestead, which was built in 1905 and is now on the National Register of Historic Places. The inside walls are papered with fascinating old *Saturday Evening Post* clippings, while the history of the cabin is detailed in interpretive signs. If you want to enjoy a longer visit, the upstairs loft and the porch are good spots to lay out your sleeping bag for the night.

> **Warning:** *South of Bernard Creek the Snake River Trail gets less use than it does to the north, so it is even more overgrown with grasses and poison ivy. In places the poison ivy is hard to avoid. If you are particularly allergic, you might want to stop at Bernard Creek.*

To continue on to Granite Creek, follow the trail up the little slope just south of McGaffee cabin and gradually gain about 200 feet before dropping back to the river. You pass prominent Saddle Creek, coming in on the Oregon side, then enter another narrow section of the canyon. Sheer cliffs on the Oregon side force the trail in that state to make a difficult detour some 1500 feet above river level, but your trail makes it through this section very easily with almost none of the usual ups and downs. About 3 miles from Bernard Creek, you go right (downhill) at a potentially confusing fork (the left fork just

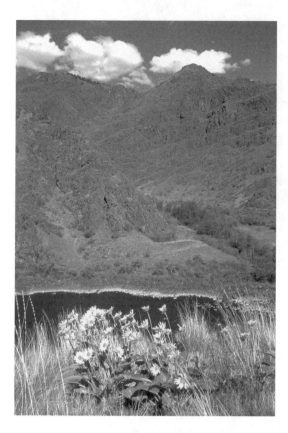

View west to Saddle Creek

deadends) and come to a grassy flat with possible campsites. The trail loops to the right around a boggy area here, then climbs briefly to Three Creek, which is a good source of water if you camp at the flat.

You splash across Three Creek, then go up and down past Granite Creek Rapids and through a 0.5-mile section that stays very close to the river's waters. Near the south end of this section the trail crosses an overhanging rock face, where it must have taken lots of dynamite to blast the trail into the rock. Immediately after this rock face, the path crosses a small flat area with possible camps just before you reach swift-flowing Granite Creek. The Snake River Trail goes a short distance up Granite Creek through an area of unusually lush riparian vegetation, then comes to a meadow and a junction.

If you are interested in the canyon's history, bear left at this junction and hike a little less than 1 mile up the Little Granite Trail to an old homestead, whose history is detailed in the interpretive material at McGaffee cabin.

> **Warning:** *Although the homestead is worth exploring, the trail to it is overgrown with poison ivy and has an unusually high concentration of rattlesnakes.*

If you are looking for a good campsite, turn right at the junction, cross Granite Creek on a sturdy bridge, and almost immediately come to a grassy flat with nice campsites.

Granite Creek is the recommended turnaround point for this trip. Some hikers continue another 2 miles to Butler Bar, but at that point the maintained trail ends. An old trail keeps going another 4 miles to Brush Creek, but the Forest Service cautiously describes this unmaintained section as "not really a trail anymore," partly because of periodic flooding by water releases from Hells Canyon Dam. So, unless you have arranged for some kind of boat transportation, it's time to turn around and hike back the way you came.

VARIATIONS The canyon's topography severely limits your options for changing this basic hike, but if you've got the money and the imagination you can spice things up by including some non-hiking activities. For example, if you don't want to make the long drive to Pittsburg Landing, you can use boat transportation instead. The best plan is to pay a jet boat operator to take you either upstream from Lewiston or downstream from Hells Canyon Dam to a drop-off point somewhere along the river. From Lewiston, most commercial operators will take you as far as Johnson Bar. From there, you can walk the trail back to Pittsburg Landing, where you have pre-arranged for another jet boat to pick you up and take you back to Lewiston. This requires reservations and it is expensive, but it saves you from having to backtrack on the trail and it avoids the long drive to Pittsburg Landing. One reliable company that provides this service is Beamers Hells Canyon Tours, (800) 522-6966.

For the best of all worlds, hike upstream to a point where you have prearranged to meet a whitewater rafting party. From there, simply hop aboard the rafts and float back to your car. This way you can experience the canyon at the relaxed pace of a pedestrian and enjoy the excitement of a rafting adventure all on the same trip. One good company for the rafting services is Northwest Voyageurs, (800) 727-9977.

POSSIBLE ITINERARY

	Camp	Miles	Elevation Gain
Day 1	Little Bar	11.5	1400
Day 2	Bernard Creek	10	800
Day 3	Bernard Creek (dayhike to Granite Creek)	11	1100
Day 4	Little Bar	10	700
Day 5	Out	11.5	1300

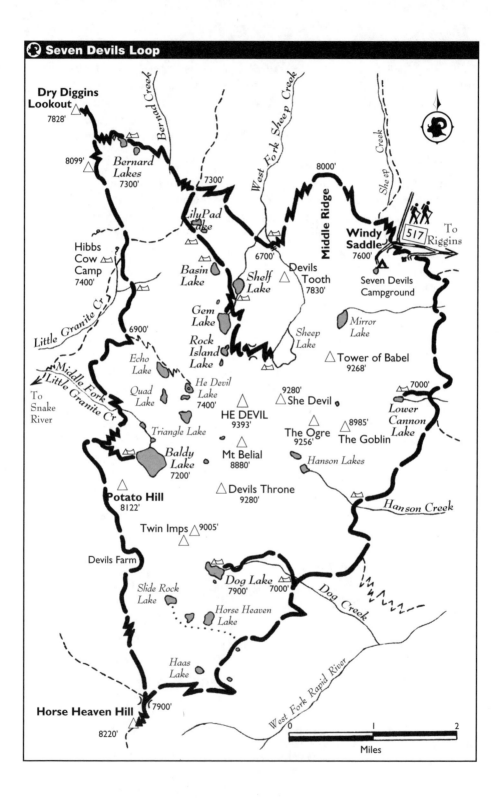

Seven Devils Loop

Dry Diggins Lookout 7828'

8099'

Bernard Creek

Bernard Lakes 7300'

7300'

LilyPad Lake

Hibbs Cow Camp 7400'

West Fork Sheep Creek

Basin Lake

Shelf Lake

8000'

6700'

Devils Tooth 7830'

Middle Ridge

Sheep Creek

Windy Saddle 7600'

To Riggins

517

Seven Devils Campground

Little Granite Cr

6900'

Gem Lake

Rock Island Lake

Sheep Lake

Mirror Lake

△ Tower of Babel 9268'

Echo Lake

He Devil Lake 7400'

9280'
△ **She Devil**

7000'

Middle Fork Little Granite Cr

To Snake River

Quad Lake

HE DEVIL 9393'

The Ogre 9256'

8985'
The Goblin

Lower Cannon Lake

Triangle Lake

Baldy Lake 7200'

△ Mt Belial 8880'

Hanson Lakes

△ **Potato Hill** 8122'

△ Devils Throne 9280'

Hanson Creek

Twin Imps △ 9005'

Devils Farm

Slide Rock Lake

Dog Lake 7900'

7000'

Dog Creek

Horse Heaven Lake

Haas Lake

West Fork Rapid River

Horse Heaven Hill 7900'

8220'

0   1   2

Miles

8 Seven Devils Loop

RATINGS (1–10)			MILES	ELEVATION GAIN	DAYS	SHUTTLE MILEAGE
Scenery	Solitude	Difficulty	28	4400	2-4	N/A
8	6	5	(43)	(8500)	(3-6)	

MAP USFS - Hells Canyon National Recreation Area.

USUALLY OPEN Late June to October.

BEST Late June to early August.

PERMITS None.

RULES Maximum group size of 8 people and 16 stock animals.

CONTACT Hells Canyon National Recreation Area, Riggins Office, (208) 628-3916.

SPECIAL ATTRACTIONS Good mountain scenery; great views from Dry Diggins Lookout.

PROBLEMS Rough access road; numerous fire-scarred areas.

HOW TO GET THERE From New Meadows, drive 34 miles north on U.S. Highway 95 to a junction exactly 0.3 mile south of the Hells Canyon National Recreation area office in Riggins. Turn left (west) on a gravel road, following signs to Seven Devils Campground, and go 1.8 miles to an unsigned fork. Turn left and begin climbing on Forest Road 517, a good gravel road that is suitable for passenger cars, but which is also narrow, steep, and bumpy, so camping trailers and recreational vehicles are not recommended. After 9.8 miles, go right (uphill) at a fork, where the route abruptly deteriorates to a slow, rocky dirt road. Exactly 4.8 miles later is another unsigned fork, where you veer right (uphill) and drive a final 0.5 mile to a junction at Windy Saddle. Turn left and go 100 feet to the well-signed trailhead parking lot on the right.

INTRODUCTION The alpine meadows, green forests, and towering crags of the Seven Devils Mountains provide a welcome high-elevation contrast to the stark, bunchgrass-covered slopes of Hells Canyon. Unlike that sun-baked landscape, these high peaks provide all the usual mountain pleasures, including flower-covered meadows and trout-filled cirque lakes, plus the more unusual benefit of awe-inspiring views into the canyon's depths. A good trail goes all the way around the Seven Devils Mountains, but since the main loop bypasses almost all of the high lakes and many of the best viewpoints, you'll want to schedule extra time for plenty of side trips.

These mountains lie west of the great Idaho Batholith, so the geology of the Seven Devils is different from other mountains in central Idaho. Instead of the usual granite, these mountains are composed of dark-colored basalt, which has been uplifted and spectacularly eroded by water and glaciers into a wildly contorted assortment of cliffs, crags, and cirque basins.

DESCRIPTION Most people hike this loop counterclockwise, but I prefer a clockwise tour as this saves the best scenery for last. So, go east across the dirt road directly opposite the trailhead parking lot and start hiking on Boise Trail #101, which makes a downhill traverse across a grassy slope. In July, this dry slope is brightened by colorful wildflowers like buckwheat, yarrow, aster, and paintbrush, while 4-foot-tall coneflower and groundsel are found in the wetter areas. In addition to the flowers, these meadows provide excellent views east to the endless, rolling mountains of central Idaho and southwest to the dark crags of the Seven Devils Mountains.

You descend two quick switchbacks to the bottom of the meadows, then go through a gate and pass a Forest Service guard station.

▲ All in a Name ▲

The intriguing name "Seven Devils" comes from a Native American legend about a lost Indian brave. While traversing this craggy terrain, the brave is said to have encountered a devil, which he fled from in fear only to come across a series of six more devils before finally making his way to safety. In honor of this legend, the highest peaks in this range carry sinister-sounding names such as He Devil, She Devil, Devils Tooth, Devils Thumb, Tower of Babel, The Ogre, and The Goblin. Fortunately, the landscape is much more appealing than those ominous names would suggest.

Look for small signs stating simply TRAIL that guide you past the buildings and over the dirt access roads of this facility. After the station, you descend through open forests mostly of lodgepole pines and subalpine firs to the wilderness boundary at another gate and a junction with the little-used Silvers Trail. You go straight, pass through the gate, and walk downhill for about 200 yards beside a tiny creek.

The trail finally levels off, curves to the right (south), then for the next 2 miles maintains a nearly level course by zigging into side canyons with trickling creeks and zagging out to ridgelines with good views. Most of the way is through forests and large burn areas, where wildflowers like

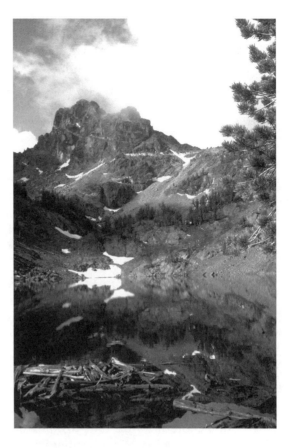

Tower of Babel over Mirror Lake

birchleaf spiraea, fireweed, and pearly everlasting have taken advantage of the sunlight to put on an impressive display of color. This display should continue for many years, because the regrowing lodgepole pines are still only a few feet tall. The burn areas provide good habitat for several species of woodpeckers, which pound away at the decaying snags looking for grubs and insects. For hikers, these open areas provide nice views of the Tower of Babel, a distinctive high point with a dark, squared-off summit.

A little over 3 miles from the trailhead is a signed junction with the Cannon Lake Trail. This 0.75-mile side trail makes a moderately steep climb up a fire-scarred hillside to small Lower Cannon Lake, a lovely mountain gem rimmed with pink-blooming spiraea. The lake has several good campsites and excellent views of Tower of

Babel and its surrounding crags. Mountain goats are often seen on these crags, their white bodies contrasting nicely with the dark rock.

Warning: The Hells Canyon National Recreation Area map shows lots of ups and downs along the next several miles of the Boise Trail. The actual alignment is really very gentle. Do not rely on this map to calculate elevation gains and losses.

You go straight at the Cannon Lake junction, hop over Cannon Creek, then climb a bit to a ridgeline, where there is a junction with the Wurl Trail, which forks to the left. Your trail goes slightly right and for the next 2 miles remains nearly level as it travels through more burn areas and scattered patches of standing, green trees. At the end of this section, you pass a good campsite on the right just 75 yards before you step across the meager, but reliable, flow of Hanson Creek.

Tip: Off-trail enthusiasts can scramble about 1 mile up this creek to the high cirque basin that holds the two Hanson Lakes, which are set impressively beneath the heights of The Ogre and Mt. Belial.

After Hanson Creek, you climb a bit through another burn area on the north side of a spur ridge. In mid-August you should plan on making slow progress during this climb, because huckleberries are abundant here and you won't be able to resist stopping to pick and eat the juicy treats. You round the top of the ridge, then turn right and contour for 0.5 mile to a junction with the Dog Ridge Trail. Go straight and continue on the level to yet another burn area and a crossing of small Dog Creek. There is a good campsite just after the crossing in a tiny patch of unburned spruce and fir trees west of the trail. A superb side trip follows a steep, unmaintained bootpath up Dog Creek to beautiful Dog Lake, which has a couple of decent campsites and excellent views of the cliffs below Twin Imps.

Warning: Dog Creek is the last reliable water source on the main trail for over 9 miles, so stock up here and carry at least two quarts.

The Boise Trail continues south from Dog Creek, climbs to the top of another spur ridge, then does some lazy ups and downs through yet another large burn area. Although rather stark and completely shadeless, these fire-ravaged areas have an eerie sort of beauty. This is especially true in July and early August, when the black and silver snags are mixed with vivid displays of fireweed and pearly everlasting. After leaving this burn area, the trail traverses a south-facing hillside with good views to craggy Monument

Peak and Black Imp in the southern Seven Devils, then comes to usually dry Horse Heaven Creek. An unsigned track heads uphill beside this dry creek toward Horse Heaven and Slide Rock lakes in the remote talus-rimmed basin to the west.

Immediately after Horse Heaven Creek, the trail passes just above a shallow pond, which typically dries up by midsummer, then comes to the base of a jumbled rockslide. Here you turn southeast, make an uphill traverse to the top of yet another spur ridge, then turn sharply west and climb across the south side of the ridge through flower-spangled meadows with excellent views. The

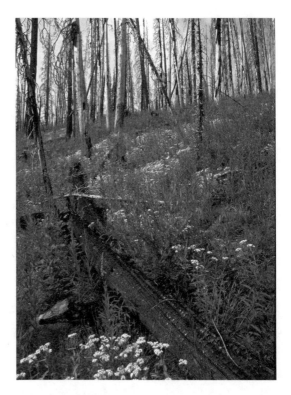

Flowers in burn area

traverse ends with four switchbacks that go up a large talus slope to a four-way junction in a high saddle at the southern end of your loop.

Views from this saddle are restricted by trees, so take the time for a side trip to the old lookout site at Horse Heaven Hill. To reach it, go left (south) and climb four switchbacks in about 0.5 mile to a quaint log cabin at the top of Horse Heaven Hill. If you like great views, then this spot will be heaven for more than just horses. To the north are the contorted peaks of the Seven Devils Mountains, dominated by the distinctive pinnacle of He Devil, while to the south are Carbonate Hill and tall Monument Peak. The most impressive view, however, is to the west of the distant Wallowa Mountains in Oregon and down into the gaping chasm of Hells Canyon, which drops fully 6700 feet from the top of Horse Heaven Hill to the Snake River. Bring your lunch and schedule extra time to do plenty of gawking.

To continue the loop trip, return to the junction in the saddle north of Horse Heaven Hill and go north, following signs to Hibbs

Cow Camp. The well-graded trail begins with a gradual climb across steeply sloping meadows filled with brushy Douglas' knotweed and the silvery snags of a very old burn. You top out on a side ridge with fine views down the canyon of Devils Farm Creek, then descend four switchbacks on a very rocky and exposed hillside. At the bottom of these switchbacks, you contour across a burned-over hillside, then go through Devils Farm, a rocky and waterless little basin below the towering ramparts of a ridge south of Twin Imps. The trail then makes a gradual, 250-foot climb that turns out to be nothing but a waste of energy, because you immediately lose all of that elevation (and more) on a long downhill traverse of a partially burned-over slope on the west side of Potato Hill.

At the bottom of the traverse, the trail goes around a wide ridge and comes to a fork. The trail to the right goes uphill to large Baldy Lake. This side trip is well worth doing, because the lake has a choice of excellent campsites and features superb views across the water to the dark mass of Devils Throne. The main trail veers left at the Baldy Lake junction and winds down through an old burn area that is now filled with regrowing pines.

At the bottom of this descent, you use stepping stones to cross two branches of Middle Fork Little Granite Creek, then make two switchbacks and a lengthy traverse up a sun-exposed hillside, where you are treated to outstanding views west to Oregon's Black and Bear mountains and down to the Snake River at Granite Creek. You then go up and down around a ridge and across a wooded basin to a small culvert over a seasonal creek. A few hundred yards past this creek is a junction with the deadend trail to Echo and He Devil lakes, yet another good side trip.

The main trail goes straight and climbs steadily for about 1 mile through a pleasant mix of forests and view-packed meadows to a very good campsite just after you step over the trickling headwaters of Little Granite Creek. A short uphill then takes you to a junction. About 100 yards west of this junction is Hibbs Cow Camp, where there is a good (but horsy) campsite, a trickling creek, and the chimney of a burned-down old cabin. A signed trail descends from this camp to the Snake River at Granite Creek.

You go straight at the junction and walk 0.5 mile up an increasingly dusty and horse-pounded trail to another junction in a sparsely vegetated hilltop meadow. The fastest way to complete the loop

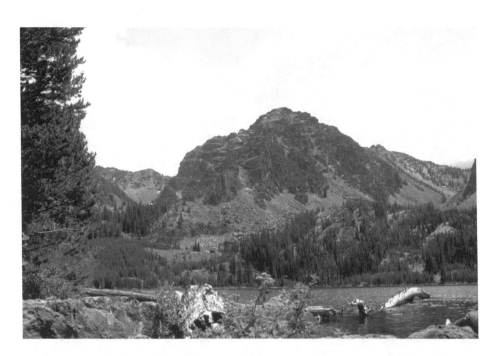

Baldy Lake

is to go right, but if you do that, you'll miss Dry Diggins Lookout, which has perhaps the best views in the state of Idaho. So bear left and walk slightly downhill for about 0.2 mile to an unsigned fork with a horse trail that goes left to an outfitter camp. You go straight and gradually gain elevation through forests and lovely meadows filled with the colorful blossoms of lousewort, yarrow, valerian, lupine, Jacob's ladder, and larkspur to a rocky viewpoint near the top of an 8099-foot peak. There are superb views here, especially back to the peaks of the Seven Devils Mountains.

But the best views are yet to come, so follow the trail as it steeply descends from Peak 8099 in three switchbacks to a junction just below a grassy saddle. Drop your pack here, grab your lunch and a camera, and take the trail to the left. In 0.5 mile this wildly scenic path winds up to the lookout building atop Dry Diggins. Although it has not been used for decades, this sturdy building is still in remarkably good condition and provides a nice platform for taking in the scenery.

And what scenery! Any credible list of America's greatest viewpoints *must* include Dry Diggins. The expected view southeast to

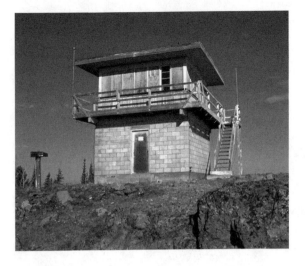

Dry Diggins Lookout

the craggy summits of the Seven Devils Mountains is outstanding, as is the distant vista southwest to Oregon's snowy Wallowa Mountains. But the real breath-stealing highlight is the look seemingly straight down over 6500 feet to the raging whitewater of the Snake River at the bottom of Hells Canyon. It's one of those scenes that words, and even photographs, cannot adequately convey. You have to see it for yourself. Sharing the view with you may be a small band of surprisingly tame mountain goats, which wander around on the crags near the lookout.

After spending as much time at Dry Diggins as your schedule will allow, return to the junction 0.5 mile from the lookout and take the trail that goes downhill to the east. This path descends several rocky switchbacks, initially in meadows and then through forests, to Bernard Lakes. The first of this group of three lakes is only a pond, but it is immediately followed by a much larger body of water. Both of these lily-pad-filled lakes have good views of Dry Diggins to the west and craggy Peak 8099 to the southwest.

Tip: The best camps are above the north shore of the third, least scenic lake, which is a short distance downhill from the second lake.

After the third Bernard Lake, the circuitous trail winds down through more forests and past a small, marshy pond to a usually dry gully at the head of Bernard Creek. From there, you walk through lush meadows and ascend nine moderately steep switchbacks to a prominent four-way junction in a large burn area.

A little used trail goes left (north) along Dry Diggins Ridge, while the heavily used trail that bears slightly left (east) is your return route to Windy Saddle. First, however, take the time for a terrific side trip past a string of scenic, fish-filled mountain pools to spectacular Sheep Lake. To do so, turn right on a dusty trail and walk less than 0.5 mile to a trail fork, where you bear left and go past aptly named Lily Pad Lake to a small, very green meadow with a good campsite near its north end. The trail then goes southeast, heading directly toward the ominous mass of He Devil, the highest point in the Seven Devils, and several lesser peaks that flank him on either side. Together they form an impressive skyline.

You soon pass just below Basin Lake, which has good campsites and a nice setting, then cross the lake's trickling outlet creek and almost immediately turn left at an unsigned fork (the right branch just deadends at Basin Lake). You climb two switchbacks, then ascend a bit more on a rocky tread to a ridge a little above lovely Shelf Lake. This lake is a step up in both elevation and scenery from Basin Lake. A side trail drops left to some good campsites near the southwest shore of Shelf Lake.

More twists and turns in the trail take you up to an unsigned junction immediately before you cross a small creek. The trail to the right goes steeply uphill for about 250 yards to deep and well-named Gem Lake, which features outstanding views of He Devil to the southeast and an unnamed craggy ridge to the west.

But don't stop here, because the array of ever-more-impressive lakes is not yet over. The main trail goes left at the unsigned junction, crosses the small creek, and climbs the rocky hillside east of Gem Lake to tiny but gorgeous Rock Island Lake. From there, you make a few more long switchbacks up to a wide saddle, where you can look southeast over the basin of Sheep Lake to the hulk of She Devil and east to the more dainty Tower of Babel. The trail then switchbacks down to some excellent, but rather popular, camps on Sheep Lake's southwest shore.

Tip: The best and most photogenic views of Sheep Lake are from its north end, which you can reach on a rough angler's path.

After this lengthy and rewarding side trip, return to the four-way junction north of Lily Pad Lake and turn right (east). The trail descends six irregularly spaced but well-graded switchbacks to the bottom of a large talus slope, then goes up and down across a heavily forested basin. An abundance of huckleberries provide tasty treats if you are visiting in August or early September.

You splash across the bubbling creek that drains from Shelf Lake, then take a log over West Fork Sheep Creek to a very good campsite just below a lovely cascading waterfall. In the next couple

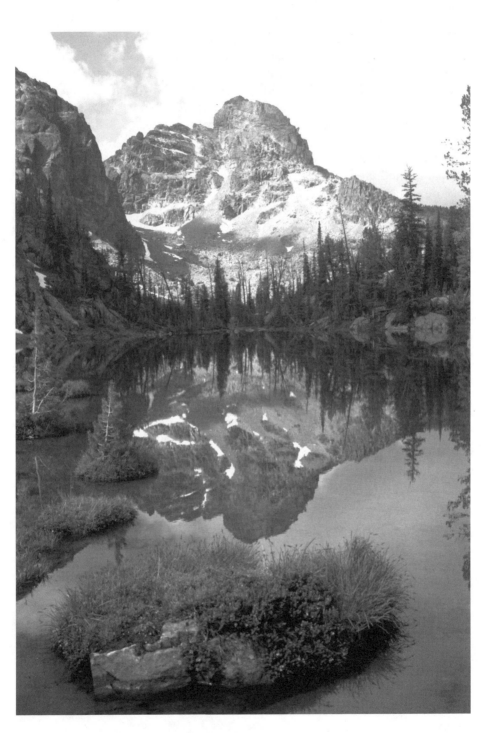

He Devil over tarn near Sheep lake

of miles the trail gains some 1300 feet, beginning with four short switchbacks and then a long traverse across a talus slope.

Tip: *As you climb, be sure to look behind you for great views of the sharp pinnacle of Devils Tooth.*

The next 10 uphill switchbacks have long northward legs and short southward legs, so by the time you finally reach the top of the ridge you are at least 1 mile north of the falls on West Fork Sheep Creek. After completing this gently graded but tiring ascent, the trail rounds the north side of wide Middle Ridge just above some impressive cliffs, from the top of which are fine views east to Heavens Gate Lookout and north down the rugged canyon of Sheep Creek.

You now make two gentle, downhill switchbacks and a long, curving traverse that take you to a junction near the base of a large rock formation. You go straight, then climb five rounded switchbacks to Windy Saddle and your car.

POSSIBLE ITINERARY

	Camp	Miles	Elevation Gain
Day 1	Dog Creek (with side trip to Lower Cannon Lake)	8	600
Day 2	Baldy Lake (with side trips to Dog Lake and Horse Heaven Hill)	12	2800
Day 3	Sheep Lake (with side trip to Dry Diggins Lookout)	13	3000
Day 4	Out	10	2100

VARIATIONS For a shorter trip, stick to the more scenic (and crowded) trails on the northern part of this loop, around the main highlights of Sheep Lake and Dry Diggins.

For the adventure of a lifetime (although with complicated transportation logistics) do the northern part of the loop, then take the trail down Little Granite Creek from Hibbs Cow Camp to the Snake River. From there, either walk down the Snake River Trail to Pittsburg Landing (see Trip 7), or arrange for a raft to pick you up and float the river to Pittsburg Landing or Lewiston.

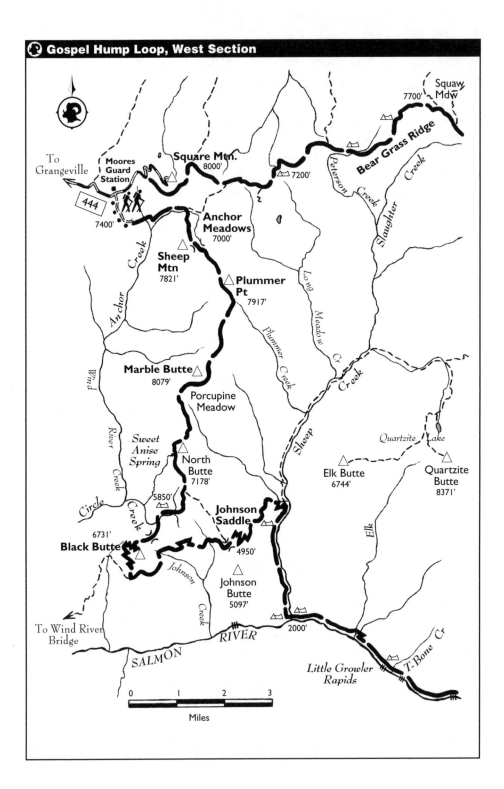

To Grangeville

Moores Guard Station

444

7400'

Square Mtn.
8000'

7200'

Bear Grass Ridge

7700'

Squaw Mdw

Peterson Creek

Slaughter Creek

Anchor Meadows
7000'

Sheep Mtn
7821'

Anchor Creek

Plummer Pt
7917'

Long Meadow Cr

Marble Butte
8079'

Plummer Creek

Sheep Creek

Porcupine Meadow

Wind River Creek

Sweet Anise Spring

North Butte
7178'

Quartzite Lake

Elk Butte
6744'

Quartzite Butte
8371'

5850'

Circle Creek

6731'

Johnson Saddle

4950'

Black Butte

Johnson Creek

Johnson Butte
5097'

Elk Creek

To Wind River Bridge

SALMON RIVER

2000'

Little Growler Rapids

T-Bone Cr

0   1   2   3

Miles

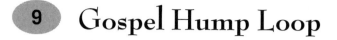

9 Gospel Hump Loop

RATINGS (1–10)			MILES	ELEVATION GAIN	DAYS	SHUTTLE MILEAGE
Scenery	Solitude	Difficulty	68	12,600	5-8	N/A
7	8	10	(70)	(13,600)	(5-8)	

MAP USFS - Gospel Hump Wilderness.

USUALLY OPEN July to October.

BEST Early-to-mid July, if you can stand the sometimes intense heat in the Salmon River Canyon, otherwise September.

PERMITS None.

RULES Maximum group size of 20 people and 20 stock animals.

CONTACT Red River Ranger District, (208) 842-2245 and Salmon River Ranger District, (208) 839-2211.

SPECIAL ATTRACTIONS Solitude; great views of the Salmon River Canyon; whitewater rafters to watch.

PROBLEMS Rattlesnakes and poison ivy in the Salmon River Canyon; some brushy and poorly maintained trails.

HOW TO GET THERE From U.S. Highway 95 in Grangeville, turn east onto State Highway 13 and drive 1.0 mile through town to a junction directly across from the Nez Perce National Forest headquarters. Turn right (south), following signs for Snow Haven Ski Area, and drive 0.8 mile on this good paved road to a junction, where you go straight. Just 1.5 miles later, veer right at another junction and stay on this paved road as it goes past the ski area and enters national forest land, where it becomes Forest Road 221. At 24.2 miles from the Grangeville turnoff is a four-way junction, signed as Four Corners. Turn left, staying on paved Road 221, and drive 6.8 miles to a junction, where you turn left again, following signs to Gospel Hump Wilderness and Sawyer Lookout.

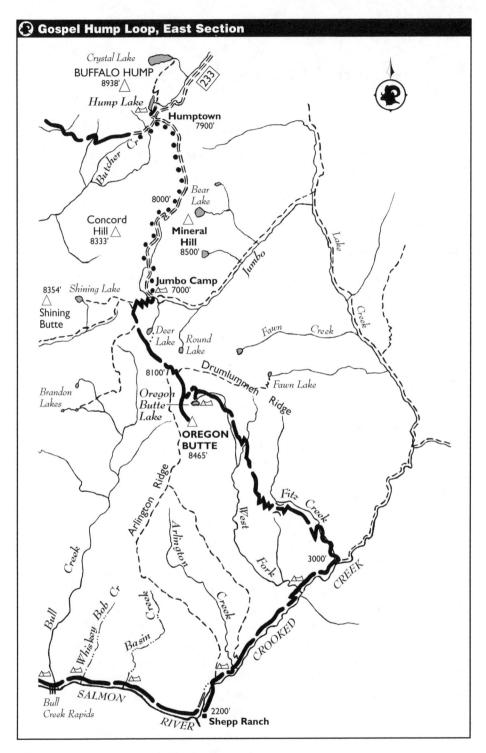

Crystal Lake

BUFFALO HUMP
8938'

Hump Lake

233

Humptown
7900'

Butcher Cr.

Bear
Lake

8000'

Concord
Hill
8333'

Mineral
Hill
8500'

Jumbo

Jumbo Camp
7000'

8354'   Shining Lake

Shining
Butte

Deer
Lake

Round
Lake

Fawn   Creek

Lake   Creek

8100'   Drumlummen

Fawn Lake

Brandon
Lakes

Oregon
Butte
Lake

Ridge

OREGON
BUTTE
8465'

Fitz Creek

West

Arlington Ridge

Arlington   Creek

Fork

3000'

Bull   Creek

Whiskey Bob Cr.

Basin   Creek

CROOKED   CREEK

SALMON

Bull
Creek Rapids

RIVER

2200'
Shepp Ranch

You are now on Forest Road 444, which is steep, but is otherwise a good gravel road with a relatively smooth surface. As will soon become apparent, this road is also wildly scenic, with outstanding views that make it one of the most spectacular drives in Idaho. After 6.0 miles the surface gets rougher, but it remains a reasonably good gravel and dirt road that passenger cars can easily travel. There are several signed trailheads along the road. The one you want is 11.8 miles from Road 221, directly opposite the single log building of the Moores Guard Station.

INTRODUCTION Diversity is the defining characteristic of Gospel Hump Wilderness, with its amazing variety of landforms, vegetation, and wildlife. This ruggedly difficult loop samples all of the wilderness' diverse scenery including view-packed subalpine ridges, high mountain lakes, and the great depths of the Salmon River Canyon. The flora along the route is equally diverse, with everything from subalpine forests and wildflower meadows at higher elevations to parched grasses and scattered ponderosa pines in the near desert at the bottom of the Salmon River Canyon. Wildlife is common in all of these environments, including black bears, elk, moose, and bighorn sheep. Except for boaters on the Salmon River, however, your chances of seeing very many *people* on this hike are slim.

This hike is unabashedly difficult, with many steep ups and downs over extremely rugged terrain. Take this hike only if you are in top physical condition, and even then you will need to take it slow.

DESCRIPTION The trail begins as a narrow jeep track that gradually descends through lovely beargrass meadows in a high-elevation forest of subalpine firs. You soon cross a small burn area and come to the end of the road, where you bear right on a foot trail and drop to a crossing of a trickling tributary of Anchor Creek. From here, you contour through pleasant forests to a junction at the east end of Anchor Meadows, a beautiful group of small, subalpine meadows that are covered with wildflowers in July. You bear right, hop over the main stem of small Anchor Creek, then go up a moderately steep incline for about 1 mile to a grassy saddle on the east shoulder of Sheep Mountain. The trail then descends to another small meadow before climbing rather steeply to the top of a ridge that extends south from 7917-foot Plummer Point.

About 2 miles south of Plummer Point, the rolling trail takes you across burned-over slopes on the east and south sides of rounded Marble Butte a little above small Porcupine Meadow, where you actually stand a better chance of seeing deer or elk than porcupines. The trail then descends 700 feet through a lovely forest untouched by the fire to small but reliable Sweet Anise Spring, where there is good water, but no campsite.

After the spring, you make a steady downhill through lodgepole-pine forests to a junction with the Johnson Butte Trail. By taking this steep route you can shorten the loop distance by about 5 miles, but you'd also miss some terrific canyon scenery and the view from Black Butte. So I recommend that you turn right, go fairly steeply downhill for 0.5 mile, then travel up and down through an area of large erratic boulders to a very good campsite about 200 yards beyond the crossing of tiny Circle Creek. More steep little ups and downs then take you to a second creek crossing, where there is a much smaller campsite with room for only a single tent.

The trail makes a short but very steep climb away from Circle Creek to a viewless saddle on the east side of Black Butte, followed by an uphill traverse of the densely forested north side of the peak. At the end of this traverse is a junction with the short and not-to-be-missed spur trail to the top of Black Butte. This side trail makes 10 short switchbacks to the brushy summit, which is graced with a sturdy-looking, but unstaffed, wooden fire lookout building that sits atop a solid stone base. The view from this lofty grandstand is stupendous, especially south to the gaping Salmon River Canyon, which drops fully 4700 vertical feet to the raging river. You can also look northeast over the forested mountains, ridges, and canyons of the Gospel Hump Wilderness, and north to Square Mountain and the Gospel Peaks near where you started this hike.

Back on the main trail, the elevation rapidly falls and the temperature quickly rises as you switchback steeply down the relatively dry and sunny southwest side of Black Butte. The vegetation changes to suit the new environment, with lots of brushy ceonothus bushes beneath open stands of fire-scarred ponderosa pines. A little over 1 mile down from the Black Butte Lookout Trail is a junction with a trail that heads west (right) to the Wind River Bridge and the Lower Salmon River Road. You veer left and make a long, view-packed, up-and-down traverse of the steep slopes of the Salmon River Canyon. Views down into the canyon and up to several granite rock outcroppings above the trail are almost constant and always outstanding. The rugged, 3-mile traverse ends at Johnson Saddle and a reunion with the Johnson Butte Trail.

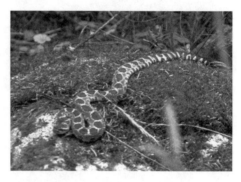

Rattlesnake

Warning: *Rattlesnakes are abundant in the Salmon River Canyon. Although they are not aggressive, they will defend themselves if they feel threatened or if you inadvertently get too close. Few hikers make it through this section without seeing at least one or two of these chunky, venomous reptiles.*

Brace your knees now, because it's all downhill from Johnson Saddle as the trail makes several, often steep switchbacks and long traverses that take you down 2500 feet in 3 miles to an unsigned fork just above rushing Sheep Creek. Your trail veers right (downhill), switchbacks a few more times, then turns downstream and follows a brushy and somewhat overgrown course beside large Sheep Creek. You soon pass a good campsite with a rock-lined fireplace, after which the steep-sided canyon gets increasingly scenic with impressive walls and an interesting forest of ponderosa pines and Douglas-firs. The poorly maintained trail through this area stays on the west bank of the stream, alternating between traveling beside the water, where you have to fight through areas of thick brush, and traversing drier hillsides above the creek, where the going is much easier. In a few places the trail has been blasted into

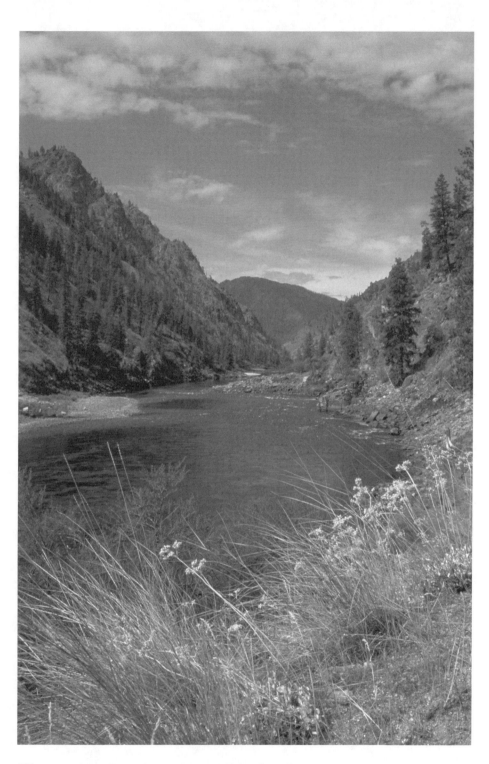

114   *Salmon River Canyon near Bull Creek*

steep rock faces several dozen feet above the water. About 2.5 miles down this trail is a large wooden bridge over Sheep Creek, just before the creek's confluence with the Salmon River. There are some very good, boater-oriented campsites on either side of the bridge.

The trail turns left (east) and goes up the Salmon River's scenic canyon, generally staying on open, rocky slopes with scattered ponderosa pines, bunchgrass, and late-summer-blooming sunflowers. The wetter, north-facing slopes on the opposite side of the river have more trees, but they also show evidence of large fires with many burned-over areas.

Warning: Poison ivy is very common along this section of the trail, so despite the often hot temperatures, shorts are a poor clothing choice.

It won't be easy for you to concentrate on avoiding ground-level menaces like poison ivy and rattlesnakes, because your attention will naturally be drawn to the scenery. Of particular interest are the river's numerous sandy beaches, which are covered with water in early season, but that make great lunch spots or campsites in late summer. At other points, the trail climbs to rocky overlooks about 100 feet above the river, where the views up and down the river corridor are outstanding.

About 1.5 miles from Sheep Creek you make an easy ford of Elk Creek, then walk past Little Growler Rapids to a good campsite at small T-Bone Creek. The rapids come fast and furious above this point, as you walk past four major rapids in the next 3 miles. It is fun to spend some time in this section watching whitewater rafters struggle through these rapids, especially when so many of them get wet or overturned in the process.

Warning: The canyon's wild character is often disturbed by noisy jet boats. Fortunately, these boats go by quickly and the canyon soon resumes its quiet appeal.

The next major landmark is Bull Creek, a good-sized tributary that flows out of an impressive side canyon. There are several good campsites near the log crossing of this creek, the best ones being on the west side. The river has fewer rapids above Bull Creek, as the greenish water flows through gentle riffles and quiet eddies for the next 4 miles. There are two good campsites along the way, the first just before the crossing of often-dry Whiskey Bob Creek and the second, 1 mile later, near also-dry Basin Creek. This very scenic section ends where the trail enters the mouth of the large canyon of Crooked Creek.

The trail goes a few hundred yards up Crooked Creek Canyon to the south end of a small landing strip, where the route turns right and crosses a segmented bridge to privately-owned Shepp Ranch, a comfortable-looking guest facility. **Note:** The area around this ranch, and for about 1 mile up Crooked Creek, is private property. Hikers are allowed to walk through, but not to camp.

After crossing the bridge, you turn left, walk past the ranch's horse pens, then take a jeep road that parallels Crooked Creek. When the road ends, you make a knee-deep ford of the creek, then pick up the foot trail heading up the canyon.

> *Tip:* To avoid this ford, instead of crossing the bridge at Shepp Ranch, simply walk to the north end of the landing strip, then wander through open forests to the trail.

Shortly after the ford is a junction with the trail up Arlington Ridge, where you go straight and soon pass a sign identifying the end of private land. Less than 0.5 mile later, you splash across small Arlington Creek near a fair campsite on a small flat beside Crooked Creek.

You climb briefly to a junction with Trail #202, where you go straight, then walk slowly uphill on the open, ponderosa-pine-studded hillside a little above Crooked Creek. After about 2 miles, the trail descends from the hillside and follows the stream to a log crossing of West Fork Crooked Creek. There is a good campsite on the north side of this crossing.

Not quite 1.5 miles from West Fork Crooked Creek, the trail enters an area devastated by fire, then comes to a junction just 50 yards after crossing small Fitz Creek. You turn left and head up the canyon of this tributary stream on a miserably brushy trail that crosses the creek five times in the next mile.

> *Tip:* Be sure to fill your water bottles at the last crossing, because it's 4 tough miles, and almost 3000 feet up, to your next water source.

After the last crossing, the trail leaves the dense shrubbery near Fitz Creek, goes up two switchbacks on a fire-scarred hillside, then makes a steep uphill traverse on the northeast side of a forested ridge. The traverse ends at a ridgetop saddle, where you can rest for a while to enjoy the view. You'll need that rest, because the ascent is far from over, as the trail now winds steeply up burned-over and sun-baked slopes on the southwest side of the ridge. The climb is long and very tiring, but rewards you with a fine view south to the

Salmon River Canyon and the forested hills of the distant Frank Church-River of No Return Wilderness.

The seemingly endless climb goes through more charred areas of blackened snags and lots of deadfall as the ridgeline completes a long curve to the north. This curve causes the trail to lose its view of the Salmon River Canyon, but it gains a new perspective to the northwest of Oregon Butte with its distinctive, white lookout building on top. The poorly maintained trail leaves the ridgecrest near a charred trail sign and makes a tough, up-and-down traverse on the west side of the ridge.

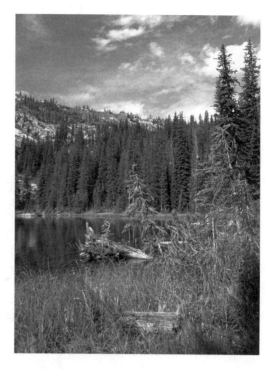

Oregon Butte Lake

Warning: *Careful navigation is important here, because it is very easy to lose the route amid all the tough-limbed brush and deadfall.*

After a little over 0.5 mile of this difficult traverse, you hop over a tributary of West Fork Crooked Creek (your first water since Fitz Creek), then switchback steeply over a small rocky ridge. The trail reenters unburned forest here and follows the main stem of West Fork Crooked Creek up a woodsy canyon. Although the trail is still maddeningly brushy in places, at least it's mostly in the shade and reasonably easy to follow.

You soon make a rock-hop crossing of the creek, then go steeply uphill for another mile. Exactly 160 yards after you cross the second of two tiny, trickling creeks, look for an orange survey tape tied to a small tree on your left that marks the start of a terrific side trip to Oregon Butte Lake. Although not an officially maintained trail, this faint angler's path is marked with orange survey tapes, so it's reasonably easy to follow. The 500-yard trail travels around a meadow, then through dense woods to a great campsite beside the small lake,

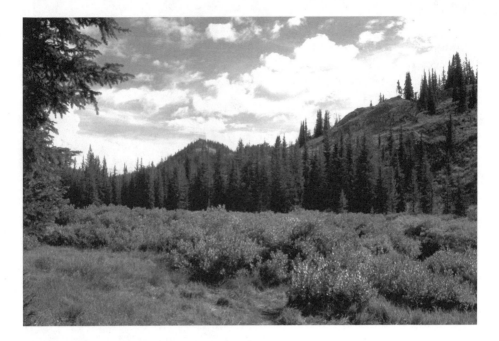

Lush meadow at Jumbo Camp

where you can enjoy both good trout fishing and a great view of Oregon Butte.

Back on the main trail, another 0.5 mile of moderately steep uphill through increasingly open forests takes you to the junction with the trail to Oregon Butte Lookout and another recommended side trip. This side trail goes left and ascends a rocky ridge for a little over 0.5 mile to the staffed lookout building. The views from this facility are outstanding and include virtually all of the route of this hike as well as seemingly endless numbers of peaks and ridges in all directions.

The main loop trail goes right and wanders gradually uphill through lovely forests and meadows in a subalpine environment. Several side trails meet your route in this area and many are worth exploring. The first side trail goes to the right and follows Drumlummen Ridge to remote Fawn Lake, which is a favorite hangout for moose. The main trail makes a short, steep climb away from this junction to a meadow-studded ridgeline, then goes about 100 yards down from the top of this ridge to a junction with the Arlington Ridge Trail.

You go straight and wander generally downhill on this beautiful, view-packed ridge to a sign pointing to Deer Lake, which you can reach by following a hard-to-find angler's trail. The next junction is with the Brandon Lakes Trail, an obscure path that goes about 3 miles to these tiny and rarely visited lakes. You bear slightly right (downhill) and, a few hundred yards later, reach the junction with the Sheep Creek Trail. About 0.5 mile down this trail is the junction with a scenic side trail to lovely Shining Lake, which has lots of big fish, although they are hard to catch.

Your route goes straight at the Sheep Creek junction, then winds steeply down several short switchbacks to a log over clear and slow-moving Jumbo Creek. Immediately past this log the trail ends at Jumbo Camp, a remote campground at the end of a primitive, four-wheel-drive road. There is an outhouse here as well as several nice (but often buggy) campsites, which you only rarely have to share with car campers.

To continue past Jumbo Camp, go north on the narrow and very rocky jeep road that goes up-and-down past lovely meadows and several isolated miner's cabins. (**Note:** These cabins are private property. Stay on the public roadway and do not trespass near the buildings.) The road climbs above the end of a large meadow, then makes a high traverse across the west side of Mineral Hill, where you'll have outstanding views northwest to Buffalo Hump and west to distant Square Mountain and the Gospel Peaks. Even though this is technically a road walk, something I try to avoid, the road is so primitive and the views are so exceptional you will not find the walk in the least bit tedious. About 4.5 miles from Jumbo Camp is the former site of Humptown, in a wide, meadowy saddle with great views of massive Buffalo Hump. A signed jeep road goes left (downhill) here on its way to Hump Trail #313 and the continuation of your loop.

Before going that way, however, take some time for a scenic side trip to nearby Hump Lake and, if possible, on to larger Crystal Lake. To get there, stay on the main road for 50 yards, then turn left on a jeep road. About 200 yards down this road is a very nice log cabin, from which you can saunter a short distance north to the shore of long, meadow-rimmed Hump Lake. There are some exceptionally photogenic views across this lake to imposing Buffalo Hump.

Tip: Look for moose browsing near the shore of this lake.

To make the 1.5-mile hike to Crystal Lake, follow the unsigned trail that goes around the east shore of Hump Lake, walk past a mine, then go steeply down a ridge to the east end of Crystal Lake.

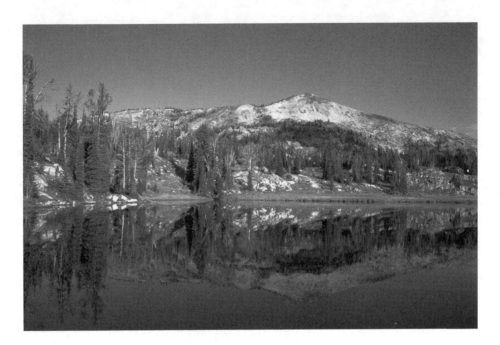

Buffalo Hump over Hump Lake

To complete the loop, return to the site of Humptown and hike 0.5 mile along the previously mentioned side road to the wilderness boundary and the start of Hump Trail #313. You will follow this scenic route for the remaining 13.5 miles of your hike, generally staying on a high ridgeline that goes constantly up and down through lovely subalpine meadows and forests. Although there is plenty of elevation gain and loss, the grade is rarely steep, in part because much of the way follows segments of a long-abandoned jeep road.

The first mile gradually descends to a tributary of Butcher Creek, then you climb around the edge of some rocky bluffs, where there are great views of Concord Hill and Quartzite Butte to the south. Immediately after this uphill, you leave the rocky old road and angle downhill to the left on an obvious foot trail. This trail takes you to a step-over crossing of the headwaters of Slaughter Creek and down to a reunion with the old road. You follow this road as it contours briefly, then climbs to an unsigned fork near the scattered openings of Squaw Meadow. You veer left, staying on the more obvious route, and, less than 0.5 mile later, come to the unsigned junction with Boundary Creek Trail.

You go straight and gradually curve to the southwest along the gentle, open slopes of appropriately named Bear Grass Ridge. After 1.5 miles, you pass a good campsite beside a tiny, shallow pond, then do more ups and downs and follow the trickling headwaters of Peterson Creek. You hop over the creek shortly before a decent campsite, then gradually pull away from the water to the signed junction with faint Trail #315 to Johns Creek. Go straight, make a moderately steep ascent to a high point on the ridge, then go down to a small meadow with a (really) tiny trickle of water and a nice campsite. Another moderate uphill (this trail never stays level for long) takes you to a cairn marking a junction that is not shown on the wilderness map. You go straight (uphill) and do still more ups and downs for about 1 mile to a signed junction.

The main trail goes left and returns to the trailhead via Anchor Meadows. For a different route that provides better views with almost no added mileage, go straight, descend to a little meadow, then climb fairly steeply up the east side of Square Mountain to a junction with Square Mountain Trail #383. You bear left and finish the hike with a scenic traverse across the view-packed slopes on the south side of Square Mountain. The trail ends at a gravel road, where you turn left and walk downhill to the Moores Guard Station.

VARIATIONS You can also access this hike from the Wind River trailhead off the Lower Salmon River Road out of Riggins. From there, it's a long, tough, often hot climb to the junction below Black Butte Lookout.

POSSIBLE ITINERARY			
	Camp	**Miles**	**Elevation Gain**
Day 1	Circle Creek	12	1500
Day 2	Salmon River at Sheep Creek (with side trip to Black Butte Lookout)	11	1200
Day 3	Arlington Creek	11	1800
Day 4	Oregon Butte Lake	10	4900
Day 5	Hump Lake (with side trip to Oregon Butte Lookout)	11	2000
Day 6	Out	15	2200

CENTRAL IDAHO SHUTTLE SERVICES

The mountains and canyons of central Idaho form a vast wilderness complex that covers an area larger than the state of New Jersey. Lovers of true wilderness delight in the fact that no paved roads cross this area and trailhead access is often limited to long drives on rugged dirt roads. From U.S. Highway 12 in the north to State Highways 21 and 75 in the south, a distance of 150 miles, only one rutted, dirt road crosses central Idaho. For wildlife, this allows for unrestricted travel without the disturbance of highways. For people, however, this situation has a downside, because circling around from a trailhead on one side of the wilderness to a different trailhead on the other side entails a tedious and time consuming drive of as much as 300 miles. This means that on point-to-point backpacking trips your hiking time will be shortened by two full days, because you have to shuttle cars back and forth at each end of your trip.

One way to avoid a long car shuttle is to take a loop hike, several of which are recommended on the following pages. Since this is not always feasible, you might want to look into other alternatives. Commercial car-shuttle services cannot make enough money if they cater only to hikers, but whitewater rafters floating down Idaho's famous rivers need transportation as well, and these people are numerous enough to keep shuttle companies in business. Hikers can use these services as well, and many companies will gladly take you not only to and from river put-in and take-out sites, but also to most area trailheads, whether or not the stop is on their regular itinerary. It isn't cheap, but many hikers think that it is well worth it.

One reliable company is River Shuttles, located in Salmon, (800) 831-8942. They will happily transport you to any reasonably accessible trailhead in the Sawtooth National Recreation Area, the Salmon River country, or along the Selway River. Another advantage is that they keep your car at their facility, which is more secure than a trailhead, and only take it to your planned exit point on the day you are scheduled to return. You must have reservations for this service, and it is fairly expensive, but by spreading the fee among your entire group the cost becomes reasonable.

Another option for getting into or out of the backcountry is by bush plane. There are dozens of remote airstrips scattered around the wilderness

Continued

(continued)

where you can be dropped off and left to hike out to your car. Alternatively, you can hike in and be picked up on a prearranged date, or pay for two plane rides and hike from one airstrip to another. Two good companies that operate throughout Idaho, but which specialize in the wilderness areas in the central part of the state, are McCall Air Taxi (800) 992-6559 and Arnold Aviation (208) 382-4844. The price of a trip depends on the size of the plane required to transport your group, how much gear you have, and the distance of the flight(s). A typical trip that transports two people and their backpacks to one of the remote airstrips along the Middle Fork Salmon River will set you back almost $400, as of 2004. That is expensive, but you have to weigh that cost against the time saved, the unique views you'll enjoy from a small plane, and the hair-raising fun and excitement of landing or taking off in a small plane from one of these tiny dirt airstrips.

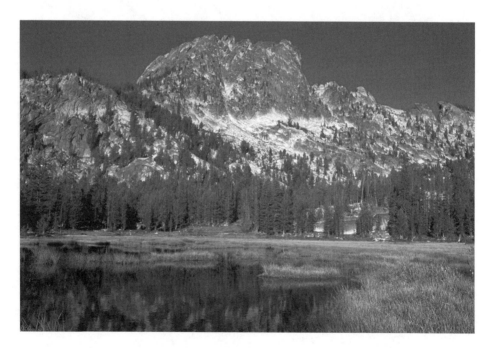

Pond below Cathedral Rock, Bighorn Crags, Trip 11

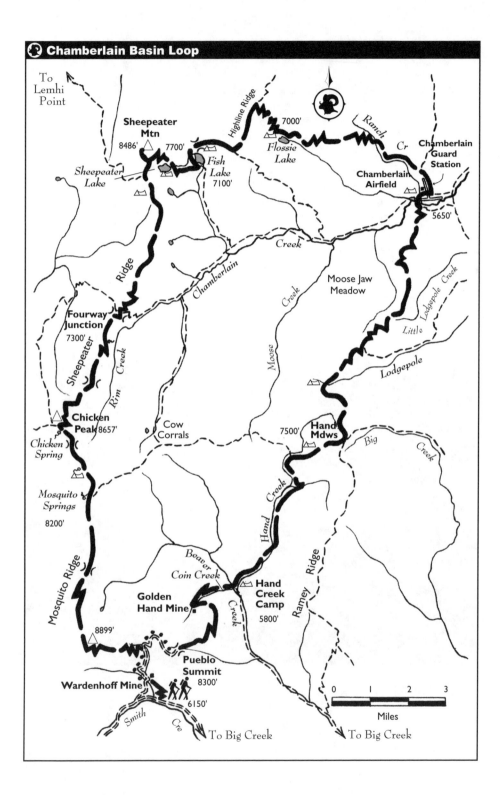

Chamberlain Basin Loop

To Lemhi Point

Sheepeater Mtn
8486' 7700'

Sheepeater Lake

Highline Ridge

7000'

Flossie Lake

Ranch

Cr

Chamberlain Guard Station

Fish Lake 7100'

Chamberlain Airfield

5650'

Chamberlain

Creek

Little Lodgepole Creek

Moose Jaw Meadow

Moose Creek

Ridge

Fourway Junction

7300'

Sheepeater

Rim Creek

Lodgepole

Chicken Peak 8657'

Chicken Spring

Cow Corrals

7500'

Hand Mdws

Big Creek

Mosquito Springs

8200'

Hand Creek

Ramey Ridge

Mosquito Ridge

Beaver

Coin Creek

Golden Hand Mine

Creek

Hand Creek Camp

5800'

8899'

Pueblo Summit

8300'

Wardenhoff Mine

6150'

Smith Cre

To Big Creek

To Big Creek

0   1   2   3

Miles

10   Chamberlain Basin Loop

RATINGS (1–10)			MILES	ELEVATION GAIN	DAYS	SHUTTLE MILEAGE
Scenery	Solitude	Difficulty	50	10,300	4-7	N/A
5	7	7	(51)	(10,600)	(4-7)	

MAPS USGS - Big Creek, Chicken Peak, Lodgepole Creek, Meadow of Doubt, Mosquito Peak, Sheepeater Mountain, Wolf Fang Peak.

USUALLY OPEN Mid-June to October.

BEST Mid-July to September.

PERMITS None.

RULES Maximum group size of 20 people and 20 stock animals; fires must be in approved fire rings near Chamberlain Airfield.

CONTACT Krassel Ranger District, (208) 634-0600.

SPECIAL ATTRACTIONS Wildlife; solitude.

PROBLEMS Long, rough road access; extensive burn areas.

HOW TO GET THERE There are several possible approaches to this trailhead, all of which require long drives on bumpy gravel roads. The most direct access starts from a junction on State Highway 55, 27 miles south of McCall or 0.8 mile north of Cascade. Turn east onto Warm Lake Road, which becomes Forest Road 22, and drive 34.8 miles on this winding, paved road past Warm Lake (where the road becomes Forest Road 579) and over Warm Lake Summit to the junction with Johnson Creek Road just before the pavement ends. Turn left (north) onto Forest Road 413 and go 25.4 miles on this sometimes bumpy gravel road to a junction at the isolated mining settlement of Yellow Pine. Turn right (east) onto Forest Road 412, following signs to Big Creek Station, and, after 4.9 miles, turn left (north) onto Forest Road 340, following signs to Big Creek. Drive 18.4 miles on this narrow gravel road over Profile Gap and down to a junction with Forest Road

371, where you turn right. Follow this moderately rough road for 2.7 miles to the signed Big Creek trailhead, which is a possible alternate starting point if your car does not have good ground clearance.

To reach the recommended starting point, drive through the Big Creek trailhead parking area, cross a bridge, then follow rough and bumpy Smith Creek Road. This primitive road is badly rutted and has some big rocks, but it remains passable for most cars if you go slowly. After 3.7 miles look for a tiny brown sign on a tree on your left stating SMITH CREEK CUTOFF TRAIL. Park here.

INTRODUCTION Close your eyes and try to picture what the American mountain west looked like 200 years ago. You know what I mean: One of those scenes sometimes pictured in western movies showing vast forests, an endless series of lonesome ridges and peaks, pristine lakes, and lots of wildlife. Now open your eyes and head for the Frank Church-River of No Return Wilderness to see how well you did. There is no better place in America to run this experiment, because this is the second largest wilderness area in the contiguous 48 states and it is perhaps the last place where you can still hike for days, weeks, or even months, and never even come close to a road.

The hike into Chamberlain Basin, actually a high, forested plateau, is one of the more enticing trips in this wilderness, because it has a particular abundance of wildlife, several good-sized lakes, excellent views, and reasonable trail access. Of course, "reasonable" is not the same as "easy" — it's still a long walk — but at least you don't have to start your trip under a back-bending load of two or three weeks worth of supplies, which is necessary for most other trips in this huge wilderness.

Although reasonably good, the scenery on this hike does not compare to the grandeur of most of the other trips in this book. Instead, this trip's appeal lies in the feeling of being in a true wilderness, a quality that does not show up in pretty pictures.

Warning Much of this hike goes through fire-scarred areas with little or no shade. It can be very uncomfortable during hot weather.

DESCRIPTION The Smith Creek Cutoff Trail heads north (uphill) from the small parking area, passes two broken-down log cabins, then makes 11 short, steep switchbacks up a wooded slope. At the top of these switchbacks, you enter an area with an unusual abundance of beargrass, which in some years puts on an impressive show of tall, white blossoms in early-to-mid July. Later in the year you may catch sight of a black bear digging up the roots of this grasslike lily, which was named after the hungry bruins.

After a short traverse, you come to a jeep road and the still-occasionally-occupied buildings of the Werdenhoff Mine. (**Note:** If you have a rugged, high clearance, four-wheel-drive vehicle it is possible to drive to this point, but for most people it's better to be on foot.) You bear right (uphill) on the rough jeep road, cross a small creek, and, immediately thereafter, reach a fork. Veer right and steadily climb the jeep road for a little over 1 mile to a hunter's camp and the start of the poorly signed Mosquito Ridge Trail, which angles off to the left. This is the beginning of your loop.

In order to avoid a long, tough uphill at the end of your trip, and to save the better scenery for the end, I recommend doing the circuit counterclockwise. So go straight, staying on the jeep road as it crosses trickling North Fork Smith Creek and gradually climbs for another mile to the wilderness boundary at Pueblo Summit, where the road ends at a gate.

The view from Pueblo Summit is inspiring. As far as the eye can see to the north and east there are rolling, forested mountains and canyons with no roads or any other signs of man. This is the perfect place to test how well you did on that visualization experiment I suggested earlier.

Stepping out now into true wilderness, you go around the gate and follow an abandoned jeep track that has now deteriorated into a wide, rubbly trail. For the next 2 miles this old track slowly descends through forests of subalpine firs and lodgepole and limber pines to the interesting old buildings and remains of the Golden Hand Mine, which are worth investing some time to explore.

The old jeep road goes right (downhill) at an unsigned junction beside the mine's largest building, crosses small Coin Creek, then traverses a hillside for several hundred yards to an unsigned junction. You leave the old jeep road here and take an obvious foot trail that switchbacks downhill to the right and steeply descends for about 1 mile along Coin Creek. At the bottom of the downhill you cross Beaver Creek on a log just downstream from a horse ford, then walk 150 yards up the opposite bank to a junction with the well-used Chamberlain Trail. Bear

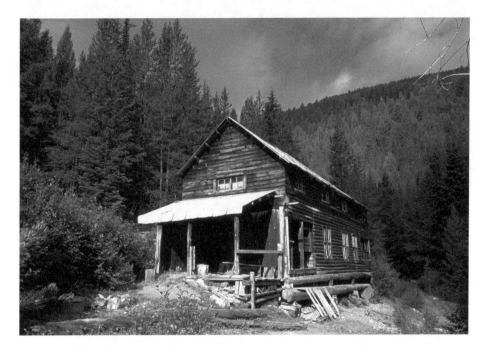

Deteriorating remains of Golden Hand Mine

left and, a few yards later, come to spacious Hand Creek Camp, which has room for at least a dozen tents if you have a large party.

From Hand Creek Camp, you go 80 yards northeast on the Chamberlain Trail to a small sign identifying the Ramey Ridge Trail, which, according to the wilderness map, heads off to the right, although there is virtually no evidence of this unmaintained route on the ground. The Chamberlain Trail goes straight and, for a little over 1 mile, wanders uphill through viewless but pleasant forests to a crossing of Hand Creek. In early summer this ford is chilly and calf-deep, but by mid-August the water will barely get above the tops of your boots. The trail steadily ascends from the ford and follows a pleasant course under the shady canopy of Douglas-firs and Engelmann spruces. The trail never takes you far from Hand Creek, so you can count on the soothing sound of "river music" as a constant companion.

Eventually, the pace of your climb quickens and the forest cover thins as lodgepole pines come to dominate at higher elevations. These more open forests have less shade, but reward you with frequent views of the forests and rock outcroppings on the ridge west of Hand Creek. Not quite 2 miles from the ford, the trail takes a little wooden bridge over a tributary stream. This is a lovely spot to rest or eat lunch, which gives you the time to appreciate the groundsel, grass of parnassus, Queen Anne's lace, wild carrot, and other colorful wildflowers that grow on the banks of the little creek.

The trail follows the tributary creek briefly, then makes one switchback and returns to its course beside larger Hand Creek. The climbing abates 0.5 mile later, after which you lazily wander through open pine forests above a grassy area bordering Hand Creek to a signed junction with the Crane Meadows Trail. Bear right and, about 250 yards later, pass a very good, but easily overlooked, campsite below you on the left just above a small meadow on Hand Creek.

Now the trail, which has been significantly rerouted from what is shown on the wilderness map, makes a long and very unsatisfying climb through viewless forests on the hillside to the northeast. This realignment was done so the trail would bypass lovely but fragile Hand Meadows, which was once a scenic highlight of this trip and a good place to see wildlife. Unfortunately, the new trail stays in less attractive forests and burn areas and misses the meadows altogether.

After topping a woodsy ridge, the trail skirts the edge of an old burn area, then curves to the right and makes a downhill traverse to a four-way junction. You go slightly left, staying on the Chamberlain Trail, and for the next 2.5 miles make a rather monotonous and shadeless passage through a large burn area. Deadfall is a constant problem here, and in most of the other burn areas along this trail. Not quite 2 miles into this burn area is a fair campsite beside a trickle of water at the head of Lodgepole Creek.

Tip: Refill your water bottles here, because this is the last water for the next 5.5 miles, and the majority of that distance has no shade.

For the next few miles the trail gradually descends along a wide, rolling ridge. The route includes a couple of lazy switchbacks, but for the most part it's a straightforward downhill. Most of the distance goes through a fascinating mix of old fire scars, recent burn areas, and some pockets of trees that have, so far, been totally untouched by flames. In a wide saddle about 2 miles from Lodgepole Creek is a sign pointing to the very faint trail that goes to your right down Little Lodgepole Creek.

Biology of a Burn

The scenery is a perfect classroom for studying the effects of natural fire on a wild forest. Although some areas were completely scorched from ground to tree top, most of the forest looks more like a patchwork quilt. Some trees, seemingly at random, were left unscathed, while their neighbors, just a few inches away, are now blackened snags. Many trees had their trunks singed, but their crowns are still intact.

The different fire ages on display here allow you to observe the stages of how a forest recovers from a fire. Initially, only grasses poke up through the charred remains. After this, wildflowers like fireweed and beargrass take over, to be followed a few years later by young evergreens. The first trees to grow are usually lodgepole pines, because the cones of this evergreen require the heat of a fire to release their seeds, an evolutionary adaptation that gives the young pines an advantage in capturing the sunlight in a new fire scar. As for wildlife, elk are especially common in the most recent burn areas, feeding on the succulent young grasses that grow in disturbed areas.

Tip: *The wilderness map also shows a trail that goes left to Moose Jaw Meadow, but there is no sign of this trail on the ground.*

You go straight on the main trail, descend two gentle switchbacks, then go up and down along the top of the wide, fire-scarred ridge. About 1 mile from the Little Lodgepole turnoff, the rolling section of the ridge ends and the trail goes more consistently downhill. In this area you will probably begin to hear the occasional sound of small airplanes taking off and landing at the Chamberlain Airfield. This is an unusual sound for most designated wilderness areas, but it is fairly common in the large wilderness areas of Idaho, where several active landing strips provide access to these remote regions.

The ridge gradually peters out and drops off more steeply, but the trail compensates with a couple of well-graded switchbacks, so the downhill is never overly steep. Soon after the trail levels off, you come to a junction with the Cold Meadows Trail, which goes to the right. About 200 yards from this junction is a bridge over large Chamberlain Creek (actually the size of a small river), where you can restock your water supply or spend a few hours trying to catch some of the creek's hungry trout.

Tip: *The only approved campsites in this area are on the south side of the airfield, a few hundred yards north of the creek. Do not camp near the bridge.*

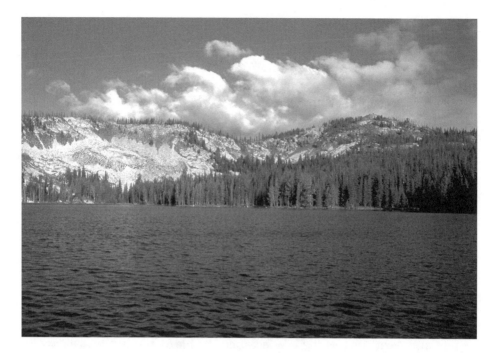

Sheepeater Lake

On the top of the low bank north of Chamberlain Creek is a poorly signed junction just before the long, east-west landing strip at Chamberlain Airfield. Go straight, cross the dirt landing strip, then walk a short distance through forests to an unsigned junction. You bear right, cross the clear waters of small Ranch Creek, and soon come to the scattered buildings of the Chamberlain Guard Station. The two isolated Forest Service personnel who spend their summers here are happy to provide a friendly greeting.

To continue the hike, go east across a north-south landing strip in Chamberlain Airfield and pick up the trail that goes north through the forest. At the end of the landing strip is a meadow where the trail splits. You veer left, following signs to Flossie Lake, and once again walk through partially burned forests. Much of the rest of the trip, in fact, is in burned areas, which is an interesting and unique ecosystem, although the scenery won't appeal to everyone.

For the next 1.5 miles the trail travels beside Ranch Creek, where lush, grassy meadows host a wide variety of wildflowers. The peak bloom is in July and early August, when the most common varieties are yarrow, aster, and cinquefoil. Later in the summer, goldenrod and gentians keep the color show going. Something else to look for in this area, and for some time to come, is the sign of wolves. These large canines find good habitat in this area and you will probably see the scat and tracks of the small pack that calls this place home. If you are *really* lucky, you could even see the animals or hear them howling at night. One evening I lay in my sleeping bag for almost an hour listening to wolves howl – a classic wilderness experience that I will not soon forget.

You hop over Ranch Creek about 2.5 miles from the Chamberlain Guard Station, then the pace of your climb increases as eight switchbacks take you up a hillside that is badly charred by fire. After this, you wander up and down through a mix of green forests and burned woods, then make a rather long and tiring climb around a series of rounded, rocky knolls, and drop about 100 feet to shimmering Flossie Lake. This attractive lake sits in a small basin beneath a rocky butte, but the scene is less than perfect, because most of its shoreline is scarred by fire. Some of the trees on the south and west sides of the lake escaped the blaze, but in the designated camping area on the north side, which all visitors are required to use, there is nothing but blackened snags.

The trail continues slowly climbing beyond Flossie Lake, first rounding the lake's basin, then going up four switchbacks under the welcome shade of unburned spruce and pine trees. You pass a lovely little pond with a grassy shore and the appropriate name of Frog Pond, after which the rocky trail wanders up a half dozen switchbacks to a junction atop viewless Highline Ridge.

You turn left (south) and follow the wide ridgeline for a little over 1 mile to another junction on a severely fire-scarred hilltop with expansive views of Chamberlain Basin. The obscure and unsigned trail to the left heads down to Chamberlain Creek, but you turn right and walk slowly downhill through this bleak, charred landscape to a wide saddle. The trail then curves to the left (south) and makes an uneven descent to the south shore of meadow-rimmed Fish Lake. There are some excellent campsites at this lake, although they tend to be plagued by mosquitoes.

Tip: The best campsites are under some large, unburned trees near an inlet creek on the southwest shore of the lake.

Not far above the southeast shore of Fish Lake is a junction, where you turn right and go steadily uphill for 1 mile to Sheepeater

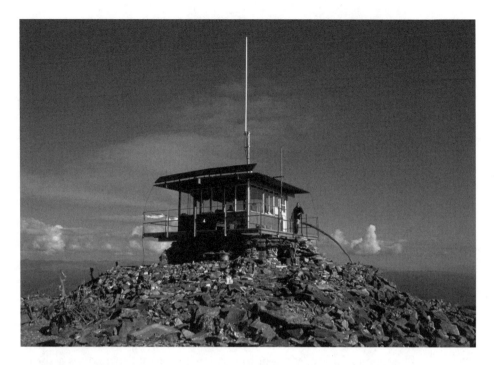

Sheepeater Mountain Lookout

Lake. This beautiful lake sits in a cirque on the side of Sheepeater Mountain and is surrounded by lovely, unburned forests and scenic talus slopes. Sharp-eyed hikers will be able to spot the lookout building atop Sheepeater Mountain to the northwest. There are excellent campsites on the north shore of Sheepeater Lake, which allows you to savor a wonderful night at this mountain gem. The name "Sheepeater" is the Anglicized version of the name for a powerful tribe of local Native Americans who called themselves "meateaters" and who preferred to hunt and eat bighorn sheep.

The trail now makes a moderately steep, 1-mile climb that winds up to a junction atop the ridge west of Sheepeater Lake. The short, not-to-be-missed trail to the right climbs 500 yards to the staffed lookout building atop Sheepeater Mountain. The friendly staffer, who told me that she has enjoyed this view for 17 summers, claims that her location is now the most isolated staffed fire lookout in the lower 48 United States (as measured by its distance from the nearest road). In an average year she logs about 50 visitors, a number which she considers makes the place overly crowded.

To continue the hike, head south along the ridge trail, following signs to Chicken Peak, and walk mostly uphill for a few hundred yards to the signed junction with the little-used, 6.5-mile trail to Lemhi Point. This rather long side trip is worth the time, because from the heights of Lemhi Point you'll enjoy a great view almost straight down into the depths of the gaping Salmon River Canyon. The main trail goes straight at the junction and wanders up and down along the gently undulating ridge. It's an easy and very enjoyable walk with frequent views, lots of beargrass, and plenty of wildlife. Keep an eye out especially for nimble bighorn sheep near the rocky areas, and shy black bears, chubby spruce grouse, and swift-running mule deer in the forests. Not quite 1 mile from the Sheepeater Mountain turnoff is a small, marshy pond on your left with permanent water and possible campsites.

About 3 miles south of Sheepeater Mountain the trail makes a steady descent to a woodsy saddle with the self-explanatory title of Fourway Junction. Go straight at the junction and climb eight short switchbacks, then begin a long, gradual ascent of the southern half of Sheepeater Ridge. Most of the way is in recent burn zones a short distance away from the rock outcroppings and cliffs on the east side of the ridge.

Tip: *Be sure to leave the trail from time to time to check out these rocky areas, both to enjoy the views and to look for bighorn sheep.*

Not quite 1.5 miles from Fourway Junction, you lose about 100 feet of elevation and come to the welcome water of a tiny spring at the base of a small rockslide. You then go up five switchbacks and make a rugged, up-and-down traverse across the rocky east face of Sheepeater Ridge, passing four more tiny springs along the way. Eventually, you climb back up to the top of the ridge at a rocky, windswept saddle. If you look southwest from here, you should be able to spot the anomalous, bright orange roof of the old lookout building atop Chicken Peak.

The trail switches to the scenic west side of Sheepeater Ridge and climbs on a rocky tread to a high point on the eastern shoulder of Chicken Peak. It's easy and well worthwhile to make the short side trip to the rapidly decaying lookout building on the summit of Chicken Peak. Although it is no longer staffed, this quaint building is worth a visit to examine the old-style architecture with its log cabin base and steeply-sloping metal roof. If that doesn't interest

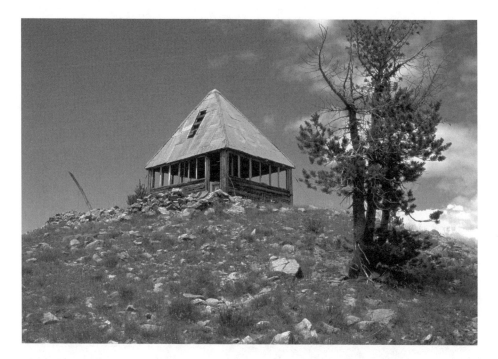

Abandoned Chicken Peak Lookout

you, then just sit back and admire the view, which includes more ridges, canyons, and mountains than I could possibly list here.

The trail makes a few lazy switchbacks down from the shoulder of Chicken Peak to a junction beside the reliable flow of Chicken Spring. Unfortunately, there is no flat ground near this spring, so camping is not a realistic option. Go straight at the junction and walk a short distance along the southwest side of the ridge, then switch to the northeast side at a little saddle. After this, you make a short, stiff climb above an intensely green meadow at the head of Rim Creek and pass a very pleasant campsite beside a couple of small springs.

> *Tip:* If you plan to camp in this vicinity, do so at these springs rather than at the smelly outfitter camp near larger Mosquito Springs, 0.5 mile ahead.

The now-gentle trail climbs a bit to an unsigned fork where a trail drops to the right to the outfitter camp at Mosquito Springs. You bear left and, just 50 yards later, come to a signed junction with a trail that goes left to a place with the uninviting name of Cow

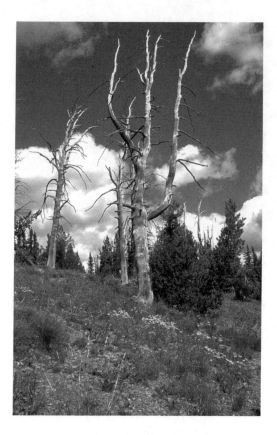
Old snag along Mosquito Ridge

Corrals. You go straight, making your way south along wide and very scenic Mosquito Ridge, and soon leave the last of the fire-damaged areas. The remainder of the hike goes through green, unburned meadows and forests that perfectly complement the excellent distant views.

The scenic tour begins with a long, gradual ascent, mostly on the partly forested west side of the ridge, where gnarled whitebark pines add a nice touch to the scenery. You go around the west side of a high, rounded knoll, then drop to a saddle and climb once again. This uphill starts with two switchbacks, then makes a long, gentle ascent on the west side of the ridge nearly to the top of an 8899-foot high point. The trail then curves to the east and descends five moderately graded switchbacks to a nice ridgetop viewpoint, where you can look all the way north to Sheepeater Mountain. The final 1.5 miles takes you down 20 more switchbacks all the way to the Mosquito Ridge trailhead. Bear right and retrace your steps down the jeep road to the Werdenhoff Mine, the Smith Creek Cutoff Trail, and your car.

VARIATIONS If you'd rather not drive the rough road to the Smith Creek Cutoff trailhead, then start your hike at the Big Creek trailhead instead. From there, walk about 3 miles down the Big Creek Trail to its junction with the Chamberlain Trail, then turn left and walk 7 miles up Beaver Creek to Hand Creek Camp and the junction with the described loop.

If you've got the money and want to avoid the long drive altogether, then charter a plane to take you to the Big Creek Airfield, which is located just 1 mile south of the Big Creek trailhead. You could then arrange to have the same plane pick you up a few days later at Chamberlain Airfield.

Yet another option is to turn this into a long, one-way adventure by continuing north on the Chamberlain Trail all the way to the Salmon River. From there, you can either have prearranged for a rafting party to pick you up and float you back to civilization, or be picked up by an airplane, perhaps from the remote Campbells Ferry Landing Field.

POSSIBLE ITINERARY

	Camp	Miles	Elevation Gain
Day 1	Lower Hand Meadows	10	3900
Day 2	Chamberlain Basin	10	400
Day 3	Sheepeater Lake	11	2700
Day 4	Mosquito Springs (with side trips to Sheepeater Mountain and Chicken Peak)	12	2800
Day 5	Out	8	800

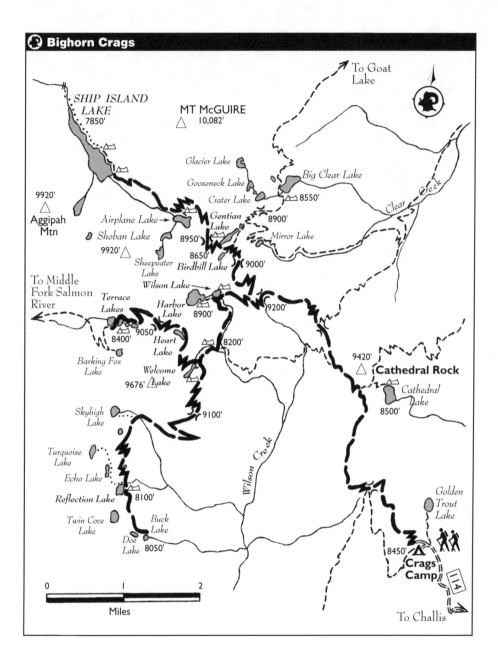

SHIP ISLAND
LAKE
7850'

MT McGUIRE
△ 10,082'

To Goat
Lake

Glacier Lake

Gooseneck Lake

Big Clear Lake

△ 8550'

Clear Creek

Crater Lake

9920'
△
Aggipah
Mtn

Airplane Lake →

Shoban Lake

8950')

Gentian
Lake

8900'

Mirror Lake

9920' △

Sheepeater
Lake

8650'
Birdbill Lake

9000'

To Middle
Fork Salmon
River

Wilson Lake

9200'

Terrace
Lakes

Harbor
Lake

8900'

9420'
△ **Cathedral Rock**

9050'
8400'

Heart
Lake

8200'

Cathedral
Lake

8500'

Barking Fox
Lake

Welcome
9676' △Lake

9100'

Skyhigh
Lake

Wilson Creek

Turquoise
Lake

Echo Lake

Golden
Trout
Lake

Reflection Lake
8100'

Twin Cove
Lake

Buck
Lake

Doe
Lake 8050'

8450'
**Crags
Camp**

114

To Challis

0   1   2

Miles

11 Bighorn Crags

RATINGS (1–10)			MILES	ELEVATION GAIN	DAYS	SHUTTLE MILEAGE
Scenery	Solitude	Difficulty	46	9000	3-6	N/A
9	4	6				

MAPS USGS - Hoodoo Meadows, Mt. McGuire.

USUALLY OPEN July to October.

BEST Mid-July to mid-August.

PERMITS None (just register at the trailhead).

RULES Maximum group size of 20 people and 20 stock animals.

CONTACT Cobalt Ranger District, (208) 756-5100.

SPECIAL ATTRACTIONS Spectacular granite domes and peaks; stunning alpine lakes; wildlife.

PROBLEMS High altitudes with no chance to acclimate; poor access road.

HOW TO GET THERE From Challis, drive 8.0 miles north on U.S. Highway 93, then turn left onto Morgan Creek Road, following signs to Cobalt. Stay on this good gravel road, which becomes Forest Road 55, for 33.2 miles as it climbs over Morgan Creek Summit and descends into the valley of Panther Creek to a junction. Turn left onto Forest Road 112, following signs to Bighorn Crags and Yellowjacket, and climb 7.1 miles on this bumpy gravel road to a saddle and a four-way junction. Turn right onto Forest Road 113, then drive carefully for 8.6 miles on this rough dirt-and-gravel route to another junction. Turn right onto Forest Road 114 and drive 2.2 difficult but passable miles to Crags Campground and the signed parking lot for the hiker's trailhead.

INTRODUCTION The Bighorn Crags feature the most spectacular peaks and lakes in Frank Church-River of No Return Wilderness. And

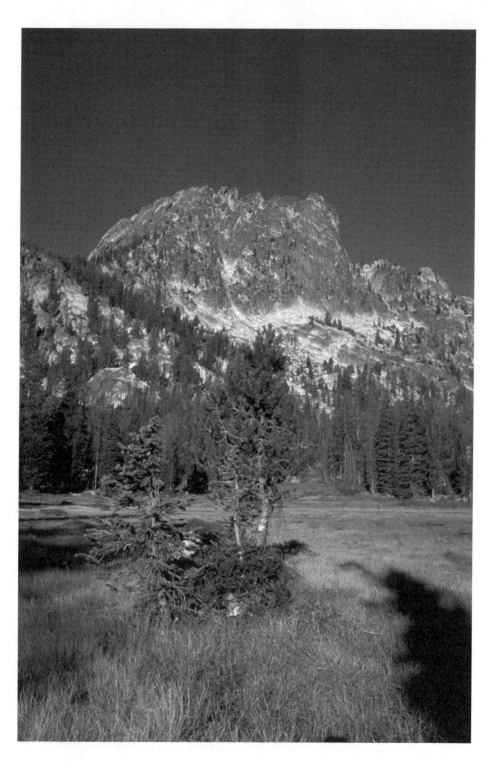

Cathedral Peak from meadow to the east

spectacular is definitely the right word. The scenery is absolutely delightful, with craggy granite spires, high peaks, and dozens of gorgeous alpine lakes tucked into glacial cirques. In addition to scenery, lucky hikers sometimes see elk, mountain goats, and bighorn sheep. The Crags, in fact, were named for a small band of nimble-footed sheep that live amid the spires.

Although uncrowded by comparison to similarly scenic back-country in other parts of the American West, by Idaho standards the Bighorn Crags get a lot of visitors. The Forest Service, therefore, asks hikers to tread lightly and follow all "no-trace" principles.

> **Warning:** *At 8456 feet, the Crags trailhead is one of the highest in the state. Those not accustomed to the altitude will have no warm-up period in which to get acclimated.*

DESCRIPTION The trail begins with a series of short uphill switch-backs, followed by a long traverse across a mostly open slope with views down to Golden Trout Lake. The high-elevation forest here, and for nearly all of this hike, consist primarily of whitebark pines and subalpine firs with a few lodgepole pines. Many of the trees are dead, creating a forest of scenic, silvery snags. After about 1 mile those dead trees help to frame a wonderful view where the trail rounds a high ridge and you get your first sweeping vistas of the many impressive granite domes, cliffs, and spires of the Bighorn Crags.

> **Warning:** *There is no water along the first 7 miles of this ridgeline trail, so you should start with at least two quarts.*

A little less than 2 miles from the trailhead is a four-way junction in a little saddle. Two trails come in from the left here — the wide stock trail from Crags Campground, and a narrower trail that leads to Yellowjacket Lake. You go straight, climb a bit, then follow a scenic ridge with lots of polished granite towers and outcroppings that rise from the ridgetop. Although the trail has many ups and downs, it is gently graded, and cool breezes often waft over the ridge, so the hiking is enjoyable.

About 2.5 miles from the Yellowjacket Lake turnoff is a junction near the base of Cathedral Rock, a prominent granite monolith. The Gant Mountain Trail goes to the right. This path drops fairly steeply for a little less than 0.5 mile to Cathedral Lake and a nearby marshy meadow with a very photogenic view of Cathedral Rock. This side

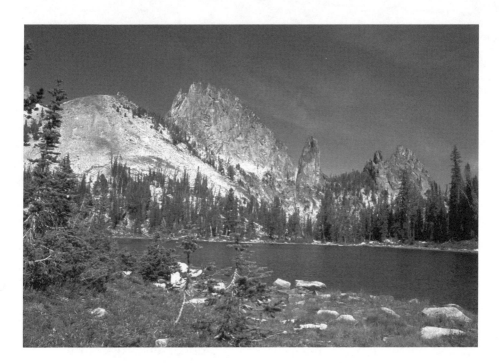

Fishfin Ridge over Harbor Lake

trip provides you with the first chance for water and possible camp-sites.

The main Crags Trail bears left at the junction at the base of Cathedral Rock, descends about 150 feet, then traverses around the south side of the Rock. The open forests here provide good habitat for Clark's nutcrackers, a striking gray, black, and white relative of the crow that is the most common bird at these altitudes. The species was named after its discoverer, Captain William Clark, of the Lewis and Clark expedition.

Not quite 0.5 mile from the Gant Mountain Trail turnoff is a junction with the Waterfall Trail, which heads left on its way to Welcome Lake and the southern Bighorn Crags. You turn right (uphill) on the shorter and more popular trail to the Crags, which quickly ascends to a saddle on a windy ridge, where you can look northeast down the forested valley of Clear Creek.

At the northwest end of the saddle is a junction with the Clear Creek Trail, where you go straight and make a fairly steep climb up the shoulder of a rounded ridge. After savoring the fine views from atop this ridge, you descend a bit, then traverse a hillside above a tiny, shimmering pond in a basin on your left. The trail makes two switchbacks up to a high, often windy pass where you get your first up-close look at the rugged Bighorn Crags. The high, jagged, and very narrow ridgeline directly to the west is Fishfin Ridge, while in a shallow, but very scenic basin to the southwest you can see Wilson and Harbor lakes. These enticing lakes are surrounded by a series of high peaks and polished granite domes.

The trail descends from the pass in one moderately long switchback to a junction just a few feet above a rocky gap in Fishfin Ridge. The Crags Trail to Ship Island Lake goes to the right, but for the nearest water and camps go straight on the Harbor Lakes Trail. This path descends one switchback, then contours to the shores of beautiful Wilson Lake. Unless you made the side trip to Cathedral Lake, this is the first reliable water since the trailhead, almost 7 miles back. There are several good campsites near the outlet and an excellent campsite hidden in the trees beside the inlet on the southwest shore.

To visit equally beautiful Harbor Lake, stay on the trail as it goes around the south shore of Wilson Lake to a switchback, then leave the official trail and go straight on an obvious footpath. This path climbs briefly through a low, grassy swale to Harbor Lake, a deep mountain gem with scenic peninsulas and shores that are rimmed with heather, grasses, and boulders.

Tip: *There are three or four very good campsites amid the subalpine firs near the lake's outlet.*

Either Harbor or Wilson lake makes an excellent central location for a base camp from which to explore the rest of the Bighorn Crags. There are enough worthwhile destinations to keep you busy for a wonderful week of exploring. The three most rewarding dayhikes are described below.

To visit Ship Island Lake, the largest and best known lake in the Crags, return to the junction on Fishfin Ridge and turn north on the Crags Trail. This well-built path descends three very gradual switchbacks on a steep talus slope to the base of the cliffs on the north side of Fishfin Ridge. From here, you traverse gradually uphill on open, rocky slopes to the top of a narrow ridge, then descend three gentle switchbacks to a junction near unseen Birdbill Lake.

The trail to the right goes past a pond below Gentian Lake, then switchbacks steeply over a pass and drops to appropriately named

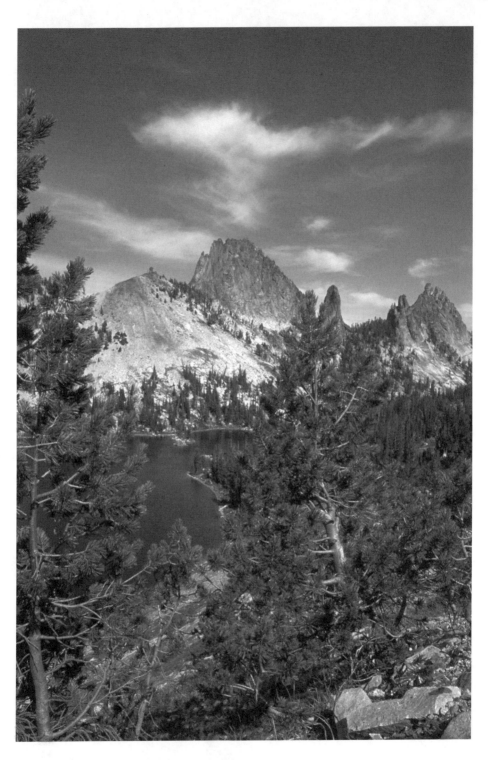

Harbor lake from ridge to the south

Big Clear Lake, a worthy destination in itself. For Ship Island Lake, however, you turn left and drop to the popular camps around Birdbill and Gentian lakes. The trail goes west, between the two lakes, then climbs seven switchbacks to a pass, where you can look northwest to Airplane and Ship Island lakes, and north to 10,082-foot Mt. McGuire, the highest peak in the Crags. The very gently graded route now goes down three short switchbacks, then turns right and descends 15 irregularly spaced switchbacks to a signed junction above unseen Airplane Lake. A short side trail goes left to some good campsites on the northeast shore of this lovely lake.

Tip: *If you are feeling adventurous, you can scramble southwest from Airplane Lake to trailless Shoban and Sheepeater lakes, which have secluded camps and good fishing.*

To continue to Ship Island Lake, hike west for 1.5 miles down a woodsy valley with lots of beargrass to some excellent campsites at the southeast end of this long and very scenic lake. The lake is surrounded by high peaks, the most dramatic being a group of tall, jagged, granite spires above the northwest shore. The lake has a small island, but it takes a lot of imagination to envision this low, forested bit of land as a "ship."

Tip: *In mid-to-late September the huckleberry bushes near this lake's shoreline turn bright red, adding a touch of color to the scenery.*

A maintained trail continues about 0.5 mile along the lake's northeast shore past some scenic peninsulas and superb campsites. Beyond this point, adventurous hikers can follow a rough game trail all the way to the lake's outlet, then carefully scramble down steep granite slabs to an impressive waterfall on Ship Island Creek.

Warning: *The granite rock face beside this falls provides good footing when it is dry, but it can be dangerously slippery when wet.*

From the top of this waterfall there are excellent views to the bottom of the Middle Fork Salmon River Canyon, almost 5000 feet below.

Another excellent dayhike from your base camp at Wilson or Harbor lake goes south to Reflection Lake and a string of smaller lakes in the southern Bighorn Crags. To visit this area, start from the switchback on the south shore of Wilson Lake and go south on the official trail. This path contours briefly, then descends a steep hillside of granite slabs where the trail is marked by small cairns and your knees take a pounding on the unyielding rock. At the base of this section is a small campsite with unreliable water. You then go fairly steeply downhill, beside a tiny creek in a slot canyon on your left, to a junction with the Waterfall Trail and a nice, woodsy campsite beside Wilson Creek.

You turn right, hop over the creek, then gradually ascend a few lazy switchbacks to a junction with the trail to the Terrace Lakes (see the recommended dayhike to them). For Reflection Lake, you go straight and, 100 yards later, pass a short, unmarked spur trail to the right. This path leads to some nice campsites beside shallow Welcome Lake, which is surrounded by large meadows and has a good view of a high, unnamed mountain to the west.

Warning: In July, this lake hosts the worst concentrations of mosquitoes in the Bighorn Crags.

To continue to Reflection Lake, bear left at the junction with the Welcome Lake spur trail and climb a series of nine, long, well-graded switchbacks to the top of a ridge. Views from this ridge extend all the way east to the mountains of Montana. As you gradually round this ridge to the right (southwest) you also gain fine perspectives of Reflection Lake and its surrounding lake-dotted basin to the southwest.

To reach this basin, you go down two very long switchbacks to a pretty meadow, then wind downhill in the trees to a small creek. You hop over the creek, then, for the next few miles, wander up and down through this forested basin on a very gradual and extremely circuitous trail. You eventually pass a small, marshy pond filled with lily pads, then climb a bit more and finally reach deep Reflection Lake, where there are a couple of good campsites.

Beyond Reflection Lake the trail goes over a minor ridge and deadends at the marvelously named family grouping of Fawn, Doe, and Buck lakes. For even more scenery, leave the trail and explore the scenic basin surrounding Reflection Lake. Of the many off-trail lakes in this vicinity, the prettiest are Twin Cove, Turquoise, and Skyhigh, all of which can be reached via reasonable scrambles for those skilled with map and compass.

Yet another outstanding dayhike from your base camp at Harbor or Wilson lake goes to the Terrace Lakes, a string of four, jewel-like bodies of water on the west side of the Bighorn Crags divide. To reach them, take the route described above to the junction near Welcome Lake and turn right (west). This trail climbs in long switchbacks to Heart Lake, a curve-shaped pool in a scenic basin, then ascends two more long switchbacks to a narrow, rocky divide where you can see the Terrace Lakes strung out in the basin to the west.

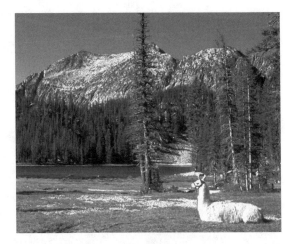

Llama at Airplane Lake camp

The recently rerouted trail makes one switchback, then a sloping traverse to another switchback, and reaches the first lake in this chain. All four of these deep lakes have fish and adequate campsites, but the final Terrace Lake is the largest and, arguably, the most scenic.

Tip: The campsites at these lakes provide more solitude than most others in the Bighorn Crags, because they are somewhat off the main trails.

If you still have some energy and are looking for a *really* secluded spot, try Barking Fox Lake. To reach it, hike south on the Waterfall Trail, which goes gradually downhill from the last Terrace Lake on its way to the Middle Fork Salmon River. After about 0.5 mile, you round the end of a ridge and come to the first switchback and a junction. Turn left here on an obvious but unsigned bootpath and follow it for about 0.1 mile to tiny, meadow-rimmed Barking Fox Lake. Once you've had your fill, return to your car the way you came.

POSSIBLE ITINERARY			
	Camp	**Miles**	**Elevation Gain**
Day 1	Harbor Lake	7	1200
Day 2	Harbor Lake (dayhike to Ship Island Lake)	11	2300
Day 3	Harbor Lake (dayhike to Buck and Reflection lakes)	13.5	2700
Day 4	Harbor Lake (dayhike to Terrace Lakes)	7.5	2200
Day 5	Out	7	600

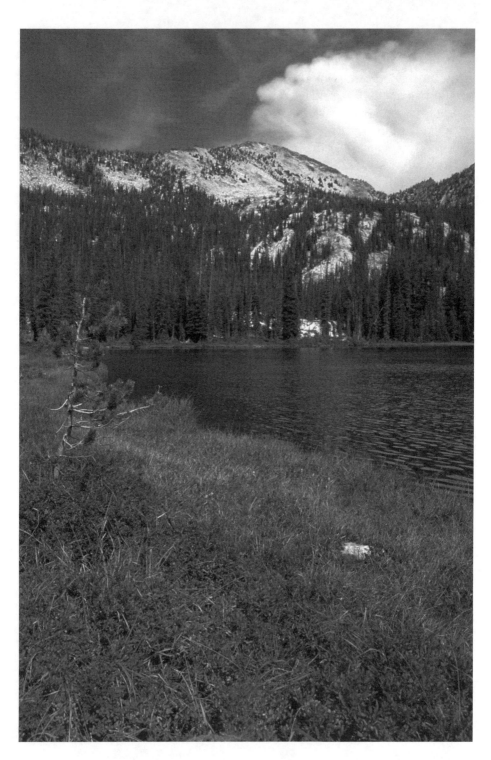

Lower Terrace Lake

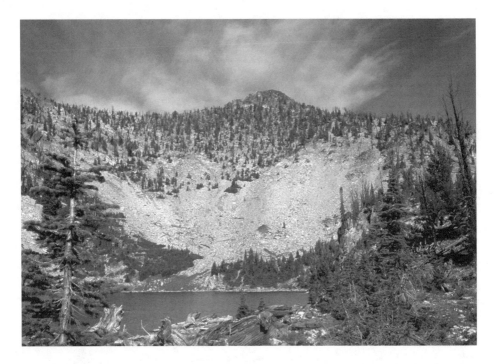

Turquoise Lake

VARIATIONS You can make a semi-loop out of this trip by returning from the southern Bighorn Crags on the Waterfall Trail, between the junction beside Wilson Creek, northeast of Welcome Lake, and the junction near Cathedral Rock.

If you want to extend this hike into an area with more solitude, then leave the main Bighorn Crags at the junction near Birdbill Lake and hike 7 miles northeast, past Big Clear Lake, to remote Goat Lake, in a scenic basin beneath Beehive Mountain.

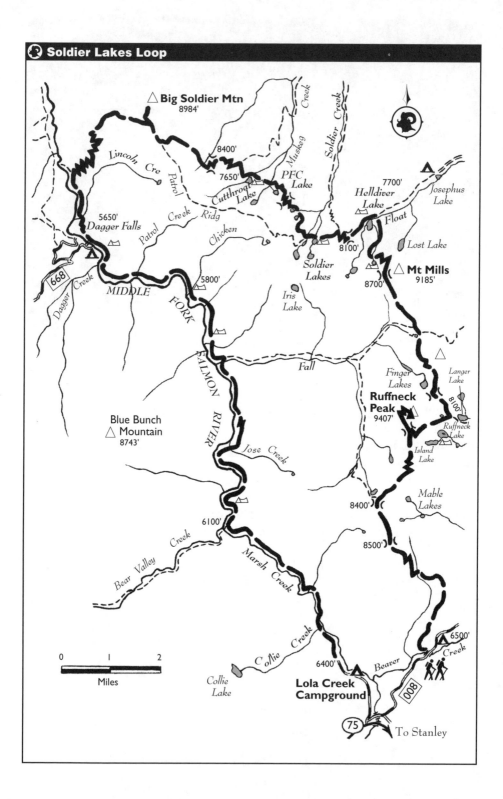

12 Soldier Lakes Loop

RATINGS (1–10)			MILES	ELEVATION GAIN	DAYS	SHUTTLE MILEAGE
Scenery	Solitude	Difficulty	40	7300	3-5	4
7	6	7	(42)	(8300)	(3-5)	

MAPS USGS - Cape Horn Lakes, Chinook Mountain SE, Greyhound Ridge SW.

USUALLY OPEN July to October.

BEST July to September.

PERMITS None.

RULES Maximum group size of 20 people and 20 stock animals.

CONTACT Yankee Fork Ranger District, (208) 838-3300; Middle Fork Ranger District, (208) 879-4101.

SPECIAL ATTRACTIONS Easy road access; lots of small but pretty lakes; fine views from lookouts.

PROBLEMS A few rattlesnakes in the Middle Fork Salmon River Canyon.

HOW TO GET THERE From Stanley, drive 18.4 miles northwest on State Highway 21 to a junction just after the highway makes a sweeping turn southwest. Turn right (north), following signs to the Seafoam Area and Lola Campground, and go just 30 yards to a junction. If you have two cars, take one of them 1.6 miles down the road to the left to the large trailhead parking lot for the Middle Fork Trail.

To reach the recommended starting point, turn right at the junction and drive 0.4 mile to a fork. Bear left, following signs to Seafoam, and proceed 1.7 miles on this smooth, oiled-gravel road to the trailhead parking lot immediately after a bridge over Beaver Creek. The trail starts next to the creek, just past a large livestock tie-off area.

INTRODUCTION This is a nice sampler of the huge Frank Church-River of No Return Wilderness, which avoids the long, bumpy drive on dirt and gravel roads that is required to reach most other trailheads in this wilderness. In addition to good road access, this loop gives you a taste of all the varied environments in the wilderness, including forested ridges, high mountain lakes, tall viewpoint peaks, and a deep river canyon. Although the loop does not take you to the *best* the wilderness has to offer of any of these features, it's a good choice if you want to get a bit of everything in one compact package.

DESCRIPTION The trail follows Beaver Creek downstream for about 100 yards, then curves to the right through a grassy meadow rimmed with lodgepole pines. The first 1.5 miles are nearly level and provide a nice warm-up that gets you into the swing of backpacking. You will need that warm-up, because the trail then makes a long climb that despite being moderately graded is quite tiring. The route takes you up a partly forested hillside, where the trees are almost all lodgepole pines, with just a few Douglas-firs sprinkled in for variety. Where the trees break at forest openings, the vegetation is dominated by grasses, sagebrush, and the blossoms of yarrow and lupine. Although the climb provides little in the way of views, you probably will see plenty of wildlife.

About 2.5 miles from the trailhead, you step over a small creek, then make a long climb up a steep hillside. Fortunately, the ascent includes a half dozen switchbacks, so the grade remains reasonable. Not quite 5 miles from the trailhead, you top out at a pass on a small ridge, from which you get your first view north to the rocky hump of 9407-foot Ruffneck Peak and several nearby mountains. The trail then makes a curving descent to a small meadow, losing about 150

Wildlife in the Wilderness

Commonly seen wildlife in the Frank Church-River of No Return Wilderness includes a large variety of birds, such as dark-eyed juncos, hairy woodpeckers, mountain chickadees, brown creepers, goshawks, and red-breasted nuthatches. You might also be lucky enough to see a pine marten, a member of the weasel family with a dark brown back and a tannish-orange belly. As their name implies, pine martens prefer coniferous forests, where they feed on small rodents such as chipmunks and voles.

feet, followed by an uneven climb to a junction at a pass on top of a second ridge.

Your trail angles to the right and makes a view-packed, slightly uphill traverse across the rocky southeast side of an unnamed knoll. The views here encompass some of Idaho's best-known and most spectacular areas, including much of the Sawtooth Range, the White Cloud and Boulder mountains, and the broad Sawtooth Valley. The views get even better when the traverse ends and two switchbacks take you up to a high ridgeline, where you can look down on several small, greenish-colored lakes in the forested basins on either side. You can also admire new vistas of the many rugged ridges and peaks in this corner of the wilderness, all of which are composed of whitish or light-tan rocks.

The trail follows the undulating ridgeline north on a course that heads directly for Ruffneck Peak. This distinctive summit is easy to recognize, because it has a gently sloping, forested west side and a much steeper, rocky east face. At a junction in a saddle just south of the peak, it's time to drop your pack and make an excellent side trip. So grab your camera and bear left on a trail that goes up three long switchbacks in a moderately steep, 0.5-mile climb to the summit of Ruffneck Peak. At the top is a green-roofed fire lookout, which despite being a bit run down is still staffed and has extensive views. In addition to the previously described views south toward the Sawtooth Valley, you can enjoy sweeping vistas north and west into the vast heart of Frank Church-River of No Return Wilderness and look east to the rugged peaks of the Yankee Fork country.

From the junction in the saddle south of Ruffneck Peak, the main trail goes right, descends two switchbacks, then makes a long downhill traverse across the rocky east face of the peak. Near the bottom of the traverse, you pass a tiny pond with a good view back up to Ruffneck Peak, then come to a junction not far above the shore of Langer Lake.

> **Tip:** It's worth your time to visit Langer Lake and to go south on obvious bootpaths to nearby Ruffneck and Island lakes, which are both backed by impressive rocky buttes and have good campsites.

You turn left at the junction and soon regain much of your previously lost elevation. The trail goes uphill at a moderately steep grade through partial forest to a pass on the northeast side of

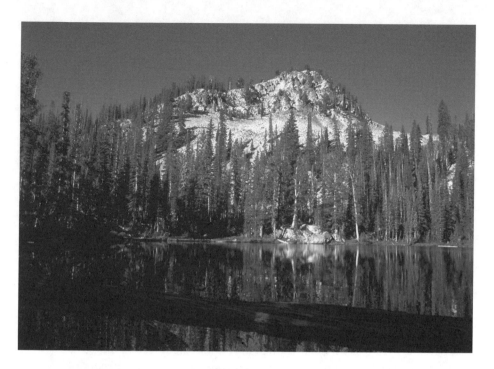

A small Soldier Lake east of Colonel Lake

Ruffneck Peak, from which you can see the lookout on the top of the peak and a deep, blue lake in the basin to the west.

The trail, which has been significantly rerouted from the one shown on the USGS and Forest Service wilderness maps, descends a bouldery slope on the northwest side of the pass to a murky, tea-colored pond. From there, you steeply lose about 200 feet on a rocky tread, then go up and down across the west flank of an unnamed peak. Eventually, you pass just above a good-sized spring and, 100 yards later, reach a junction with the trail to Seafoam Creek. You go straight and descend to a second junction, where you once again go straight and tackle the next climb, a 700-foot, 1.5-mile ascent to a high pass on the west shoulder of Mt. Mills. Most of this climb is evenly graded, but the final 150 feet are quite steep.

You make two moderately steep switchbacks down from the pass, then wind down to a scenic little lake near the base of a rockslide. There is an excellent campsite a little above the lake's northeast shore.

Tip: Although this lake is too shallow for fish, the campsite here is much more private than those at popular Helldiver Lake, ahead.

You hop over the lake's trickling outlet creek, then turn downstream and follow the intermittent flow through an open forest. After crossing the creek a second time, you descend to a log crossing of small Float Creek and almost immediately reach a junction. Turn left and soon come to lovely Helldiver Lake, which has several good campsites and nice views of Mt. Mills.

Warning: This lake is accessible by a short, 2-mile walk from a trailhead at Josephus Lake, so it is fairly crowded, especially on weekends.

From Helldiver Lake, the trail climbs 400 feet to a heavily forested divide, then goes down seven short switchbacks to a junction beside a marshy pond. You turn left and traverse a slope with about an even mix of subalpine-fir woods and talus fields to an excellent, but rather crowded campsite beside the first of the Soldier Lakes. For more privacy, take an unsigned angler's path to an isolated campsite on the lake's southwest shore.

This lovely subalpine pool will naturally generate an appetite to see more lakes and, happily, there is plenty nearby to satisfy that hunger. The most attractive destinations are the two largest and most scenic Soldier Lakes. Although these lakes are off trail, they can be reached by rugged angler's paths that head south and southwest from the first Soldier Lake. In addition to better scenery and good fishing, these lakes provide more privacy than the first lake.

The main trail goes less than 0.5 mile from the first lake to a junction shortly after you cross the cascading outlet of Colonel Lake, a narrow gem with nice campsites. Here you have a choice. If you're looking for views, then turn left and take the high route along Patrol Ridge, where you'll enjoy magnificent panoramas down into the Middle Fork Salmon River Canyon and over the rugged peaks and ridges of the southern part of Frank Church-River of No Return Wilderness. Since that trail passes no water or campsites, however, most people will prefer to follow the right fork. This rocky, up-and-down route soon goes past a pair of scenic, unnamed lakes, both of which sit below impressive rock outcroppings, then climbs three switchbacks to a low divide. From here, you descend past a pond at the base of a talus slope, then continue downhill to an obvious side trail that leads to P.F.C. Lake. This deep lake sits beneath the crags of Patrol Ridge and, despite having a lower rank than the other Soldier Lakes, is arguably the most spectacular member of the troop.

After P.F.C. Lake, the trail switchbacks down to a log over Muskeg Creek, then goes up and down for 0.5 mile to Cutthroat Lake. True to its name, this lake has some nice-sized cutthroat trout, as well as good campsites and excellent views of jagged Patrol Ridge. After crossing the outlet creek of Cutthroat Lake, the trail curves to the right and climbs fairly steeply to a junction. You turn left and go gradually uphill past a shallow pond, then switchback twice and go up a hillside with a mix of flower-filled meadows and open, high-elevation forests. The climb ends with five steep switchbacks that take you up to at saddle at the top of a spur ridge. The grade eases here as the trail goes up and down through a lovely alpine meadow below the main line of Patrol Ridge.

Tip: Fill your water bottles at one of the two small creeks in this meadow, because this is your last water source until Lincoln Creek, at the bottom of the Middle Fork Salmon River Canyon about 6 miles ahead.

Once the trail leaves the meadow, it climbs across the top of a huge talus field, then steeply ascends to a ridgetop junction amid a field of August-blooming lupines. This is where you reunite with the trail along Patrol Ridge.

You turn right, contour around the southwest side of a rounded knoll, then come to a rather faint junction. The continuation of your loop goes downhill to the left. The rewarding side trip to Big Soldier Mountain begins here.

To tackle the long descent to the bottom of the Middle Fork Salmon River Canyon, make a rather gentle downhill on a spur ridge, where whitebark pines thrive and alpine wildflowers such as pink heather brighten the slopes. The trail then gets very steep as it goes down through a shadeless burn area, quickly leaving the high-elevation environment in favor of mid-elevation grassy slopes and forests of Douglas-firs and lodgepole pines.

Warning: The trail here has lots of dangerously loose rocks and pebbles that require careful footing.

The steepness of the descent lessens briefly, then resumes on a relentless downhill that requires plenty of rest stops for sore knees and jammed toes. The difficulty is increased because the trail receives only sporadic maintenance, so there are usually significant

Big Soldier Mountain Side Trip

To visit Big Soldier Mountain, go straight at the junction on Patrol Ridge and walk 0.5 mile up the view-packed ridgeline to the mountain's abandoned lookout building. The historic old wooden building is interesting to look at, but the walkway around it is so deteriorated it's probably not safe to walk on. The view, however, remains unimpaired and is glorious. The enormity of Frank Church-River of No Return Wilderness spreads out to the north, west, and east, while to the southeast ·you can look over much of the rugged terrain that you have already tra-

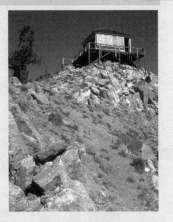

versed on this loop. To the southwest you can look 3400 feet down to the bottom of the Middle Fork Salmon River Canyon, your next destination.

amounts of deadfall along the way. Also, there are relatively few switchbacks to relieve the steep grade and most of those that do exist are concentrated near the bottom.

Tip: Going up this steep, waterless slope is extremely arduous, which explains why I recommend a counterclockwise loop.

The trail abruptly levels off on the flats near the Middle Fork Salmon River and comes to a junction. You turn left, following signs to Dagger Falls, and soon climb away from the crystal-clear river, then make a rough traverse of a talus-and-scree slope well above the water. A little over 1 mile from the junction, you cross small but very welcome Lincoln Creek, where you can finally refill your water bottles and soak your tired feet in cool water.

The trail now makes a series of short but very steep ups and downs for 0.5 mile to a junction beside a large bridge over the Middle Fork Salmon River just above rampaging Dagger Falls. You go straight, staying on the east side of the river, and soon pass an inviting riverside campsite.

The now-gentle trail spends most of the next few miles either crossing nearly level riverside benches peppered with lodgepole pines and quaking aspens, or contouring across dry slopes with lots of sagebrush and wildflowers. The two most showy flowers here

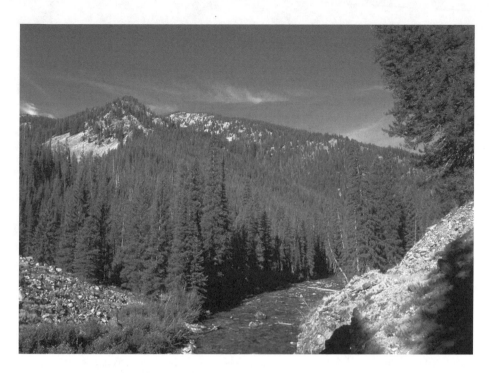

Along lower Marsh Creek

are balsamroot, which blooms yellow in June and early July, and rabbitbrush, which also blooms yellow, but not until mid-August and September. Just 2 miles above Dagger Falls the trail crosses small Patrol Creek on a wooden bridge, then does more gentle ups and downs as it follows the curves of the meandering river. About 2 miles past Patrol Creek is a bridge over Chicken Creek and a very good, large camp just past the bridge.

For the next few miles the trail crosses several small side creeks on bridges, climbs over rock outcroppings with canyon views, and goes across forested flats about 50 to 100 feet above the river. The hiking isn't spectacularly scenic, but it's easy and attractive, especially in the cool of the morning.

Warning: *On hot afternoons you will often be bothered by large horse flies, which follow you for miles and are almost impossible to swat.*

A little less than 1 mile from Chicken Creek is a good riverside campsite just below a well-preserved log cabin. As in so many similar old cabins, the doorway into this one is only about 4 feet high, which leaves you to wonder about the stature of all those early pioneers and miners.

You go a short distance into the major side canyon of Fall Creek and soon reach a junction with the Fall Creek Trail. Go straight, cross the creek on a large bridge, then return to your course above the river. The trail soon goes through a recent burn area, then makes a long climb through forests and up a talus slope to an overlook about 400 feet above the river. From this high point, you gradually descend back to river level, then go through a particularly dramatic section where the trail has been blasted into the rock just a few feet above the water.

Tip: Excellent fly-fishing opportunities abound in this area.

As the trail climbs away from the river, it passes two fine campsites, then climbs over a rocky overlook and comes to a fork.

The trail to the right goes up Bear Valley Creek, but your trail goes left and follows Marsh Creek. It is the merging of these two large creeks that forms the Middle Fork Salmon River. Above this point the canyon is wider and the slopes are less steep than it was further downstream, which allows Marsh Creek to meander lazily over gravel bars and through small meadows. The trail is also gentle, spending most of its time climbing gradually through forests and crossing small tributaries. About 3 miles from the Bear Valley Creek turnoff is a large bridge over Marsh Creek, after which you take a bridge over Collie Creek, then make a gentle, 1-mile walk to the Middle Fork trailhead. If you were not able to leave a car here, then you will either have to hitchhike or make the easy, 3.7-mile road walk back to your car.

POSSIBLE ITINERARY

	Camp	Miles	Elevation Gain
Day 1	Ruffneck Lake (with side trip to Ruffneck Peak Lookout)	9	3500
Day 2	Cutthroat Lake	10.5	1800
Day 3	Chicken Creek (with side trip to Big Soldier Mountain Lookout)	12	2100
Day 4	Out	10.5*	900*

* This excludes the 3.7-mile road walk to close the loop.

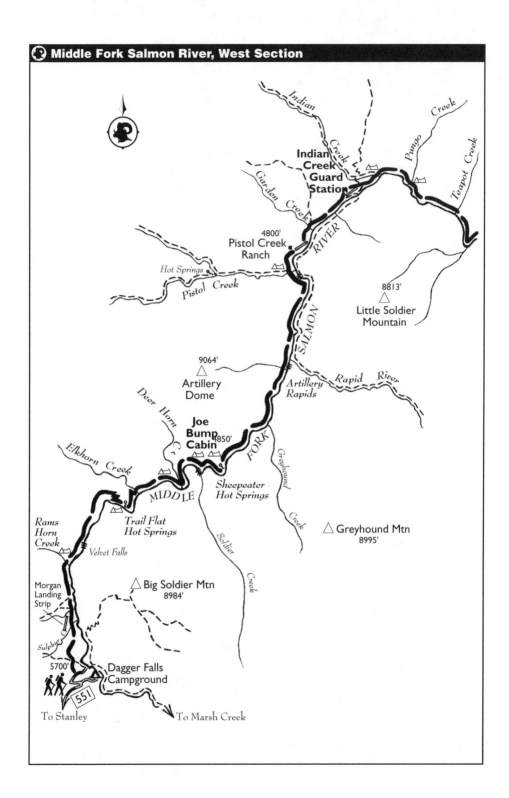

Indian Creek

Pungo Creek

Teapot Creek

Indian Creek Guard Station

Garden Creek

4800'
Pistol Creek Ranch

RIVER

Hot Springs

Pistol Creek

SALMON

8813'
△
Little Soldier Mountain

9064'
△
Artillery Dome

Rapid River

Artillery Rapids

Deer Horn Cr.

Joe Bump Cabin 4850'

Elkhorn Creek

FORK

Greyhound Creek

Sheepeater Hot Springs

MIDDLE

△ Greyhound Mtn
8995'

Rams Horn Creek

Trail Flat Hot Springs

Soldier Creek

Velvet Falls

Morgan Landing Strip

△ Big Soldier Mtn
8984'

Sulphur

5700'

Dagger Falls Campground

551

To Stanley

To Marsh Creek

13 Middle Fork Salmon River

RATINGS (1–10)			MILES	ELEVATION GAIN	DAYS	SHUTTLE MILEAGE
Scenery	Solitude	Difficulty	67	4200	6-8	89
7	6	6				

MAP USFS - Frank Church-River of No Return Wilderness - South Half.

USUALLY OPEN May to November.

BEST September and October.

PERMITS None.

RULES Maximum group size of 20 people and 20 stock animals; all fires within 0.25 mile of the Middle Fork Salmon River must be in fire pans; you are required to pack out all human waste from a corridor 0.25 mile on either side of the Middle Fork Salmon River (easy enough for boaters, but not realistic for backpackers).

CONTACT Middle Fork Ranger District, (208) 879-4101.

SPECIAL ATTRACTIONS Whitewater rafters to watch; terrific canyon scenery; numerous excellent hot springs.

PROBLEMS Long car shuttle; rattlesnakes; hot summer temperatures; rough road access to the eastern trailhead.

HOW TO GET THERE To reach the recommended exit point, drive 13.2 miles northeast of Stanley on State Highway 75 to a junction just before a bridge over Yankee Fork Salmon River. Turn left (north) onto Yankee Fork Road and drive 8.7 miles on this paved (then good gravel) road past an interesting assortment of mining equipment and exhibits to a fork just after the bridge over Jordan Creek. Turn left onto Forest Road 172 and drive 4.4 miles to an unsigned fork. Go straight (uphill) and proceed 16.0 miles over scenic Loon Creek Summit and down to the Loon Creek Guard Station. Continue 0.7

mile past the guard station to a fork, where you bear right and drive the final 4.4 miles to the good-sized parking lot for the Loon Creek trailhead at the end of the road.

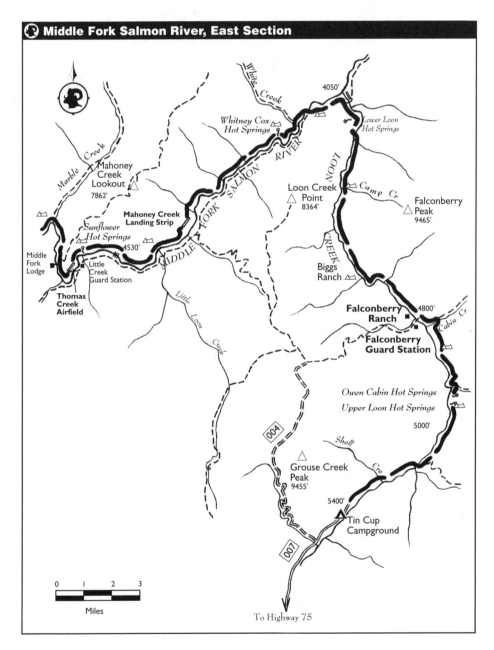

Middle Fork Salmon River, East Section

White Creek

4050'

Whitney Cox Hot Springs

Lower Loon Hot Springs

Marble Creek

Mahoney Creek Lookout
7862'

Loon Creek Point
8364'

Camp Cr

Falconberry Peak
9465'

Mahoney Creek Landing Strip

MIDDLE FORK SALMON RIVER

LOON CREEK

Sunflower Hot Springs
4530'

Middle Fork Lodge

Little Creek Guard Station

Biggs Ranch

Thomas Creek Airfield

Little Loon Creek

Falconberry Ranch
4800'

Cabin Cr

Falconberry Guard Station

Owen Cabin Hot Springs

Upper Loon Hot Springs

5000'

004

Shell Cr

Grouse Creek Peak
9455'

5400'

Tin Cup Campground

007

0 1 2 3
Miles

To Highway 75

Warning: The road from the unsigned fork before Loon Creek Summit all the way to the trailhead is rocky and quite rough. Passenger cars can make it, but you must drive slowly and carefully.

To reach the starting point, return to Stanley and drive 21.8 miles northwest on State Highway 21 to a junction just before Banner Creek Campground. Turn right, following signs to Cascade and Bruce Meadows, and drive 9.6 miles on gravel Forest Road 198 to a prominent junction. Turn right, following signs to Dagger Falls and Boundary Creek Campground, and proceed 9.8 miles to a fork, where you bear left and go 0.6 mile to the large trailhead parking area.

INTRODUCTION Over countless millions of years the Middle Fork Salmon River has been busy carving a spectacular, deep canyon into the granite rock of central Idaho. From the top of the canyon looking down, this massive gash in the Earth is impressive, but it pales in comparison to the awe-inspiring views enjoyed by visitors at the bottom of the canyon who look up at towering walls that rise thousands of feet above the remarkably clear river. One hundred years ago, most of the people who saw these views were trappers and prospectors who established remote homesteads in the canyon. In recent years, the vast majority of visitors have been rafters and kayakers, who are drawn not only to the scenery but also to the challenge of one of America's most legendary whitewater rivers.

Hikers are only beginning to discover the wonders of this canyon, but their numbers are sure to increase as word gets out about the excellent scenery and the canyon's other great attribute, its hot springs. The trail passes numerous excellent hot springs, ranging

 Timing is Everything

Although it isn't a desert, the Middle Fork Salmon River Canyon is noticeably hotter and drier than the surrounding mountains. As a result, the area's spring wildflowers soon wilt under the relentless sun and trees are scarce in the lower reaches of the canyon. During July and August it can be oppressively hot in the canyon, so this trip is best done in the "shoulder" seasons of spring and fall. Spring is beautiful, but in May and June the river is often crowded with boaters. On the other hand, September is idyllic, because most of the boaters have gone home for the season and you will generally have the canyon and its hot springs all to yourself.

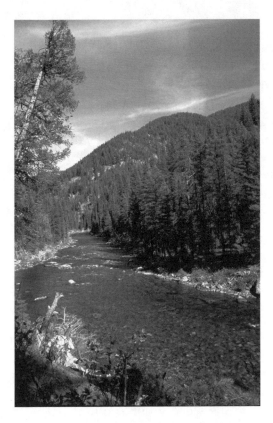

Middle Fork Salmon River Creek

from tiny seeps to huge springs where large volumes of hot water come bubbling out of the ground. Almost all of the springs provide excellent bathing opportunities, which makes the Middle Fork Salmon River Trail perhaps the best extended backpacking trip for hot-springs lovers in the American West.

Tip: *The Middle Fork Salmon River is managed as a catch-and-release fishery; single barbless hooks are required and no live bait is allowed.*

DESCRIPTION You set off on a wide and dusty trail in an old burn area that is now covered with a regrowing forest of lodgepole pines, a few quaking aspens, and some Douglas-firs. The trail goes up and over a minor ridge, then drops to a junction with a trail to the Boundary Creek boat launch. Just 100 yards later, you meet lightly-used Trail #215, which angles left. The main trail goes straight at both junctions and wanders up and down through forest well away from the Middle Fork Salmon River for the next 1.5 miles. As the trail slowly gets closer to the river, it skirts the privately owned Morgan Landing Strip, which is prominently labeled with several NO TRESPASSING signs.

At the end of the private property, the trail crosses good-sized Sulphur Creek on a sturdy, metal bridge, then comes to an easy rock-hop crossing of small Prospector Creek and a junction with the trail of the same name. You bear right and walk a short distance to a second junction, this time with a lower spur of the Prospector Creek Trail. You go straight, cross a forested shelf about 30 feet above the river, then hop over a tiny creek a little before the wooden bridge over Rams Horn Creek. There is a good (but very small) campsite about 50 yards past this bridge.

Downstream from Rams Horn Creek the trail closely follows the lovely, green-tinted river as it cascades merrily along past rock outcroppings, steep hillsides, and talus slopes. The trail goes around these obstacles with numerous ups and downs on the forested hillside above the river. Individually, these sections aren't particularly difficult, but together they add up to a fair amount of elevation gain and loss. A prominent rocky ridge soon forces the river to make a wide turn to the southeast. The trail follows suit, although in a more rugged fashion than the river, as you are forced to climb over a high rock outcropping, then switchback down a rough talus slope back to river level. Just before the river turns north, there is an excellent, large camp area above Trail Flat Hot Springs, an inviting group of pools at the edge of a rocky gravel bar by the river. Like all of the hot springs in this canyon, this is a great place to spend some time soaking sore muscles and enjoying the scenery. Bring a swimsuit if you're concerned about modesty.

The trail climbs gradually away from the hot springs, then makes three downhill switchbacks to a bridge over rushing Elkhorn Creek. After this, it's more up and down near the river as the canyon becomes increasingly narrow with steeper walls and lots of rough talus slopes. In addition to getting steeper, the terrain also gets drier, so the forests are less dense and consist almost entirely of Douglas-firs and ponderosa pines. You pass a nice campsite where the winding river makes a sharp bend to the right, and, shortly thereafter, rock-hop over tiny Deer Horn Creek. More curves in the river then lead you through a particularly steep-walled part of the canyon to several good campsites on a lightly forested flat near small Joe Bump Cabin.

Just 100 yards beyond Joe Bump Cabin is a tiny wooden sign pointing to Soldier Creek, soon followed by the gravesite of Elmer "Set-Trigger" Purcell, whose headstone informs you that he was a prospector and trapper who died in 1936. About 1 mile later is the excellent camp area

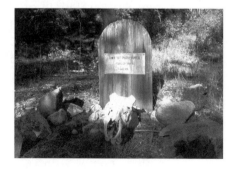

Grave of Elmer Purcell

beside the wonderfully warm waters of large Sheepeater Hot Springs. The "rotten egg" smell from sulfur in the water makes camping here a bit aromatic, but the opportunity to luxuriate in such warm water more than makes up for the unpleasant odor.

Tip: Since Sheepeater Hot Springs is often crowded, especially during the boating season, you might prefer to set up your tent at a good boater's camp about 0.5 mile past the hot springs.

For the next several miles the trail crosses increasingly barren and brushy slopes that are exposed to the sun and can be very hot in midsummer. Fortunately, although you rarely have easy access to the river, there are several small side creeks along the way, so finding water is never a problem. The next significant landmark is the narrow canyon of Rapid River, which joins the Middle Fork just below Artillery Rapids. A trail comes down that canyon, but instead of crossing the Middle Fork here, that trail follows the river downstream, paralleling your route for the next several miles. The trail on your side of the river spends most of those miles traveling through a partial burn area, where many of the trees are either dead or fire-scarred, so shade is at a premium.

About 3 miles past Rapid River you take a large bridge over Pistol Creek to a junction near several good campsites on the creek's north bank.

Tip: For a nice side trip, turn left and hike 3 miles up the Pistol Creek Trail to a secluded hot springs.

The main trail goes right and soon takes you past the log buildings and private landing strip at Pistol Creek Ranch. Several confusing jeep roads cross the trail near the ranch. To find the correct route, walk straight through the ranch property to the northeast end of the landing strip, where a sign saying INDIAN CREEK WAY marks the resumption of the trail.

The gentle trail now takes you to a rock-hop crossing of small Garden Creek and, immediately thereafter, a junction with the trail to Big Baldy Lookout. You bear slightly right (staying level) and closely follow the river for 1 mile to a fork just before the Indian Creek Landing Strip. The main trail goes right, but if you want to visit the Indian Creek Guard Station, bear left and soon reach the isolated station, with its quaint log buildings, friendly personnel, and piped water.

The trail goes through the guard station property, then continues to the end of the landing strip, where you reunite with the trail that bypassed the station. Another 0.5 mile of gentle walking takes you to a good campsite just before the bridge over large Indian Creek. Immediately after this bridge you turn right at an unsigned junction and walk 1 mile to small Pungo Creek, which has several good campsites on either side of the hop-over crossing.

The Middle Fork Salmon River Trail now wanders merrily along at an gentle grade, slowly going down into an ever-drier and increasingly barren landscape. The only trees here are a few ponderosa pines, while twisted big sagebrush grows

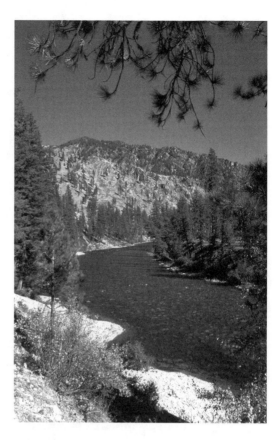

Middle Fork Salmon River near Pistol Creek

near the water, and the higher canyon slopes are covered with nothing but bunchgrass and rocks. In early summer these slopes support wildflowers such as balsamroot and skyrocket gilia, but by later in the season they dry out and take on a golden-brown appearance.

About 1.5 miles from Pungo Creek you hop over splashing Teapot Creek, then go around a sharp bend in the river to a large and excellent campsite on a ponderosa-pine-dotted flat just above the river. Shortly after this campsite is a junction, where you turn right and immediately cross a bridge over Marble Creek. The trail then heads south, following another of the river's many twists and turns, to a junction with a faint trail that goes uphill and left on its way to Mahoney Creek Lookout. Immediately after this junction is a large bridge across the Middle Fork Salmon River that provides access to Middle Fork Lodge. This modern guest lodge comes complete with several cozy bungalows, a manicured lawn, and views from the porch that will take your breath away.

The bridge is open only to lodge guests, so others must stay on the east side of the river and follow a narrow road around a bend in the river to the Thomas Creek Airfield. The trail goes around the right side of the landing strip and soon comes to a split. To the right is Trail 001.1, which crosses the Middle Fork on a bridge, passes Little Creek Guard Station, then follows the south bank of the river for 10 miles before rejoining the main trail at White Creek Bridge. You go left on Trail 001, staying on the north side of the river, pass the end of the landing strip, and soon come to a good campsite beside a picturesque log cabin. Just 150 yards beyond this cabin is Sunflower Hot Springs, which bubbles out of the ground and invites an extended stay.

The canyon is largely devoid of trees below this point, so summer temperatures can be oppressive on these sun-exposed slopes. A more comfortable season is late August and September, when temperatures start to fall and the blossoms of sunflowers and rabbitbrush add spots of yellow to the increasingly desert-like environment.

Warning: Rattlesnakes are very common in this dry environment, so watch your step.

About 2.5 miles from Sunflower Hot Springs is a good campsite directly opposite where Little Loon Creek joins the Middle Fork. After this, you make a moderate, 300-foot ascent to the Mahoney Creek Landing Strip, which rarely receives many airborne visitors. About halfway down the airstrip the Middle Fork Salmon River Trail angles left at an unsigned but obvious foot trail.

The canyon scenery remains impressive as the trail goes over barren slopes, crosses a few trickling side creeks, and passes high overlooks with outstanding views of the river and canyon. Almost 5 miles from the Mahoney Creek Landing Strip is your next chance to ease tired muscles at small Whitney Cox Hot Springs. Here you'll find a couple of rock-lined pools and several good campsites about 300 yards past the springs.

Not far from Whitney Cox Hot Springs you hop over small White Creek and immediately bear right at an unsigned junction. The trail then goes over White Creek Bridge – a large, metal span across the Middle Fork Salmon River – and reunites with Trail 001.1. You turn left at this junction and walk downstream across a north-facing slope that supports many more trees than the drier environment on the other side of the canyon. You soon pass a good campsite, then continue another mile to the mouth of Loon Creek Canyon.

The trail goes several hundred yards up Loon Creek Canyon to a junction, where the Middle Fork Salmon River Trail turns left and immediately crosses a bridge over boisterous Loon Creek. Your route goes straight and heads up the narrow, partly forested canyon for 0.5 mile to Lower Loon Hot Springs. These springs are the perfect temperature for hours of soaking, but you'll have to pull yourself out of the water well before sunset, because there is no flat ground nearby for camping. A little over 1 mile

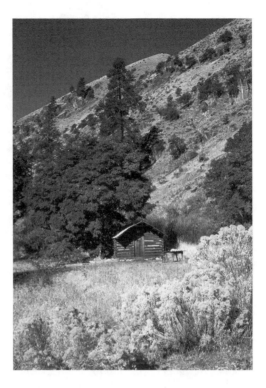

Cabin at Sunflower Hot Springs

upstream from Lower Loon Hot Springs the trail takes a bridge over Loon Creek, then begins an uneven, 2-mile ascent to a nice campsite on a small flat near the hop-over crossing of Camp Creek.

Above Camp Creek, the trail goes through a dramatic gorge, where cascading Loon Creek has carved a deep chasm with towering rock pinnacles and impressively tall cliffs. After the canyon widens, you make an easy, 1-mile walk, then pass a grassy flat on the opposite side of the creek that was once the site of Biggs Ranch. The only thing left of this old homestead is the dilapidated remains of a log cabin, but the grassy flat still has plenty of good places to camp, if you don't mind making the cold, calf-deep ford of Loon Creek to get there.

About 1 mile above Biggs Ranch the trail goes through another dramatic, cliff-walled chasm, then the canyon widens once again and you walk across a hillside overlooking a mile-long grassy flat that is on the southwest side of Loon Creek. At the southeast end of

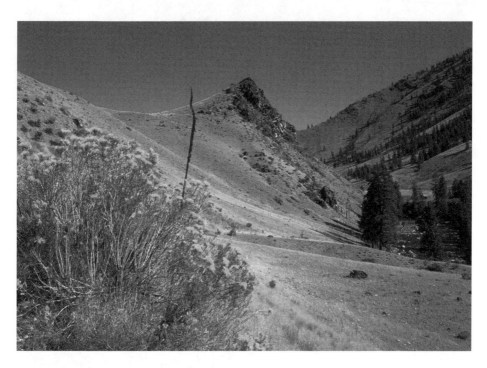

Middle Fork Salmon River near Mahoney Creek

this flat you pass an old landing strip and recently abandoned Falconberry Ranch. Soon you come to a junction with a trail that takes a bridge over the creek to Falconberry Guard Station.

You go straight, staying on the northeast side of Loon Creek, and go a short way up the brushy canyon of Cabin Creek to an unsigned and easy-to-miss junction. The main trail seems to go straight along the north bank of Cabin Creek, but you turn right and make a rock-hop crossing of the creek. The trail then crosses a grassy flat, passes above an excellent campsite (complete with a seemingly out-of-place picnic table), and climbs steadily to a bridge over Rock Creek. It's another 2 miles from here to a junction just before the bridge over large Warm Springs Creek. You bear right, cross the bridge, and, 300 yards later, reach Owen Cabin Hot Springs, which is followed less than 0.5 mile later by Upper Loon Hot Springs, the last of the hot springs you pass on this trip. The best campsites and bathing pools are near an old log cabin at Upper Loon Hot Springs.

About 1.5 miles beyond Upper Loon Hot Springs is a junction with the Cottonwood Trail, where you go straight and soon cross a bridge over Loon Creek. The trail's final 3 miles take you gently to an easy hop over Shell Creek, followed by a passage through an impressive, steep-walled gorge to the Loon Creek trailhead.

POSSIBLE ITINERARY

	Camp	Miles	Elevation Gain
Day 1	Trail Flat Hot Springs	8	600
Day 2	Pistol Creek	13	700
Day 3	Sunflower Hot Springs	13	300
Day 4	Whitney Cox Hot Springs	9	400
Day 5	Camp Creek (after a long soak in Lower Loon Hot Springs)	7	600
Day 6	Upper Loon Hot Springs	12	1100
Day 7	Out	5	500

VARIATIONS This trip lends itself nicely to several imaginative variations. If you have only one car, consider turning this into a huge 120-mile loop by hiking back from the Loon Creek trailhead via Loon Creek Guard Station, Trail-Beaver Divide, Beaver Creek, and Marsh Creek. This loop involves some road walking and adds three full days of hiking to an already long trip, but the scenery is good throughout.

Another option is to skip the Loon Creek Trail and keep hiking downstream on the Middle Fork Salmon River Trail to the Big Creek Pack Bridge. From there, you can either hike out via the 26-mile trail up Big Creek (see Trip 30) or climb the Waterfall Trail and exit via the Bighorn Crags (see Trip 11).

For a *really* exciting alternative, arrange to have a bush plane fly you out of the canyon from a remote landing strip. The Taylor Landing Field, about 5 miles up the Big Creek Trail, is probably the most logical choice.

Finally, you can prearrange to have a rafting party pick you up partway down the canyon and make an exciting float trip to a take-out on the main Salmon River.

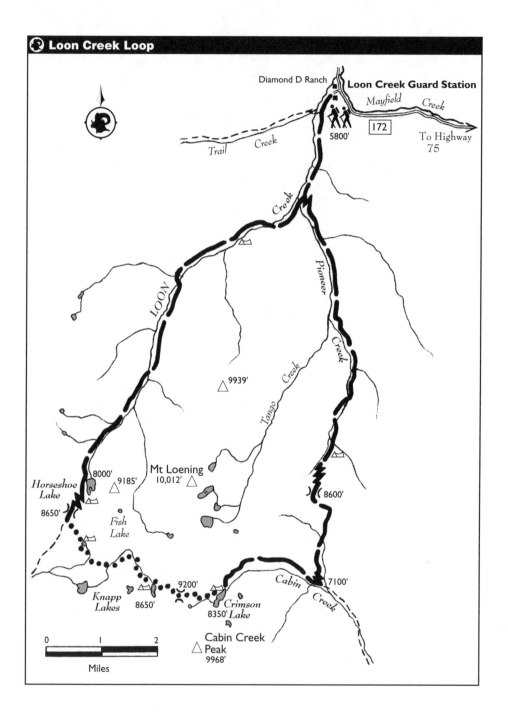

Loon Creek Loop

Diamond D Ranch
Loon Creek Guard Station
Mayfield Creek
172
5800'
To Highway 75

Trail Creek

Creek

LOON

Pioneer Creek

△ 9939'

Tango Creek

Mt Loening
10,012' △

8000'
△ 9185'
Horseshoe Lake
8650'

Fish Lake

8600'

Knapp Lakes
8650'
9200'
Crimson Lake
8350'

Cabin Creek
7100'

Cabin Creek Peak
△ 9968'

0   1   2
Miles

14 Loon Creek Loop

RATINGS (1–10)			MILES	ELEVATION GAIN	DAYS	SHUTTLE MILEAGE
Scenery	Solitude	Difficulty	27	6100	3-4	N/A
8	8	7				

MAPS USGS - Casto, Knapp Lakes, Mt. Jordan, Pinyon Peak.

USUALLY OPEN July to October.

BEST Mid-July to September.

PERMITS None.

RULES Maximum group size of 20 people and 20 stock animals.

CONTACT Middle Fork Ranger District, (208) 879-4101.

SPECIAL ATTRACTIONS Solitude; colorful mountain scenery.

PROBLEMS Fairly long and moderately difficult cross-county section; rough road access; rough trail through burn area.

HOW TO GET THERE From Stanley, drive 13.2 miles northeast on State Highway 75 to a junction just before a bridge over Yankee Fork Salmon River. Turn left (north) on Yankee Fork Road and drive 8.7 miles on this paved (then good gravel) road past an interesting assortment of mining equipment and exhibits to a junction just after the bridge over Jordan Creek. Turn left onto Forest Road 172 and drive 4.4 miles to an unsigned fork. Go straight (uphill) and proceed 16.0 miles on this narrow road as it climbs over scenic Loon Creek Summit and down to the Loon Creek Guard Station. The road from the unsigned fork before Loon Creek Summit all the way to the guard station is rocky and quite rough. Passenger cars can make it, but you must drive slowly and carefully. There is no parking allowed inside the guard station property, so park near the fence outside.

INTRODUCTION Although mining roads separate the protected headwaters of Loon Creek from the rest of Frank Church-River of No

Return Wilderness, this small appendage contains some of the most scenic terrain in the entire wilderness. The jagged peaks here rise above 10,000 feet and are made up of a stunningly beautiful collage of gray, white, and reddish rocks. When you add this colorful geology to the area's cirque lakes, clear streams, and flower-covered meadows, you have a great place to go for a backpacking vacation.

DESCRIPTION To locate the unsigned trailhead, walk past the guard station and go through a gate at the southwest corner of the property. You then walk diagonally 250 yards to the southwest corner of a livestock enclosure, where there is another gate and a trail register box. The trail starts on the other side of the gate. The trail is in good shape and easy to follow, although it's a bit dusty due to horse use out of the adjacent Diamond D Ranch.

The trail goes about 500 yards across a nearly level plain, only populated by scattered sagebrush and a few Douglas-firs and lodgepole pines, to the signed junction with the Beaver-Trail Creek Trail. You go straight, briefly descend to the willow thickets beside Loon Creek, then climb back up to the plain and pass through a mile-wide burn area. After this, the trail does some small ups and downs to a fork and the start of your loop.

The trip is easier to navigate if you go counterclockwise, so bear right at the fork and immediately drop to Pioneer Creek. The trail crosses the creek on a log, then heads southwest up the scenic canyon of Loon Creek, following that stream for about 0.5 mile before coming to a knee-deep ford of the cold, clear water. You climb the opposite bank, then walk through a partially burned area where deadfall is often a problem, but which affords your first good views of the steep and rugged walls on either side of the canyon.

> **Warning:** About 0.5 mile past the ford the trail appears to cross the creek, but this is actually just a side path that goes to a campsite on the other side of the creek.

Your trail remains on the northwest side of the stream and slowly climbs under the shade of a relatively dense Douglas-fir forest. The trees block any decent views, but the trail is never tedious and you stand a good chance of seeing elk. After 2 miles, you rock-hop an unnamed tributary creek, then ford the main stem of now-somewhat-smaller Loon Creek.

The canyon soon curves to the south and the forest cover changes to relatively small and widely-spaced lodgepole pines, which allows you to catch tantalizing glimpses of the surrounding mountains. Those glimpses become unobstructed views about 1 mile later, when you cross an avalanche chute with lots of wildflowers and stunted quaking aspen trees. You reenter forest, then come to another crossing of Loon Creek, this time on a convenient log. After this crossing, the trail climbs at a noticeably steeper grade for 1 mile to where a tall, pointed mountain splits the canyon in two.

Tip: The Forest Service wilderness map shows a primitive trail going up the left fork of the canyon to tiny Fish Lake, but there is no sign of this trail on the ground.

You stick with the main branch of cascading Loon Creek and climb fairly steeply for 2 miles until the grade levels off not far before large and shallow Horseshoe Lake. This scenic pool has pleasing views of a rocky ridge to the east and some good campsites near its southwest shore.

From Horseshoe Lake, the trail winds steeply uphill for about 1 mile to 8650-foot Loon-Knapp Divide, from where there are wonderful views northeast over the Horseshoe Lake Basin. On the other

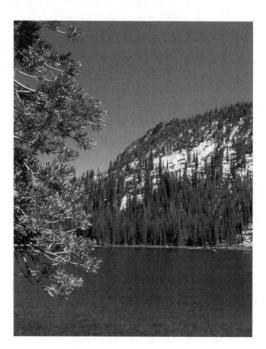

Horseshoe Lake

side of the divide you descend for 300 yards to a small, waterless gully, then look for a sketchy path that angles uphill to the left. This is where you leave the trail and rely on your skills with map and compass. The open forests make the walking relatively easy, but trees block the views, so navigation can be difficult. Occasional game paths help keep you on course and you may even find a few cut logs indicating sections of a long-abandoned trail. Nonetheless, novice hikers should not attempt this section without experienced leadership. On the other hand, veteran route-finders will find it fairly easy and enjoyable. Of necessity, the description here is rather general, but those who are good at cross-country travel need only a general description.

The best route goes southeast gradually losing elevation for about 0.5 mile to a lovely, meadow-rimmed lake with a good campsite on its northwest shore. You then follow this lake's seasonal outlet creek to the second of two shallow ponds, veer left, and climb over a tiny divide. From here, you angle downhill to a small creek, then turn upstream and follow this intermittent creek past a series of very scenic ponds and small lakes that are collectively called the Knapp Lakes. At the top of the drainage you come to the highest of the Knapp Lakes, a long, kidney-shaped pool that sits beneath a craggy ridge of light gray and tan rock. There is plenty of flat ground around this lake, so you have a choice of very good campsites with almost guaranteed solitude. Unfortunately, there are no fish in any of these lakes.

The cross-country travel to this point has been relatively easy, but now you must make a short, very steep, and quite difficult climb. Your goal is a low point in the ridge due east of the lake at the top of a long, tannish-orange scree slope. The easiest way to reach the pass is to avoid the loose rock of the scree slope and head instead up a hillside just north of the pass, where the soil is stabilized by scattered whitebark pines. It's only a 600-foot climb, but plan on taking at least 1 hour to accomplish this steep ascent.

> **Warning:** Do not go over the inviting lower pass south of the lake. It leads to a small, unnamed lake that is worth visiting, but there is no reasonable access beyond that to Crimson Lake.

Things get a lot easier at the pass, as you descend a moderately steep slope of rocks and alpine wildflowers, where you soon catch sight of Crimson Lake in the basin to the east. The route down goes past a scenic tarn in an area of highly colorful rocks, then follows this tarn's dry outlet creek all the way down to large and irregularly shaped Crimson Lake.

The name of this lake obviously does not refer to the color of the water, but it *does* accurately describe the bright reddish-orange rocks and mountains that surround the lake. In addition to views of these colorful summits, the lake features fine reflections of the gray spires of Cabin Creek Peak to the south. There is an excellent campsite on the west shore of Crimson Lake, and another one at the

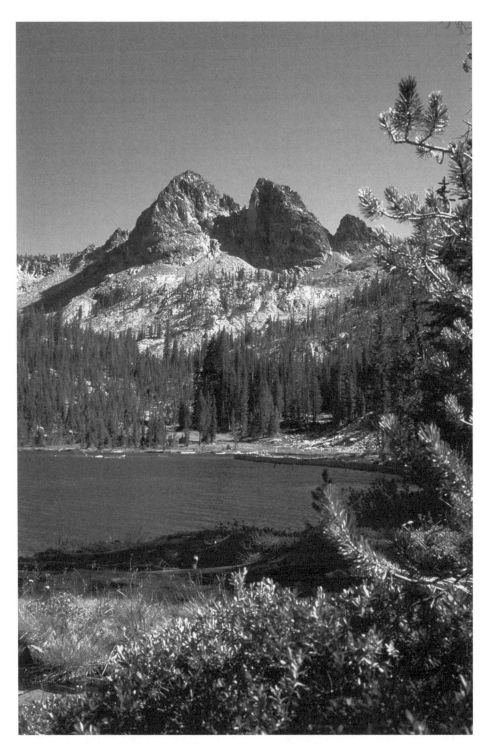

Cabin Creek Peak over Crimson Lake

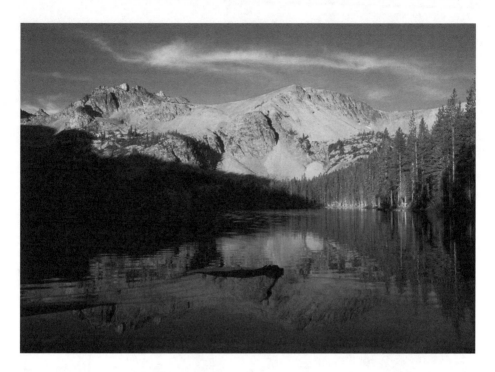

Early morning calm at Crimson Lake

northeast end near the lake's outlet. The continuation of your loop leaves as a maintained foot trail from just above the outlet creek.

> **Tip:** *If you have the time, spend an extra day or two scrambling up to several, scenic, trailless lakes in the colorful cirque basins south and north of Crimson Lake.*

It's all downhill from Crimson Lake, both figuratively in terms of scenery, and, for a while at least, literally in elevation. The trail first goes over a rounded knoll, then drops very steeply down a rocky hillside. At the bottom of the hill, you hop over a small side creek in a gully, then do a little more steep downhill until the trail's grade eases off. For the next 1.5 miles the trail goes through open forests, crosses avalanche chutes, and travels over rockslides in the canyon of Cabin Creek. Most of the way is downhill, but there are also a few short, uphill pitches to keep things interesting. About 2.5 miles from Crimson Lake is a junction with the Pioneer-Cabin Creek Trail.

You turn left, make two uphill switchbacks, then begin a long, stair-step ascent where short, nearly level stretches are interspersed with moderate-to-steep uphills. This pattern continues all the way to a high pass, where there is a good view to the south of the striking, red-topped pyramid of Red Mountain.

From this pass, the trail steeply descends six switchbacks, then goes more moderately downhill through subalpine-fir forests to a good campsite just before you hop over a clear tributary of Pioneer Creek. About 0.5 mile below this camp, you cross Pioneer Creek on a log, then closely parallel the creek downstream for several hundred yards to a flood-damaged area where part of the creek flows directly down the bed of the trail. It's very easy to lose the route here, so you'll probably have to bushwhack. To relocate the trail, look on the opposite (east) bank about 200 yards downstream from the start of the flooded area.

The next mile is a relatively straightforward downhill walk through the forest above Pioneer Creek until the trail is obscured again, this time by both flood damage and by a fire scar with large amounts of blowdown. You'll have to fight your way through this short section to where the trail becomes obvious again.

Below this point, the trail makes a rocky, sometimes steep descent through intermittent burn areas. The rugged and difficult trail is constantly in need of maintenance and should probably be rebuilt, but at least it's mostly downhill. Along the way you pass the impressive side canyon of Tango Creek, coming in from the southwest, then do another 2 miles of rough and, frankly, not-much-fun hiking to a rock-and-log crossing of a moderate-sized side creek. You close the loop by contouring for about 0.5 mile, then descending four switchbacks to the reunion with the Loon Creek Trail. To finish the trip, turn right and retrace the 2 miles back to the Loon Creek Guard Station.

POSSIBLE ITINERARY

	Camp	Miles	Elevation Gain
Day 1	Horseshoe Lake	8	2300
Day 2	Crimson Lake (most of this distance is cross-country)	6	1800
Day 3	Out	13	2000

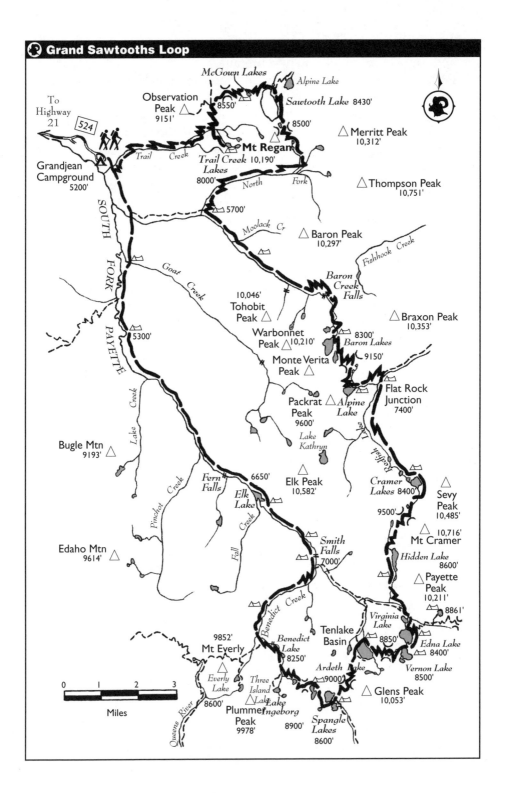

Grand Sawtooths Loop

McGown Lakes

Alpine Lake

Observation
Peak △
9151'

8550'

Sawtooth Lake 8430'

△ Merritt Peak
10,312'

To
Highway
21

524

8500'

Trail   Creek

Mt Regan
Trail Creek 10,190'
Lakes
8000'

△ Thompson Peak
10,751'

Grandjean
Campground
5200'

North   Fork

5700'

Moolack Cr

△ Baron Peak
10,297'

Fishhook Creek

SOUTH

Goat   Creek

10,046'
Tohobit
Peak △

Baron
Creek
Falls

FORK

△ Braxon Peak
10,353'

Warbonnet
Peak △10,210'

8300'
Baron Lakes

PAYETTE

5300'

Monte Verita
Peak △

9150'

Flat Rock
Junction
7400'

Lake   Creek

Packrat △
Peak
9600'

Alpine
Lake

Bugle Mtn △
9193'

Lake
Kathryn

Pinchot   Creek

Fern
Falls

6650'

Elk Peak
10,582'

Cramer
Lakes 8400'

△
Sevy
Peak
10,485'

Elk
Lake

9500'

Edaho Mtn △
9614'

Fall   Creek

Smith
Falls
7000'

△ 10,716'
Mt Cramer

Hidden Lake
8600'

△ Payette
Peak
10,211'

8861'

Virginia
Lake

9852'
Mt Everly

Benedict   Creek

Benedict
Lake
8250'

Tenlake
Basin

8850'

Edna Lake
8400'

0   1   2   3

Miles

Everly
Lake

Three
Island
Lake

Ardeth Lake
9000'

Vernon Lake
8500'

8600'
Plummer
Peak
9978'

Lake
Ingeborg
8900'

Spangle
Lakes
8600'

△ Glens Peak
10,053'

Queens River

15 Grand Sawtooths Loop

RATINGS (1–10)			MILES	ELEVATION GAIN	DAYS	SHUTTLE MILEAGE
Scenery	Solitude	Difficulty	63	12,200	5-9	N/A
9	3	6	(65)	(12,700)	(6-10)	

MAP Earthwalk Press - Hiking Map and Guide: Sawtooth Wilderness.

USUALLY OPEN July to October.

BEST Mid-July to mid-August.

PERMITS Yes (free at the trailhead).

RULES Maximum group size of 12 people and 14 stock animals; all fires must be in fire pans or on fire blankets; no fires allowed at Sawtooth Lake or Alpine Lake; dogs must be on leash from July 1 to Labor Day.

CONTACT Sawtooth National Recreation Area, (208) 727-5000.

SPECIAL ATTRACTIONS Gorgeous ridgetop wildflower gardens; outstanding mountain scenery; good fishing.

PROBLEMS Relatively crowded in places.

HOW TO GET THERE From Boise, take exit 57 off Interstate 84 and drive northeast on the Ponderosa Pine Scenic Highway (State Highway 21) to a junction near milepost 93 just before a large snow gate used to close the highway in winter. Turn right onto Forest Road 524, following signs to Sawtooth Lodge, and drive 8.0 miles on this good gravel road to the signed backpacker trailhead near Grandjean Campground. The trail starts next to a large signboard and permit station at the east end of the parking area. A parking pass is required at this trailhead. You can buy them from any ranger station and most outdoor stores in Boise or Stanley.

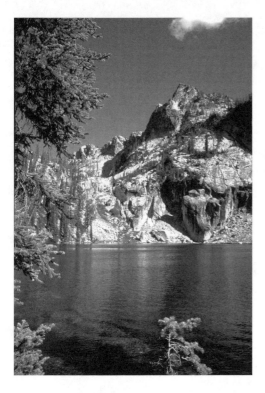

Lower Trail Creek Lake

INTRODUCTION The Sawtooth Mountains contain some of Idaho's most beautiful scenery. Although the famous views from the road are superb, if you really want to appreciate all that this range has to offer you have to leave your car and hit the trails. This long and magnificent loop takes you to many of the range's most outstanding locations and is the premier backpacking tour of the Sawtooth Mountains. It is possible to shorten this hike at several points, but since every part of the trip is glorious, it would be a shame to miss even one mile of this circuit.

DESCRIPTION You start by walking 80 yards to an unsigned junction with a horse trail, which begins at a separate equestrian trailhead and loading ramp. You turn right, walk 120 yards to a bridge over Trail Creek, then come to a junction and the start of your loop.

Hikers who want to shorten this trip should go straight on the South Fork Payette River Trail for 1.5 miles, turn left onto the Baron Creek Trail, then climb 2 miles to a junction with the North Baron Creek Trail. Unfortunately, this shortcut misses some of the finest scenery in the Sawtooth Mountains, so if you have the time, it's better to take the longer route up Trail Creek.

The Trail Creek Trail goes left at the junction and switchbacks up a dry slope of grasses and low brush punctuated with a few scattered ponderosa pines, quaking aspens, and Douglas-firs. As the elevation increases the ponderosas are replaced by lodgepole pines, and these are later joined by Engelmann spruces and subalpine firs. About 1 mile from the South Payette junction, you cross Trail Creek on a narrow log, then gradually ascend an open, south-facing slope, which supports a huge population of unusually large crickets. The steady uphill continues for the next few miles, but several dozen short switchbacks ensure that the grade is never overly steep. Along the way you make three easy crossings of Trail Creek, each time using rickety logs to keep your feet dry. About 4 miles, and 2400 feet up, from the trailhead is a junction with a trail to the spectacular Trail Creek Lakes, a highly recommended side trip.

To visit these lakes, turn right at the junction, contour briefly, then hop across a small creek. From here, the rocky trail climbs steeply for a little less than 1 mile to the shore of Lower Trail Creek Lake, a picturesque mountain pool tucked in a steep-walled cirque at the base of a craggy granite peak. The lake is surrounded by scenic talus slopes and open subalpine-fir forests, with several good-to-excellent campsites near the lake's outlet and more good camps along the north shore.

Although the maintained trail ends at this lake, it's worth the effort to visit an equally scenic lake in the upper basin. To make this steep cross-country scramble, climb the slopes east of the lower lake and follow the terrain as it naturally leads you to a trickling creek and a small pond just below Upper Trail Creek Lake.

To resume the loop, return to the Trail Creek Trail, turn right, then ascend a series of short, well-graded switchbacks to a four-way junction in a little notch.

Tip: For a fun side trip to a fine viewpoint, turn sharply left and climb 1 mile to the top of aptly named Observation Peak, where views extend over the entire northern Sawtooth Mountains.

You bear right at the four-way junction and climb several gentle switchbacks through open, high-elevation forests to the top of a small ridge. From there, you descend about 150 feet, climb over a second low ridge, then enter the lovely basin holding several bodies of water that are collectively called the McGown Lakes. After passing several ponds, you reach the last lake, which is the largest, the most scenic, and has the best campsites of the McGown chain.

Tip: The campsites here are much less crowded than those at popular Sawtooth Lake, which is just over the next pass.

From the final McGown Lake, you make a relatively easy ascent to a high pass just below timberline, where you gain your first view of Sawtooth Lake, the largest alpine lake in the range. No single superlative could do justice to this spectacular lake, but it's safe to say that it is one of the most beautiful and photogenic alpine lakes in North America. Several towering granite peaks rim the deep, azure waters, but Mt. Regan, which rises directly above the lake's southwest shore, commands the spotlight. The route down to the lake starts with a gradual traverse across a view-packed, rocky slope north of the lake. The trail then descends two fairly long switchbacks and enters an open forest of twisted whitebark pines that frame countless great views. Finally, the path winds down to the lake's outlet, where there are some badly overused campsites that really should be avoided, and a junction with a trail that is heavily used by dayhikers coming in from the east.

You go straight, hop across the lake's bubbling outlet creek, then climb to a rocky overlook. For the next mile, the trail goes up and down across an open talus slope above the east shore of Sawtooth Lake. At the southeast end of the lake you climb through a low, grassy saddle and pass a small lake below the steep slopes of Mt. Regan. You then go over a rocky pass and descend a bouldery slope to a tiny basin holding two small, unnamed lakes with mediocre campsites.

Now you begin the long descent into the canyon of North Fork Baron Creek. The downhill starts by wandering through the forest beside the new-born stream, then makes a dozen short, woodsy switchbacks to an easy crossing of the creek, which cascades down a steep slope on your right. After splashing across the creek, you descend a hot, south-facing slope that is covered with sagebrush and stunted trees kept small by frequent avalanches. At the bottom of this deep canyon, you enter a shadeless 1990s burn area and wind down to a crossing of North Fork Baron Creek. The trail crosses the creek on logs and rocks, then descends several switchbacks through unburned forests and grasslands to a junction with the Baron Creek Trail. This is where you meet the shortcut route from the South Fork Payette River Trail mentioned above.

> **Tip:** If you are looking for a campsite, there are two excellent ones about 70 yards to the right, where the trail fords North Fork Baron Creek, and a good one about 50 yards to the left, in the shade of some large fir trees.

To continue the trip, turn left and hike up the canyon of Baron Creek on a gradual trail that travels through open forests and grassy meadows. Not quite 1.5 miles from the North Fork junction, you

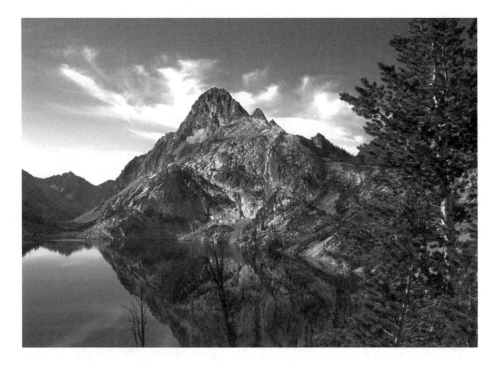

Mt. Regan over Sawtooth Lake

hop over small Moolack Creek, then walk another 0.5 mile to an excellent campsite beside Baron Creek. In early-to-mid July the open, parklike meadows near this campsite support a wealth of wildflowers, especially spiraea, which features aromatic clusters of tiny pink blossoms. Above this campsite you climb gently past Tohobit Falls, which cascade down the canyon wall on your right, and soon reach your first good view of veil-like Baron Creek Falls, dropping over a cliff in front of you.

Near the base of Baron Creek Falls, the trail curves left and begins a series of 22 tiring switchbacks. The first few switchbacks are under the shade of a pleasant forest, then the next several go up a brushy slope covered with ceanothus bushes. The remainder of the switchbacks ascend a sun-baked talus slope, where your frequent rest stops are rewarded with excellent views across the canyon to the jagged granite spires of Tohobit and Warbonnet peaks.

Tip: *Try to tackle this long climb in the cool and shade of the morning.*

A final set of four short switchbacks takes you around the base of a bulbous granite knob near the top of Baron Creek Falls. The trail then levels off and goes gently up the scenic upper valley of Baron Creek. It is interesting to observe how the granitic rocks in this upper valley display the smooth, polished surface typical of rocks shaped by the movement of glaciers. Apparently the ice did not reach the lower valley, because the rocks down there do not show this aspect.

You cross the creek on a bridge, then wind uphill for about 0.5 mile to a second crossing, this time on narrow logs. Immediately on the other side of the creek is a superb campsite.

Tip: If you prefer solitude for the night, stay at this scenic campsite, because it is less crowded than the camps at Baron Lake.

Above the campsite you climb several gentle switchbacks, then cross the creek a final time on a bridge and come to the shores of dramatic Baron Lake. Views are superb across this deep lake, especially of towering Warbonnet and Monte Verita peaks, with their numerous granite spires and cliffs. There are several large but usually rather crowded camps near the outlet of the lake.

The trail crosses a log jam at the outlet of Baron Lake, follows the east shore for a short distance, then veers away from the lake and climbs past good viewpoints to smaller Upper Baron Lake. Although very attractive, this pool will seem rather tame in comparison to the spectacular lower lake, and the single campsite here is less inviting as the ones at Baron Lake. After skirting the east shore of Upper Baron Lake, the trail climbs 30 short, moderately steep switchbacks to the top of 9150-foot Baron Divide, where a rest stop and lots of gawking are in order.

Views from this grandstand extend over much of the central and eastern Sawtooth Mountains. To the west and northwest are Monte Verita Peak, the Baron Lakes, and the valley you just ascended. To the east is the serrated eastern edge of the Sawtooths, an impressive display of craggy, pink granite, which looks very different from this angle than it does from the better-known Redfish Lake side, because the foreground here isn't flat with lakes, but a sea of jagged peaks and valleys. Below you to the south is the basin holding teardrop-shaped Alpine Lake, your next destination. Beyond that, to the southeast, is the upper canyon of Redfish Lake Creek.

After taking in all of these views, put your pack back on and descend a few moderate switchbacks to a small pond. Then the trail loops down to a larger, more attractive lake in a partly forested basin.

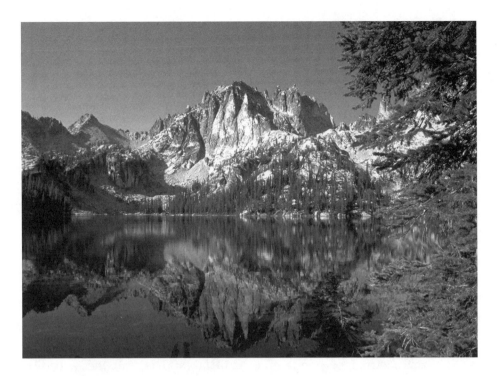

Monte Verita Peak over Baron Lake

Tip: *The campsites near this lake are usually less crowded than those at Alpine Lake.*

You descend rather steeply along this lake's outlet creek, cross it twice, then climb briefly to the top of a side ridge. Three long switchbacks then take you down to the shore of popular Alpine Lake, with its overused campsites and decent views of Packrat Peak to the west.

Beyond Alpine Lake the heavily used trail traverses a hillside above the lake's outlet stream to a nice viewpoint of Redfish Lake Creek canyon. The trail then descends a series of irregularly spaced switchbacks on a forest- and brush-covered slope to Flat Rock Junction, where you meet the trail from Redfish Lake. This trail is the source of all those white-shorts-and-tennis-shoe-wearing tourists you've been meeting, most of whom were dropped off by boat at the southwest end of busy Redfish Lake.

You turn right and soon come to a flat, sloping rock shelf over which the creek slides and which gave Flat Rock Junction its name. You cross 25-foot-wide Redfish Lake Creek here. In early summer this can be a tricky ford, but there is usually a logjam about 100 yards downstream from the ford, where you can cross more safely. On the opposite side of the crossing is a good campsite.

The path goes gently upstream, generally staying close to the sparkling creek, which gives anglers many opportunities to pull out their trusty fly rods. After 0.5 mile, the trail works away from the water and goes up the hillside to the east. You gain about 800 feet in the next mile, then level off and contour across a partly forested slope. A final short climb takes you to Lower Cramer Lake, the smallest of three beautiful alpine lakes tucked beneath the cliffs and talus slopes of Sevy Peak to the east and an unnamed pinnacle to the west. All three lakes have campsites and host lots of hungry brook trout. The best campsites are beside the two lower lakes, but Upper Cramer Lake is the largest and most scenic of the group.

Above Upper Cramer Lake the lightly used trail makes a sweeping ascent of a partly forested hillside, which provides ever-improving views of the Cramer Lakes and Redfish Lake Creek canyon. After about 0.5 mile, you hop across a little brook, then walk uphill past a string of ponds and small lakes. The trail then steadily ascends an open, rocky slope to a high pass.

Warning: *Snow often lingers on this slope until midsummer.*

From the pass, you go downhill across a talus slope above a narrow, rock-rimmed lake, then reenter forest and make a moderately steep descent to a crossing of a small creek just above the west shore of large and narrow Hidden Lake. The trail threads its way between the lake's water and steep slopes to the west all the way to the southern tip of Hidden Lake, where you'll find a couple of adequate campsites. Below the lake you pass a long, narrow pool on the outlet creek, then switchback through forest down to a junction immediately after you hop over the splashing headwaters of the South Fork Payette River.

For the most direct route back to your car, turn right and walk 18 miles down the South Fork Payette River Trail to the trailhead. Having come this far, however, don't miss the string of beautiful high lakes along an alternate trail. This route adds 9 miles and 1800 feet of elevation gain to your trip, but it compensates with lots of outstanding scenery. So, unless you are really pressed for time, turn left at the junction and slowly climb beside the "river" (nothing more than a small creek at this point) to kidney-shaped Virginia

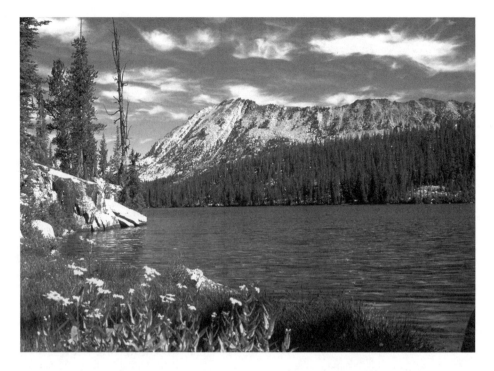

Payette Peak over Edna Lake

Lake. This forest-rimmed pool is backed by a rounded, granite butte and has good views to the north of the peaks around Hidden Lake.

Beyond Virginia Lake you ascend six quick switchbacks to 200-acre Edna Lake, which is surrounded by open, subalpine-fir forests and has outstanding views of almost nearby peak. The best campsites are near the south end of the lake, although they tend to be popular with equestrians, so expect dusty trails, horse apples, and the usual distinctive aroma. The trail follows the northeast shore of Edna Lake, then switchbacks away from the water to a junction.

The trail to the left heads east over view-packed Sand Mountain Pass, then drops to popular Toxaway Lake (see Trip 17).

> *Tip*: A side trip up this trail to either Sand Mountain Pass or the closer, off-trail goal of Lake 8861 is well worth your time. Lake 8861 is especially scenic, because it sits in a beautiful, grassy basin below the long ridge of Payette Peak. The few campsites at this lake are generally deserted and very scenic.

Back at the junction above Edna Lake, the main trail bears right, makes a few gentle ups and downs, passes a fine campsite at the

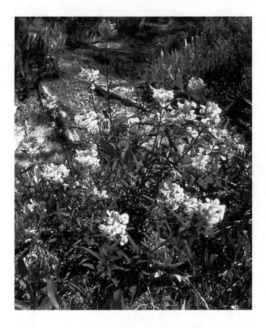

Lousewort

south end of Edna Lake, then comes to lovely Vernon Lake. This lake has good campsites along its gently sloping shores and stunning views of a triangle-shaped peak to the south.

Tip: For more solitude, try visiting the small, off-trail lake just southeast of Vernon Lake.

The trail crosses Vernon Lake's outlet creek, goes around the lake's northwest shore, then makes a series of nine uphill switchbacks. This climb takes you over a sparsely forested slope with lots of granite ledges, where you can enjoy a quick rest stop and fine views. Just before reaching a pass, you level off beside a small, island-dotted lake in a basin surrounded by subalpine firs, whitebark pines, and various alpine wildflowers.

Tip: Despite its relatively small size, this lake supports a population of good-sized brook trout. Since this lake gets less fishing pressure than nearby waters, you stand a better-than-average chance of catching dinner.

The best views at the pass are to the west over the forested Tenlake Basin, in the middle of which is large Ardeth Lake. Dominating the skyline are the rocky heights and permanent snowfields of 10,053-foot Glens Peak to the southwest. To reach Ardeth Lake, you descend 16 moderately steep switchbacks through open forest to the sparkling waters of this popular lake. There are several large and exceptionally scenic camps near the outlet and along the west shore, but be prepared to compete with horse parties for a spot.

The trail follows the northeast shore of Ardeth Lake, crosses its outlet creek, then goes another few hundred yards to a junction with a trail that goes down Tenlake Creek to the South Fork Payette River. If you want to cut the trip short, turn right at this junction and hike the 17 relatively easy miles back to your car.

Warning: In early summer you may have to exit this way, because the trail over Tenlake Divide can remain snowbound until August. Ask other hikers for the latest information.

Assuming that snow is not a concern, bear left at the junction and walk to the southwest corner of Ardeth Lake, where the trail splits. The trail to the left goes down to a spacious horse camp beside the lake's inlet. You bear right (uphill) and gradually climb through lodgepole-pine and subalpine-fir woods to a spring-fed, marshy pond with a fine view of Glens Peak. You then make eight fairly long switchbacks up a talus slope to 9000-foot Tenlake Divide. Views from this windy location are superb, especially north over the Tenlake Basin to colorful Payette Peak, Elk Peak, and Mt. Cramer.

On the south side of the divide the gently graded trail snakes down three lazy switchbacks through open woods to the shores of deep Spangle Lake. Camping here is limited, because the shoreline is quite steep and flat sites are hard to find, but there are a couple of good campsites near the northeast shore. At the southeast end of the lake is a junction with a trail down the Middle Fork Boise River. You turn right, then cross the narrow strip of rocky land between Spangle Lake and much shallower Little Spangle Lake. The small stream connecting these two lakes is easily crossed on a log jam.

You climb six short switchbacks on the hillside west of Spangle Lake and come to a very attractive little lake tucked beneath a jagged line of cliffs. The trail just barely touches this little gem, then turns right and gradually ascends a few curving switchbacks to a high, flat ridgeline with exceptional views back to Spangle Lake and Glens Peak. Also of interest here, if you can pry your eyes away from the view, are several huge boulders that provide good, up-close examples of the pink-tinted granite for which the Sawtooths are famous. A short distance past the viewpoint is deep and very scenic Lake Ingeborg, which is backed by a line of serrated peaks that are impressively streaked with snow in early summer. There are several good campsites at this lake, which allow you to spend an enjoyable evening snagging some of the lake's large brook and cut-throat trout. Sunsets are often spectacular at this lake.

The trail goes through an almost imperceptible pass west of Lake Ingeborg, then descends a long switchback to a small marshy tarn. From here, you drop to the north shore of very scenic Rockslide Lake, which gets its name from a large rockslide that drops into the lake's south shore. The trail then descends seven switchbacks, crosses the lake's outlet stream below a small, sliding waterfall, and comes to a shallow, unnamed lake, which is little more than a marsh by late summer.

Warning: Mosquitoes can be a problem here before mid-August.

At the north end of this lake/marsh is an unsigned junction with the 0.5-mile, deadend trail to Three Island Lake, which sits in a lovely basin to the south and features three tiny, rocky islets that gave the lake its name.

The main trail goes straight (north), crosses Benedict Creek on a footlog, then gradually descends a couple of long switchbacks to the grassy shores of Benedict Lake, the last of the string of high lakes along this loop. The fine views up to an unnamed, rounded mountain to the northeast will make you sorry to leave the high country behind. But leave it behind you must, so reluctantly continue down Benedict Creek past a shallow pond. You then make a series of very gradual downhill switchbacks beside a sloping waterfall to a junction with a trail that heads left (southwest) to the Queens River drainage (See Trip 16).

Tip: Hikers who have not yet had their fill of beautiful mountain lakes can bear left, climb 1 mile to a junction, then turn left to visit remote Everly and Plummer lakes. The farther of these two is only about 2 miles from the Benedict Creek Trail.

To continue on the loop, bear right at the junction and descend a short distance to log crossings of two forks of Benedict Creek. Over the next 3.5 miles the well-graded trail follows the relatively gentle canyon of Benedict Creek as that stream slowly curves northeast. The hiking is easy and pleasant, as the gentle trail passes through a series of avalanche meadows with fine views of numerous jagged peaks and plenty of wildflowers. About 1 mile from the Queens River junction is a nice creekside campsite on the right. After this, the views are blocked by trees until you get near the bottom of the canyon, where the trail makes six irregularly spaced switchbacks to a small burn area and a junction with the shortcut trail down from Virginia and Ardeth lakes.

You veer left, now on the dusty South Fork Payette River Trail, and soon pass roaring Smith Falls, a sliding cascade that is well worth a lengthy visit or even an overnight stay at the campsite just upstream.

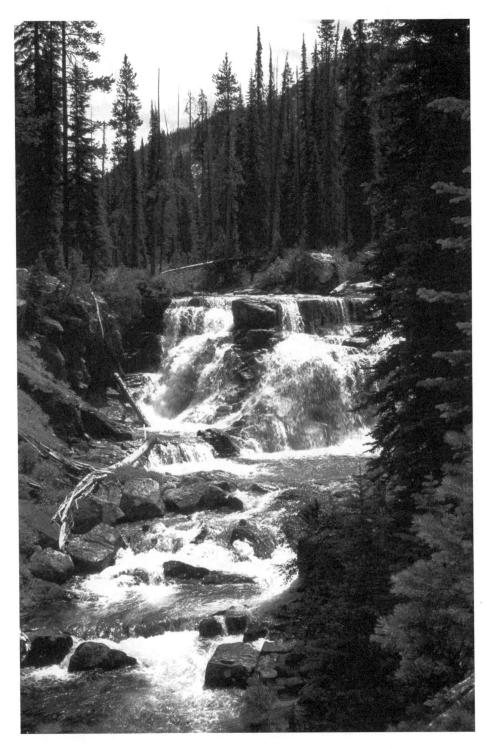

Smith Falls

Below this highlight, the trail follows the meandering stream for a little less than 1 mile to a ford of the cold, 50-foot-wide river. There is a decent campsite on the downstream side of this ford.

Warning: In early summer this crossing is can be dangerous. Wading shoes and a sturdy walking stick are recommended.

Below the ford it's a straightforward river walk all the way back to your car. The trail is never steep, so the miles are easy and go by quickly. The early miles are under the shade of stately Douglas-fir trees with an interesting mix of greenery in the understory. On your left, the river remains hidden in boggy areas bordered by nearly impenetrable tangles of willows and Engelmann spruces. These obstacles generally preclude access to the water, which is a shame, because the South Fork Payette River is one of Idaho's premier fly-fishing streams. The clear waters support both rainbow and brook trout, with opportunities for catching big fish improving as the stream gets larger down the canyon.

A little over 1.5 miles from the ford, you reach shallow and swampy Elk Lake. Except for around the campsite near its southeast end, this lake's shoreline is hidden by a tangle of spruce trees. About 1 mile past the lake you pass above a rocky gulch where the river tumbles through a narrow channel. This cascade goes by the name of Fern Falls, although calling it a "waterfall" seems overly generous.

After this "falls" the trail descends a few gentle switchbacks, then simply wanders down the widening canyon. There aren't any high peaks in view so the scenery is rather subdued, but there are woodsy ridges visible on both sides of the canyon and the nearby forests are continuously attractive. The trail is brushy in places, but the hiking is easy as you gradually descend through a mix of forests, avalanche chutes, and rockslides. The river is more accessible now, and anglers will be eager to avail themselves of every opportunity.

About 5 miles below Fern Falls the forest cover changes to lodgepole and ponderosa pines, with many of the open parklands and meadows so closely associated with the latter species. The temperatures can get uncomfortably warm at these lower elevations during the height of summer, especially since the ponderosas provide relatively little shade, but because the trail stays level or goes gradually downhill the heat is tolerable.

The river slowly curves north and splits, with the various branches wandering in wide curves and eddies through increasingly open meadows. Near the largest of these you come to the site of Deadman Cabin, where you'll find several good campsites amid the pines with easy access to the river. Even hikers who aren't interested in casting a line should take the time to explore the meadow's fine views, wildflowers, and beaver activity.

At the north end of the meadow, the often-dusty trail passes a large spring, then travels through an area of dead and burned timber to a junction with a trail that heads west up the canyon of Mink Creek. You go straight, staying on the South Fork Payette River Trail, and continue another mile to the bridgeless crossing of Goat Creek. There is a good campsite just north of the easy ford. After a refreshing rest stop here, you hike through burned forests for about 1.5 miles to a calf-deep ford of Baron Creek.

Tip: You can't see it from the ford, but there is a log across the creek about 50 yards upstream from the official crossing.

A short distance past this crossing is a junction with the Baron Creek Trail. To finish the hike, you go straight and make a gentle, 1.5-mile, up-and-down stroll back to the bridge over Trail Creek and the Grandjean trailhead.

POSSIBLE ITINERARY

	Camp	Miles	Elevation Gain
Day 1	Trail Creek Lake	5	3100
Day 2	North Fork Baron Creek	12	1500
Day 3	Baron Lake	7	2700
Day 4	Cramer Lake	7	1900
Day 5	Lake Ingeborg	12	2800
Day 6	Elk Lake	11	200
Day 7	Out	11	500

VARIATIONS If you have only two or three days for your hike, then just do the scenic loop as follows: go up Trail Creek to Sawtooth Lake, down North Fork Baron Creek, and out via Baron Creek and South Fork Payette River. Alternatively, for a five or six-day hike, skip the trail up Trail Creek and meet the loop instead where the trails along Baron Creek and North Fork Baron Creek meet.

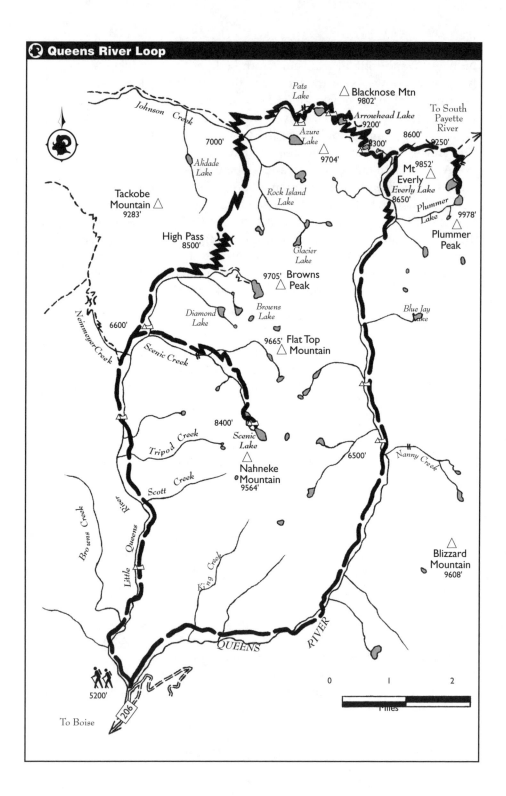

Queens River Loop

Blacknose Mtn
9802'

Pats
Lake

Johnson Creek

To South
Payette
River

Arrowhead Lake
9200'

Azure
Lake

7000'

8600'

8300'

9250'

Alidade
Lake

9704'

Mt 9852'
Everly
Everly Lake
8650'

Tackobe
Mountain
9283'

Rock Island
Lake

Plummer
Lake

9978'

Plummer
Peak

High Pass
8500'

Glacier
Lake

9705' Browns
Peak

Neimeyer Creek

6600'

Diamond
Lake

Browns
Lake

Blue Jay
Lake

Scenic Creek

9665' Flat Top
Mountain

Tripod Creek

8400'

Scenic
Lake

Scott Creek

Nahneke
Mountain
9564'

6500'

Nanny Creek

Browns Creek River

Little Queens River

King Creek

Blizzard
Mountain
9608'

QUEENS RIVER

5200'

206

To Boise

0   1   2

Miles

16 Queens River Loop

RATINGS (1–10)			MILES	ELEVATION GAIN	DAYS	SHUTTLE MILEAGE
Scenery	Solitude	Difficulty	31	5800	3-4	N/A
9	7	5	(42)	(9100)	(4-5)	

MAP Earthwalk Press - Hiking Map and Guide: Sawtooth Wilderness.

USUALLY OPEN July to October.

BEST Mid-July to mid-August.

PERMITS Yes (free at the trailhead).

RULES Maximum group size of 12 people and 14 stock animals; all fires must be in fire pans or on fire blankets; no fires allowed at Scenic Lake; dogs must be on leash from July 1 to Labor Day.

CONTACT Sawtooth National Recreation Area, (208) 727-5000.

SPECIAL ATTRACTIONS Fine mountain scenery; good lake and stream fishing; dramatic canyon scenery along the lower Queens River.

PROBLEMS Some burn areas with dense regrowing shrubbery, wear long pants.

HOW TO GET THERE From Boise, take exit 57 off Interstate 84 and drive 12.9 miles northeast on the Ponderosa Pine Scenic Highway (State Highway 21) to a junction immediately after a large bridge over an arm of Lucky Peak Reservoir. Turn right, following signs to Atlanta and Arrowrock Dam, and drive 4 miles to the end of the pavement, then settle in for a long, rather tedious drive on a bumpy gravel road. Stay on this road, which become Forest Road 268, for 63.3 miles up the canyon of the Middle Fork Boise River to a junction directly across from Queens River Campground. Turn left onto narrow Forest Road 206 and follow it for 1.8 miles to a fork, where you veer left and drive a final 0.3 mile to the Queens River trailhead.

There are a few campsites at the trailhead should you arrive late and want to spend the night before starting your hike.

INTRODUCTION The Sawtooth Mountains have an embarrassment of riches, including colorful fields of wildflowers, jagged granite peaks, and gorgeous, high-elevation lakes. This loop trip explores the southwest part of the range and includes a nice sampling of all these wonderful qualities. In addition, it takes you through the impressive depths of the lower Queens River Canyon, a spectacular rocky chasm that features scenery not normally associated with a high mountain wilderness. Because this hike avoids the most famous attractions in the Sawtooth Wilderness, visitors here enjoy a much higher degree of solitude than in the better-known and more accessible parts of the range.

DESCRIPTION The trail drops briefly from the northwest end of the parking area to a sturdy bridge over the Queens River and a junction at the start of the loop.

For a clockwise tour, bear left and head up the canyon of the Little Queens River. The open forests at these lower elevations are a pleasant mix of ponderosa pines, lodgepole pines, Douglas-firs, and Englemann spruces. Beneath these trees, the forest floor is covered with a wealth of grasses and colorful wildflowers such as goldenrod, pearly everlasting, horsemint, and three flowers that grow up to six feet tall in this area – fireweed, coneflower, and larkspur. Apart from the flowers, the scenery is pleasant but unspectacular. You travel gradually uphill on a sometimes rocky tread for 0.5 mile, then cross the river on a bridge and come to a small meadow that holds an old wooden cabin and the rusted remains of an abandoned mine. The gentle trail then continues up to an easy crossing of Browns Creek and a slightly more tricky, ankle-deep ford of the Little Queens River.

Another mile of gentle uphill takes you past a nice campsite, then on to a broken-down miner's cabin, which is interesting to explore. The slope of your ascent picks up slightly after this – although it still couldn't be described as "steep" – as you go up three switchbacks, then contour across a hillside well above the stream. Less than 1 mile from the cabin you hop over Scott Creek, then wander through a mix of forests and meadows to a log crossing of Tripod Creek. About 0.5 mile later is a very good campsite just before a rock-hop crossing of the Little Queens River.

Beyond this crossing the trail goes through rolling, sagebrush-dotted meadows to a junction with the Neinmeyer Creek Trail, which heads northwest up to an obvious saddle. You bear right and soon pass a very large beaver pond about 200 yards before a tiny sign marking the junction with the Scenic Lake Trail.

If you want to make the side trip to this lake (and how could you not want to visit a place named Scenic Lake?), then bear right and travel down to an easy crossing of what's left of Little Queens River. There is a good campsite on the right about 100 yards before this crossing and another one on the left just after the crossing. The trail climbs steadily away from the crossing through sloping meadows that in July are ablaze with the colorful blossoms of death camas, sulphurflower, paintbrush, and aster.

Warning: Horse flies are common here and can be very bothersome on a warm afternoon.

At the end of the meadows you make six moderately graded switchbacks and then an uphill traverse to the base of a small, tumbling waterfall on Scenic Creek. Four more switchbacks lead to the top of the falls and just beyond to a sign stating HORSE TRAVEL NOT RECOMMENDED BEYOND THIS POINT. The reason for this sign soon becomes apparent as the trail winds very steeply up a rocky, almost shadeless hillside that is a challenge for two-legged visitors, much less livestock. The grade eases considerably at the top of the slope, where you go up and down through open, subalpine-fir forests past a pair of small, marshy ponds.

Warning: The trail is easy to lose in this area. Look carefully for blazes and a few cut logs that provide navigational clues.

In its final mile the trail goes through beautiful meadows beside small Scenic Creek, crosses the creek once, then makes a short climb to a small but attractive lower lake, where the trail seems to stop. To reach the more spectacular upper lake, cross the outlet of the lower lake, follow its shoreline for about 150 yards, then climb steeply for 0.2 mile to your final reward at Scenic Lake.

It's not easy to live up to a name like Scenic Lake, but this beautiful mountain pool manages to do so with ease. It is set in a dramatic cirque beneath Nahneke Mountain and is backed by tall cliffs and talus slopes. The best campsites are near the outlet, and for the pleasure of a night at this beautiful lake you'll be glad that you

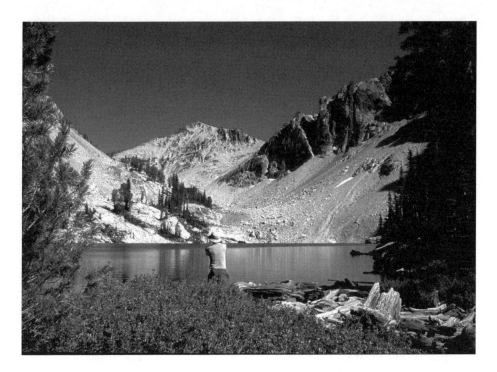

Angler at Scenic Lake

packed your heavy gear all the way up here. A bonus of camping here is that the lake has a good population of plump cutthroat trout and the fishing pressure is relatively light. Remember that fires are prohibited at Scenic Lake, so bring your cook stove.

After returning to the Little Queens River Trail, you turn right (upstream) and make a long, relentless climb at a moderate grade through spacious meadows on the rolling slopes above the river. Views improve as you climb, especially south down the valley of the Little Queens River and east up to the peaks around Browns Lake. You pass a cairn marking where an old trail comes in from the right, then make two long, rounded switchbacks to a junction with the Browns Lake Trail. The 1-mile side trail to this good-sized lake gains about 500 feet of elevation, but it's worth the effort if you have the time.

The main trail goes left at the Browns Lake junction and steadily climbs 11 switchbacks through open forests to an 8500-foot saddle with the rather unoriginal name of High Pass. The best views here are north over the drainage of Johnson Creek to Smoky Peak, and northeast to the tip of South Raker, a distinctive sharp pinnacle that peeks over the ridge west of Blacknose Mountain.

Two well-graded switchbacks and a long, gentle traverse take you down from High Pass into a sloping burn area, after which you make two more switchbacks and follow a small creek through flower-covered meadows with fine views of the nearby peaks. After following this creek for less than 0.5 mile, the trail gradually pulls away from the stream and passes through more of the burn area. A few final switchbacks take you down to a rock-hop crossing of Johnson Creek, a cascading stream that is bordered by lush riparian vegetation dominated by willows, monkshood, and Queen Anne's lace. About 200 yards after the crossing is a junction with the Johnson Creek Trail.

You turn right, following signs to Pats Lake, and climb a fire-scarred hillside, where fireweed, ceonothus bushes, and young quaking aspen trees are quickly reclaiming the blackened landscape. The shadeless climb begins with four long switchbacks followed by an uphill traverse of a little less than 1 mile. At the end of the traverse, you ascend four short switchbacks to a log over the creek that drains this high valley, then make a short, stiff climb to a second creek crossing near an intensely green meadow. The striking color of this meadow is in sharp contrast to the blackened snags all around. Only 200 yards later, you cross the creek a third time, just below a stair-step waterfall, then wind fairly steeply uphill to the top of the falls. Above the falls you make an uneven ascent to a final creek crossing a short distance below Pats Lake. The trail stays well to the north of this lake, so a short side trip is required for you to enjoy the excellent views across the water to Blacknose Mountain, northeast of the lake, and an unnamed, craggy ridgeline to the south. There are some very good campsites under a few unburned trees along the lake's northwest shore.

Above Pats Lake the rocky trail makes eight uphill switchbacks on a partly forested hillside to lovely Arrowhead Lake. This deep gem is set in a beautiful alpine basin and has lots of hungry cutthroat trout, many of them large. The few campsites here are rather exposed (the ones at Pats Lake are better), but you'll find at least one good site on a little ledge above the north shore.

The trail ascends a series of moderately graded switchbacks above Arrowhead Lake to the highest point of this trip at a wide,

9200-foot pass that sits just below timberline. The views from here are magnificent, especially southeast to pointed Mt. Everly and the upper basin of Queens River. Below the pass the trail winds down past a few weather-beaten trees and through alpine meadows, where high-elevation flowers such as Cusick's speedwell, owls clover, pink heather, bistort, aster, and pussy toes add color to the magnificent mountain scenery. The trail then goes past three small-to-medium sized lakes, all of which feature fine views of Peak 9704 to the west. There is a good campsite near the outlet of the second lake in this chain. A final nine switchbacks take you down to a junction with the Queens River Trail in a lovely meadow below the cliffs and snowfields of Mt. Everly.

The return route of this loop goes right, but I recommend that you first take the opportunity for an outstanding side trip to Everly and Plummer lakes, which are tucked in the high country on the east side of Mt. Everly. To do this excursion, turn left, climb past a pair of lovely meadows to a low pass, then wind down a fairly steep and rocky trail past the crumbling cliffs on the north side of Mt. Everly to a junction. You bear right, cross a boggy little basin with a great view of Mt. Everly, then climb steeply up to the outlet of rock-rimmed Everly Lake. To reach Plummer Lake, follow the trail around the east side of Everly Lake to where the path peters out in some meadows. From there, wander a few hundred yards south to an almost unnoticeable watershed divide, where you'll see Plummer Lake sitting in a dramatic basin beneath the dark summit of Plummer Peak.

Tip: Although very scenic, Everly and Plummer lakes have only fair campsites, so it's better to visit them on a dayhike.

Back at the Queens River junction, you turn south and begin the long descent of the dramatic Queens River Canyon. The first few hundred yards go through lovely meadows with scattered sub-alpine firs and views of several nearby granite cliffs and peaks. You then hop across the bubbling flow of the Queens River and make a moderately steep, 1-mile traverse of a mostly forested hillside to a second rock-hop crossing of the growing river. Still staying close to the water, the rocky trail winds steeply downhill through avalanche meadows that provide inspiring views of the tall peaks on either side of the canyon. At the bottom of this steep, 0.5-mile section, the trail becomes much more gentle as it goes through or beside a series

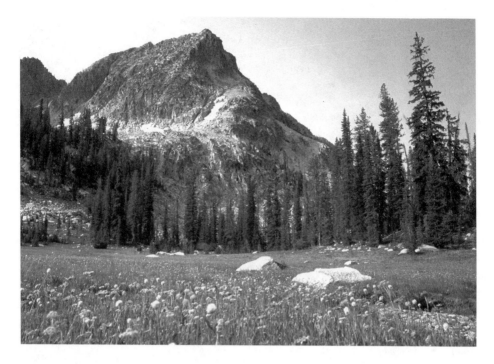

Mt. Everly from the meadow to the north

of grassy meadows to a tricky rock-hop or an easy, ankle-deep ford of the Queens River.

Warning: Confusing game paths in the meadows near this ford falsely lead you to a point that is approximately 100 feet upstream from the official trail crossing.

The next section of this very scenic trail goes through or just above some gorgeous meadows, which are bisected by the meandering Queens River and enclosed by towering granite walls and peaks that rise as much as 3000 feet above the valley floor. About 1.5 miles below the last crossing, the trail makes a seemingly unnecessary uphill detour on a hillside to the east, then goes steeply back down to river level and descends through a series of rocky avalanche meadows separated by strips of trees. These openings allow wildflowers to thrive and give hikers wonderful views of the high ridges on either side of the canyon. You pass a scenic riverside campsite in one of these strips of trees, then continue the uneven descent to a very good campsite beside Nanny Creek just before the trail crosses the Queens River. This crossing can usually be

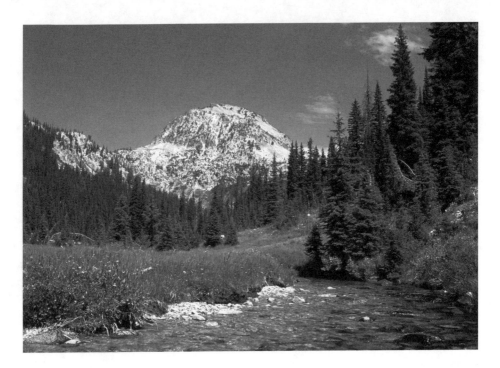

Along the Upper Queens River

accomplished on logs, but if these have been washed away, the ford is relatively easy and straightforward. The trail picks up again about 75 feet downstream from the crossing.

About 0.5 mile after this crossing, you break out of the dense forest and enter large, brushy meadows, which provide unobstructed views of the dramatic canyon scenery. The topographic map shows lots of tightly packed contour lines here and the landscape agrees with tall pinnacles and towering ramparts, especially on the right (west) side of the canyon. On your left, the river cascades along in a narrow chasm, its flow augmented by small side creeks that trickle down from the heights on either side. The scenery in this canyon is much superior to that along the Little Queens River at the start of this trip, a fact which argues in favor of a clockwise loop, so you can save the best for last. Not quite 3 miles from the last ford, you cross the river again, this time via a calf-deep ford.

Tip: *Even though there are a few logs across the stream here, they are all small and dangerously unstable, so you're better off with wet feet.*

This crossing is necessary because for the next mile the north-west (right) side of the canyon rises in steep talus slopes and tall, dark-colored cliffs that are impressive to look at but would be very hard to push a trail through. Your much easier route goes up and down on the left side of the river through Douglas-fir woods and patches of succulent thimbleberries, which ripen in August. At the end of this section is another calf-deep ford of the river.

You can put the wading shoes away now, because for the rest of the hike you remain on the north side of the now-westward-flowing river. Shortly after the last ford is a confusing area of brush and rocks, where you have to pick your way along the north bank until the trail becomes clear again. The canyon then widens and levels out as the trail leaves the river and goes through an old-growth, ponderosa-pine forest with some Douglas-firs and lodgepole pines and an understory of grasses and manzanita bushes.

Tip: The Earthwalk Press map shows a junction here with a trail that goes left up to China Basin, but there is no trail sign and no tread is visible on the ground.

The last 2 miles of your hike are nearly level, through open forests of ponderosa pines where 4-foot-tall mullein plants bloom yellow in July and August. When you reach the Little Queens River junction, turn left, cross the bridge, and return to your car.

POSSIBLE ITINERARY

	Camp	Miles	Elevation Gain
Day 1	Scenic Lake	10	3400
Day 2	Pats Lake	11	3400
Day 3	Upper Queens River (with side trip to Everly and Plummer lakes)	13	2000
Day 4	Out	8	300

VARIATIONS To extend this trip by two wonderfully scenic days, take the trail through the divide north of Mt. Everly and make a loop past the high lakes at the headwaters of the South Fork Payette River. See Trip 15 for details on this route.

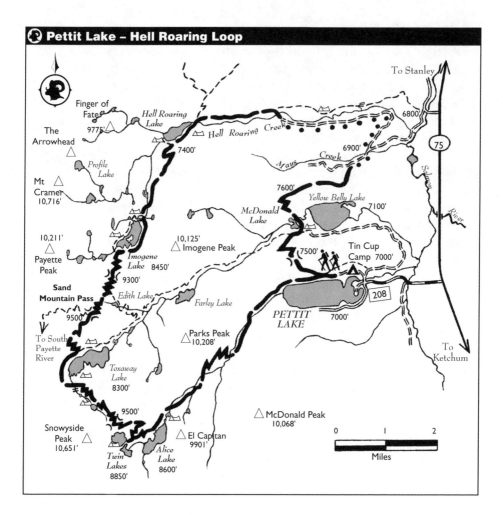

To Stanley

Finger of
Fate
9775'

The
Arrowhead

Hell Roaring
Lake

Hell Roaring Creek

6800'

75

Profile
Lake

Mays   Creek

6900'

Mt
Cramer
10,716'

7400'

7600'

McDonald
Lake

Yellow Belly Lake

7100'

10,211'

Payette
Peak

Imogene
Lake 8450'

10,125'
Imogene Peak

7500'

Tin Cup
Camp 7000'

**Sand
Mountain Pass**

9300'

Edith Lake

Farley Lake

208

9500'

To South
Payette
River

PETTIT
LAKE

7000'

To
Ketchum

Toxaway
Lake
8300'

Parks Peak
10,208'

McDonald Peak
10,068'

9500'

Snowyside
Peak
10,651'

El Capitan
9901'

Twin
Lakes
8850'

Alice
Lake
8600'

0   1   2

Miles

17 Pettit Lake – Hell Roaring Loop

RATINGS (1–10)			MILES	ELEVATION GAIN	DAYS	SHUTTLE MILEAGE
Scenery	Solitude	Difficulty	30	6000	3-4	N/A
9	3	5				

MAP Earthwalk Press - Hiking Map and Guide: Sawtooth Wilderness.

USUALLY OPEN July to October.

BEST Mid-July through August.

PERMITS Yes (free at the trailhead).

RULES Maximum group size of 12 people and 14 stock animals; all fires must be in a fire pan or on a fire blanket; no fires allowed in the Alice, Twin, or Toxaway lake basins; dogs must be on leash from July 1 to Labor Day.

CONTACT Sawtooth National Recreation Area, (208) 727-5000.

SPECIAL ATTRACTIONS Beautiful mountain scenery; lots of large mountain lakes; wildflowers.

PROBLEMS Rather crowded; mosquitoes in July.

HOW TO GET THERE From Stanley, drive 18.3 miles south on State Highway 75 to a junction just after the highway makes an angled turn to the left. (Coming from the south, this turnoff is 13.4 miles north of Galena Summit.) Turn right (west) on Pettit Lake Road, and go 1.6 miles on this washboard-riddled gravel road to a T-junction. Turn right, then drive 0.6 mile through a campground to the Tin Cup hiker's trailhead. A parking pass is required at this popular trailhead. You can buy them from any ranger station and most outdoor stores in Boise or Stanley.

If you have two cars, you can shorten this trip by leaving a second car at the Hell Roaring trailhead. To reach it, return to Highway 75 and drive 3.3 miles north to the junction with Fourth of July

Road. Turn left (west) onto Decker Flat Road and drive 0.3 mile on this rough gravel road to a bridge over the Salmon River. Immediately after the bridge is a T-junction and the trailhead.

INTRODUCTION This relatively short trip samples all of the attributes that make the Sawtooth Mountains the most popular hiking area in Idaho. The route wanders through attractive forests, goes past several beautiful mountain lakes, climbs over high passes with great views, and visits meadows with a wealth of wildflowers. Because of the excellent scenery and easy access, the trails here are some of the most popular in the state. It is, therefore, especially important that hikers be scrupulous in following all "no-trace" principles.

DESCRIPTION A wide and well-used trail heads west through open forests of Douglas-firs and lodgepole pines on the slopes beside Pettit Lake. In the open areas above the trail are lots of sagebrush and early-summer wildflowers such as lupine, fireweed, groundsel, balsamroot, and sulphurflower. Numerous short side paths lead down to the lakeshore, which is especially appealing on calm mornings when the still waters reflect McDonald and Parks peaks to the southwest.

About 200 yards from the trailhead is a four-way junction. A horse trail goes sharply right, while the path to Yellow Belly Lake angles slightly right. You will come back on the latter trail if you hike the full loop. For now, bear slightly left and stick with the rolling trail along the lakeshore. In about 1 mile you reach the end of Pettit Lake, enter Sawtooth Wilderness, and pass a registration box from which you are required to obtain a free permit.

For the next 1.5 miles you gradually gain elevation through relatively dense forests that in addition to the pines and Douglas-firs now include Engelmann spruces. The drier slopes in this area feature flowers like yarrow, paintbrush, and a particularly fetching variety of mariposa lily. The boggy areas, which are often crossed by wooden plank bridges, host thimbleberry and monkshood.

The trail passes beneath a long, craggy rock formation as it slowly ascends beside an unnamed, cascading creek. Along the way you cross the creek twice, first on convenient stepping stones, then on a log. After the second crossing, you leave the stream and make 10 well-graded switchbacks up an open slope above a marshy lake. This slope often has lots of fireweed in bloom during July. The

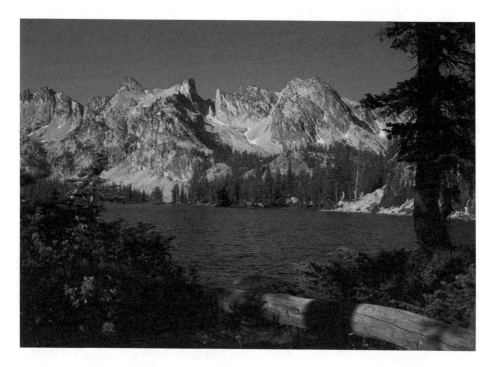

Looking southwest across Alice Lake

switchbacks take you to an attractive upper valley, where you twice rock-hop across a small creek and gradually ascend through rocky meadows and open forests. After about 0.5 mile, you climb 300 feet in lazy switchbacks and cross the creek again, this time on a bridge.

The next mile is easy and lovely as you slowly climb through open, subalpine-fir woods with good views of the many granite summits on either side of the valley. At your feet are a wealth of wildflowers, especially aster, arnica, lousewort, pussy toes, and a deep-magenta paintbrush. After a final rock-hop crossing of the creek, you pass two lovely tarns, then come to large and very scenic Alice Lake. This gorgeous lake has numerous good campsites and outstanding views west to a craggy group of unnamed summits. The most attractive campsites are near the outlet.

> **Tip:** *Alice Lake is very popular, so if you plan to camp here it is better to visit on a weekday. For a less crowded alternative, try the campsites at Twin Lakes, ahead.*

The trail follows the shore of Alice Lake for a short distance, then winds uphill on gentle switchbacks for 0.5 mile to a poorly signed fork. The trail to the left goes about 200 yards down to the strip of land between the heather-rimmed Twin Lakes. These lakes both have good campsites and feature excellent views across their tranquil waters to Snowyside Peak.

The main trail bears right at the fork and gradually climbs in long traverses and short switchbacks up an open slope. Alpine wildflowers abound here, especially Cusik's speedwell, bistort, cinquefoil, paintbrush, Douglas' knotweed, stonecrop, Rocky Mountain goldenrod, and blue beard-tongue. Views of the sparkling Twin Lakes and a group of nearby serrated peaks improve with every step. You top out at a narrow, 9500-foot pass on the northeast shoulder of Snowyside Peak.

Warning: *Snowfields often block the trail on the north side of this pass well into July.*

From the pass, you descend 19 switchbacks to a pair of small, scenic lakes with a good campsite between them, then go gradually downhill for about 1.5 miles on a sometimes rocky tread beside a small creek. The trail crosses the creek on logs just below a sloping waterfall and comes to the basin holding 1-mile-long Toxaway Lake. Although the trail stays well above this large lake, you can follow any of several bootpaths down to good campsites and fishing spots on the shore.

You hop over several small creeks feeding Toxaway Lake and, about halfway down the north shore, come to a junction. For a short, easy loop back to Pettit Lake, go straight and walk 6 miles downhill on the popular trail that goes past Farley Lake to a junction just before Yellow Belly Lake. From there, you turn right and hike over a woodsy ridge to the trailhead.

For a longer and more scenic loop, turn left at Toxaway Lake and begin a long, 1200-foot climb. The moderately steep route alternates between switchbacks and traverses on a partly forested slope with fine views back to Toxaway Lake and Snowyside Peak. You top out at a small notch in a side ridge, go around a knoll beside an orange-tinted peak, then drop a bit to a junction at Sand Mountain Pass.

Your trail bears right at the pass, climbs about 200 feet, then switchbacks down into the next basin to the north. You'll see Edith Lake below you on the right just before you come to a tiny, wet meadow with a trickling creek. Hop over the creek, then walk a short distance beneath a rocky slope to a junction beside a small pond. You go left and climb a dozen moderate switchbacks on a talus slope to a 9300-foot pass with fine views northeast to the basin holding large Imogene Lake, and north to the crags around Mt. Cramer and The Arrowhead.

The trail now descends a series of short switchbacks, first down a long talus slope, then through rolling meadows. At the bottom of the switchbacks you follow a seasonal creek to its confluence with a larger stream, which flows down from a string of unnamed and trailless lakes on the slopes of Payette Peak to the west.

Warning: Snow typically blocks this section of trail until mid-July.

The trail splits here, with the two forks forming a loop around Imogene Lake. Either trail will work and both are scenic. The old trail goes around the west and north shores of the lake and passes numerous campsites. The shorter new trail goes to the right and skirts the lake's south and east shores. On either route there are good views of the lake, its large island, and the peaks surrounding this basin.

Tip: The lake is less attractive in late summer, because it often recedes several feet, especially during dry years.

The two trails reunite at the northeast end of the lake near several more good campsites. These sites are especially appealing, because they afford fine views across the water to prominent Payette Peak. Anglers will be delighted to spend some time here trying to hook some of the lake's abundant and quite large brook and cutthroat trout.

The trail crosses the outlet of Imogene Lake, follows this creek past a couple of small tarns covered with water lilies, then veers away from the creek and makes a long, nicely graded descent in several switchbacks. Occasional openings in the tree cover along this section reward you with good views west to Mt. Cramer and north to a group of extremely rugged ridges and granite outcroppings that includes the ominously titled Finger of Fate. The final mile to Hell Roaring Lake uses numerous switchbacks to go down an old moraine that is still only lightly forested.

Tip: Just before the west end of Hell Roaring Lake, you pass an unsigned spur trail that drops to some good lakeside campsites.

The trail continues to the northeast end of Hell Roaring Lake, where there are several excellent campsites and great views to craggy

Finger of Fate on the western skyline. You cross the lake's outlet on a bridge and, about 50 yards later, come to a junction. Bear right on a heavily used trail and descend moderately for a short distance, then level off on an easy trail that travels through open forest in the lower valley of Hell Roaring Creek. Unfortunately, you rarely get close to the lovely creek, which remains out of sight on the right. About 2 miles from Hell Roaring Lake is a poorly signed junction with the old Hell Roaring Trail.

If you left a car at the Hell Roaring trailhead, then go straight and continue down the wide valley. It's a pleasant stroll that passes an excellent creekside campsite after about 1.5 miles, then goes up and down over old, rocky moraine material that is sparsely forested with lodgepole pines. You'll reach the trailhead a little over 5 miles from Hell Roaring Lake.

Those who are returning by trail to Pettit Lake will find the route is little used and a bit monotonous. Most of the way is on old jeep roads or horse trails through a monoculture of lodgepole pines that are dense enough to block the views, but not thick enough to provide much shade. The route is also outside of the protected wilderness, so you must share the trail with motorbikes and mountain bikes. Still, it's a pleasant hike and certainly more interesting than walking back on Highway 75.

To take this route, turn right at the junction with the old Hell Roaring Trail and make a knee-deep ford of the creek. You may find a log nearby, but if not, the ford is relatively easy, because the water is not swift. Almost immediately on the other side of the ford is a jeep road. Follow this road, which still gets some motorized traffic, as it stays mostly level on the south side of the valley. After about 2 miles, the road curves right around a ridge, then loses some elevation to a junction. You angle right on another jeep road and make a simple ford of Mays Creek that by midsummer probably won't even get your feet wet. You then walk 0.4 mile along the road and bear left on a trail which is no longer shown on the Forest Service map, but which still exists and is easy to follow.

The narrow trail climbs fairly steeply to the top of a viewless ridge, then turns to follow the ridgeline. After about 1 mile of undulating mostly uphill, the trail leaves the ridge and descends three switchbacks to the flat basin that holds both McDonald Lake, on your right, and larger Yellow Belly Lake, hidden by trees on your left.

You soon make an easy, ankle-deep ford across the outlet of McDonald Lake, then follow this lake's grassy shoreline, where there are good views to the west of the high peaks of the Sawtooth Range. There are no established campsites at the lake, but there's plenty of flat ground and places to set up your tent. Shortly after McDonald Lake you bear right at a junction, then walk 50 feet to a second junction, this time with the trail from Toxaway Lake.

To complete the loop, you bear left and gradually climb for almost 1 mile, gaining about 500 feet in three irregularly spaced switchbacks to the wide top of a woodsy ridge. From there, you make a gradual downhill traverse to a junction beside Pettit Lake, then turn left and retrace the final 200 yards back to your car.

POSSIBLE ITINERARY

	Camp	Miles	Elevation Gain
Day 1	Twin Lakes	7	2000
Day 2	Imogene Lake	10.5	2400
Day 3	Out	13*	1600*

* If you left a second car at the Hell Roaring trailhead, then these numbers are reduced by 3.5 miles and 1300 feet of elevation gain.

VARIATIONS For a short, two- or three-day trip, make the very popular 19-mile loop that goes past Alice and Toxaway lakes, but skips the trail to Imogene and Hell Roaring lakes.

If you want to extend the hike, consider a long side trip west from Sand Mountain Pass to Edna, Ardeth, and a string of other high lakes at the headwaters of the South Fork Payette River. See Trip 15 for details on this grand adventure.

Off-trail scramblers can take an extra day to visit spectacular Profile Lake and several other unnamed lakes set in cirque basins high on the walls of Mt. Cramer, Payette Peak, and The Arrowhead, north and west of Imogene Lake.

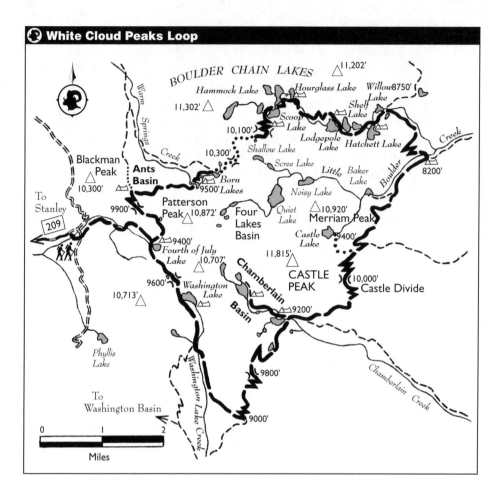

BOULDER CHAIN LAKES

△ 11,202'

Hammock Lake
Hourglass Lake
Willow 8750'
Lake

11,302' △
Shelf
Lake

Scoop
Lake

10,100'

Lodgepole
Lake

Hatchett Lake

Creek

10,300'

Shallow Lake

Scree Lake

Little
Baker
Lake

Boulder

8200'

**Blackman
Peak**
△
10,300'

**Ants
Basin**

Born
9500' Lakes

Noisy Lake

**Patterson
Peak**△10,872'

**Four
Lakes
Basin**

Quiet
Lake

△10,920'
Merriam Peak

**To
Stanley**

9900'

Castle
Lake 9400'

209

9400'
Fourth of July
Lake

10,707'

△

11,815'
△

Chamberlain

**CASTLE
PEAK**

10,000'
Castle Divide

9600'
Washington
Lake

Basin

9200'

10,713' △

9800'

Phyllis
Lake

Washington Lake Creek

Chamberlain Creek

**To
Washington Basin**

9000'

0   1   2

Miles

18 White Cloud Peaks Loop

RATINGS (1–10)			MILES	ELEVATION GAIN	DAYS	SHUTTLE MILEAGE
Scenery	Solitude	Difficulty	28	5900	3-5	N/A
10	5	8	(29)	(6200)	(3-5)	

MAPS USGS - Boulder Chain Lakes, Washington Peak.

USUALLY OPEN Mid-July to October.

BEST Late July to September.

PERMITS None.

RULES Maximum group size of 20 people and 25 stock animals; fires are prohibited within 200 yards of Scree, Shallow, Castle, and Upper Chamberlain lakes and in the Four Lakes Basin; fires are strongly discouraged in upper Boulder Chain Lakes Basin; special rules apply to tethering, watering, and feeding stock — call the Sawtooth National Recreation Area for details.

CONTACT Sawtooth National Recreation Area, (208) 727-5000.

SPECIAL ATTRACTIONS Spectacular mountain scenery; good fishing; wildlife, especially elk and mountain goats.

PROBLEMS Thin air at high altitudes; motorcycles allowed on part of the route; short but difficult cross-country section.

HOW TO GET THERE From Stanley, drive 15.0 miles south on State Highway 75 to a junction with Fourth of July Creek Road. (Coming from the south this turnoff is 16.7 miles north of Galena Summit.) Turn left (east) and stay on this bumpy gravel road for 10.2 miles to the developed Fourth of July Creek trailhead. A parking pass is required at this trailhead.

INTRODUCTION Although it would be difficult to pick a single favorite from among the dozens of mountain ranges that always draw the

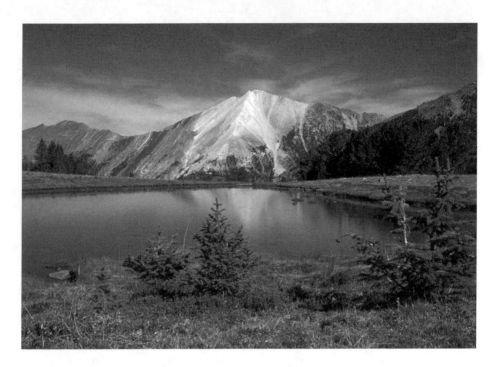

Pond in Ants Basin

admiration of Idaho hikers, you could make a strong case for the White Cloud Peaks as the best of the lot. All of the trails in this range take you through scenery that is so spectacular it simply defies description. This magnificent loop hits only a sampling of the best of these peaks. If you fall in love with this range's towering peaks and sparkling lakes, then you can expect to find yourself planning additional great adventures in the future. This loop trip requires a short but difficult cross-country scramble over a steep, rocky pass. Inexperienced hikers should consider an easier trip. Oxygen becomes noticeably scarce at the higher elevations along this trip, so it's not just the scenery that leaves lowlanders breathless. Take it slow until you get acclimated

Many of the trails in this area have been rerouted in recent years. These changes were designed to make the trails less steep and to reduce erosion. Unfortunately, the new alignments are not shown on the USGS maps, and even the more up-to-date Forest Service maps do not include the changes. The new trail alignments have also changed the distances, so the mileages shown on trail signs are no longer correct.

DESCRIPTION The well-graded trail, which to the chagrin of hikers is open to motorbikes, starts in an open forest of lodgepole pines. In the first few hundred yards the path goes over Fourth of July Creek on a little wooden bridge, crosses a rough mining road, and begins a gradual ascent. The ensuing climb takes you through Engelmann-spruce and subalpine-fir forests on the edge of some very scenic meadows. These meadows border small Fourth of July Creek, a cascading stream whose main stem and tributaries the trail crosses several times on flat-topped logs. About 1.5 miles from the trailhead the climb ends at a junction and the start of the loop.

> *Tip:* Hikers who get a late start will find a comfortable campsite above the north shore of meadow-rimmed Fourth of July Lake, about 150 yards along the trail to the right.

To start the loop, you bear left at the junction on a trail that is thankfully closed to motor vehicles. The rocky footpath climbs fairly steeply to a small, rock-lined pond. The grade then eases as you make a gradual uphill traverse on a partly forested hillside to a windy pass with great views. To the south is an unnamed brownish-orange peak rising above Fourth of July Lake. To the southwest are several gray-colored summits near the distant Champion Lakes. Finally, to the north rise the aptly named White Cloud Peaks, a line of sky-scraping mountains composed of striking whitish-yellow rock. Another prominent feature is Ants Basin, a large, green expanse directly below you to the north.

The trail briefly follows the ridge northwest of the pass, then descends seven quick switchbacks across a talus slope to Ants Basin. This nearly flat, flower-covered meadow has great views, water from trickling springs and creeks, and some possible campsites beside a tiny pond about 300 yards left of where you reach the basin floor.

The official trail across Ants Basin heads north, but it is rarely used and very hard to find. Your route follows a more obvious, unofficial bootpath that goes east and heads more directly to your destination. From where you reach the basin floor, turn right and follow this good, but unofficial path across a meadow and over an insignificant rise. The path then goes steeply downhill, makes a rolling traverse across the lower end of a rockslide, then climbs through open forest to an excellent campsite beside one of the lower Born Lakes. In a basin surrounded by brownish mountains and spires, this stunningly beautiful pool is a great location for a long lunch or a memorable night in the Idaho wilderness.

It will take some time to convince yourself to leave this idyllic spot, but once you do, follow the now-sketchy path as it goes around the west shore of the lake, then travel gradually uphill through open forest to the largest and deepest Born Lake. Here you meet an official trail, which goes northwest to Warm Springs Creek.

To continue the trip beyond the Born Lakes requires daring and experience with scrambling. Novice hikers, and all who are afraid of heights should not attempt this short but difficult cross-country section. As an alternative, these hikers can go back to Fourth of July Lake, then continue on to Washington and Chamberlain lakes. This very scenic southern part of the loop is well worth doing and stays on good trails for the entire distance.

Hikers who are up to the challenge will find that there is no easy way to get over the trailless, serrated ridge east of the last Born Lake. The most direct route goes up a very steep rocky chute, locally known as the Devils Staircase, to a tiny notch at the obvious low point in the ridge. This notch is marked by a small, needle-like rock spire. To reach this goal, you scramble over dangerously loose rocks and scree, angling slightly from left to right in order to avoid impassable cliffs on either side of your scramble route. Careful and experienced hikers will get a workout, but they should make it to the top just fine. Leave your walking stick at home. You will need both hands free for balance and to help pull yourself up.

Warning: Snow may linger in this chute or, worse, in the unseen gully on the east side of the notch through the end of July. When snow is present, the route is too dangerous to attempt.

Your troubles aren't over once you reach the pass, because you then must scramble down a very steep gully, losing about 400 feet to the base of some cliffs. It is generally easier if you stay on the left (north) side of the gully. Once you reach the bottom of the cliffs, turn left and make a relatively easy and straightforward traverse across a sloping boulder field to a prominent bench.

Tip: Although Shallow and Scree lakes in the basin on your right look inviting, do not go that way unless you want to make a side trip to explore or camp near them.

Near the northeast end of the bench is a shallow tarn with a couple of wind-whipped campsites that tend to be rather bleak in bad

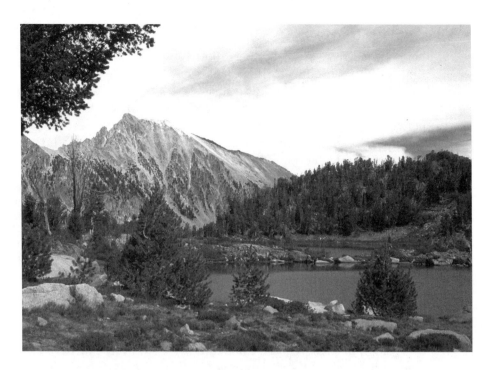

Scoop Lake in upper Boulder Chain Lakes Basin

weather. Just above the north side of the pond is a sketchy bootpath that goes northeast. You follow this indistinct route as it goes over a low rise, cuts across a scree slope, then drops to a rocky saddle, where the tread becomes more obvious. The view from this saddle is stupendous, especially east to the distant White Knob Mountains and Lost River Range, and north to the nearby Boulder Chain Lakes Basin. This spectacular basin is backed by rugged, white-granite peaks and features a string of beautiful lakes, several of which are visible from this location.

The trail into this basin follows several well-graded switchbacks that take you down a rocky slope to lovely Scoop Lake, which has several good campsites above its northwest shore. After rounding Scoop Lake and crossing its outlet, you wind down to deep Hammock Lake, which has a small island, excellent campsites, and a drop-dead-gorgeous setting. Next in the chain is Hourglass Lake, which is named for its distinctive shape.

After Hourglass Lake you descend, sometimes steeply, beside Boulder Chain Lakes Creek. The trail crosses the small creek three times during the mile-long, lakeless descent, then levels off just before it reaches very deep Lodgepole Lake. This scenic lake is the first in this basin's lower string of lakes and boasts very good campsites near both its inlet and its outlet.

The well-used trail now cuts across the narrow strip of land between Lodgepole Lake and Sliderock Lake, then goes around Sliderock's scenic south shore. From there, you descend a bit to Shelf Lake, a deep pool with several excellent campsites and more good scenery. Next is Hatchett Lake, which has a good campsite and a great view of an unnamed, jagged pinnacle to the southwest. The trail barely touches Hatchett Lake, then drops to Willow Lake, the last in the chain, and comes to a junction.

The most popular trail into the Boulder Chain Lakes comes in from the left, but your route goes right. This trail is open to motorbikes, so the tread is chewed up and rather dusty. The trail passes through a spacious, flowery meadow with a photogenic view of an unnamed peak to the north, then descends gradually through dense forest. After it breaks out of the trees, the trail descends across an open slope of sagebrush and quaking aspens on three moderately long switchbacks. In early summer, this slope hosts a good variety of wildflowers, but the most spectacular color show is in late September, when the aspens turn yellow and orange and frame outstanding views of rugged Castle and Merriam peaks to the southwest. At the bottom of the slope, the trail makes an easy ford of Little Boulder Creek and comes to a fair campsite on the south bank.

Tip: If you want to keep your feet dry, bushwhack upstream through some willows, where you can usually find a log across the creek.

About 50 yards beyond the campsite is a junction, where you turn right on a trail that is thankfully closed to motor vehicles. This path slowly climbs in forest for a little less than 1 mile to a fork that is not shown on most maps. The unsigned route to the right goes to small Baker Lake, but your trail bears left and continues the long, woodsy ascent. There are several level stretches along the way, which allow you to catch your breath and enjoy nice views through the trees. The best views feature 11,815-foot Castle Peak, the highest point in the White Clouds, and neighboring Merriam Peak, which is not as lofty but is equally rugged.

The long climb takes you to a junction with the little-used Big Wickiup Trail, which goes straight where your trail switchbacks right. About 400 yards farther, it's time to drop your heavy pack and

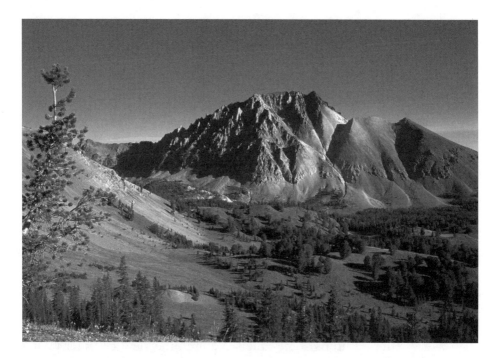

Castle Peak and Chamberlain Basin from ridge to the south

take an excellent cross-country side trip to Castle Lake, a dramatic pool tucked in a scenic cirque on the northeast side of Castle Peak. To reach it, work your way to the north end of a large, rolling basin west of the trail and look for two 3-foot-tall cairns. These mark the start of a sketchy trail that goes about 0.2 mile across a scree slope to Castle Lake. This deep, cold lake has some exposed campsites (fires are prohibited) and great views of the nearby cliffs of both Castle and Merriam peaks. In addition to the occasional awe-inspired hiker, this area is a favorite hangout for a small band of mountain goats.

Back on the main trail, you climb eight long, lazy switchbacks on an exposed slope to the top of Castle Divide, a windy, above-timber-line pass with inspiring views. The most impressive sight is nearby Castle Peak, a towering mass of contorted white rock. An obvious bootpath goes to even higher viewpoints on the ridge to the west.

To continue your loop, go fairly steeply down the gully south of Castle Divide, then descend at a more gentle grade on a recently rerouted trail. The trail winds down a series of gentle curves and switchbacks through open whitebark-pine and, later, subalpine-fir forests, then slowly curves around the south side of Castle Peak and comes to a junction with the Chamberlain Creek Trail. You go straight and soon reach a junction beside the outlet of lower Chamberlain Lake. This large, scenic lake is rimmed with meadows and has several fairly popular campsites along its east and south-east shores.

Warning: The lake's water level recedes during the summer, so it may look rather pathetic by autumn in dry years.

To visit the upper basin, take the trail along the north shore of the lower lake, climb beside a small creek, then go past a shallow pond to large and very beautiful upper Chamberlain Lake. Fish often jump from the waters of this lake, disturbing the great reflections of craggy Castle Peak, which rises directly from the lake's heather-lined shores.

Tip: The campsites at upper Chamberlain Lake are less numerous than at the lower lake, but they are also more scenic and less crowded.

After spending some time soaking in the view, consider taking the trail around the east side of upper Chamberlain Lake to another, unnamed lake, just a few feet higher in elevation.

To get back on the main loop, return to the junction beside lower Chamberlain Lake and turn south, following signs for Washington Lake. Your path wanders uphill through forests and small meadows for less than 0.5 mile to an unnamed lake. This lake can be rather unattractive by late summer in dry years, because the water level may drop 30 feet or more. Above this lake you climb to a rolling, open basin, then make one switchback and a long, uphill traverse to the top of a high ridge. This grandstand not only provides your last good view north to massive Castle Peak rising above Chamberlain Basin, but it also opens up an entirely new view south to the rugged peaks of the distant Boulder Mountains.

The trail descends two gentle switchbacks on the south side of the ridge, then goes downhill at a gradual then moderately steep grade through viewless forest. The scenery improves as the trail curves right and passes openings in the trees that provide excellent views west to the multi-colored peaks above Washington Basin. The trail then winds down a hillside to a junction with the trail to Germania Creek.

You turn right and go up and down (mostly down) across a steep slope to pretty Washington Lake Creek, then turn upstream and parallel this small creek through a pleasant mix of forests and meadows. At the prettiest of these meadows, you hop across the creek and immediately reach a trail junction. Your trail, which here is open to motorbikes, goes right and climbs steadily for another 0.5 mile to meadow-rimmed Washington Lake.

Tip: If you leave the trail and scout around a bit, you will find plenty of good campsites near the lake's southeast end. These campsites feature superb views across the water to the towering, tan-colored slopes of an unnamed peak and ridge to the north.

The trail remains in the trees, well away from Washington Lake, then angles right and touches the northwest shore. From here, you climb gradually through a low saddle with a seasonal pond, then descend through trees to scenic Fourth of July Lake. Your loop ends at the trail junction just past this lake, where you go straight and return to your car.

POSSIBLE ITINERARY

	Camp	Miles	Elevation Gain
Day 1	Born Lakes	4	1500
Day 2	Hatchett Lake	6	900
Day 3	Upper Chamberlain Lake	9	2300
	(with side trip to Castle Lake)		
Day 4	Out	10	1500

VARIATIONS For a shorter and easier version of this trip, skip the difficult cross-country section above the Born Lakes, and visit only the west half of this loop, possibly with a side trip to Washington Basin.

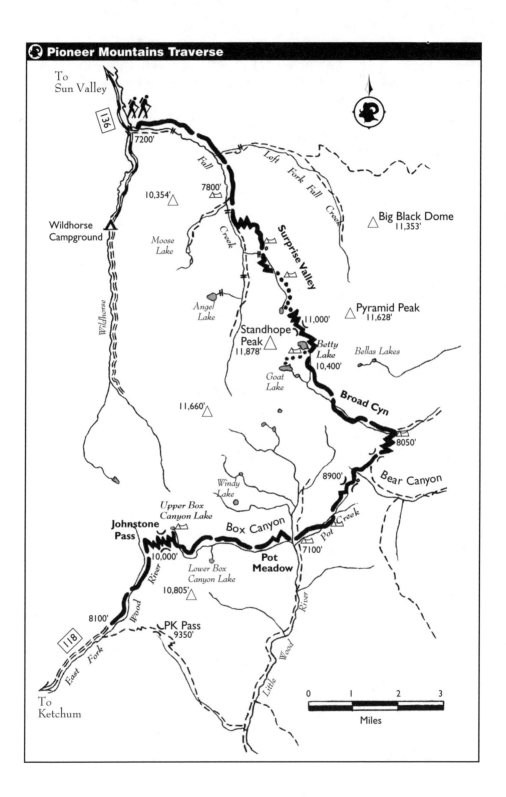

Pioneer Mountains Traverse

To Sun Valley

136

7200'

Fall

Left Fork Fall Creek

10,354'

7800'

Wildhorse Campground

Moose Lake

Creek

Surprise Valley

Big Black Dome
11,353'

Wildhorse

Angel Lake

Pyramid Peak
11,628'

11,000'

Standhope Peak
11,878'

Betty Lake
10,400'

Bellas Lakes

Goat Lake

Broad Cyn

11,660'

8050'

Windy Lake

8900'

Bear Canyon

Upper Box Canyon Lake

Johnstone Pass

Box Canyon

Pot Creek

10,000'

Lower Box Canyon Lake

Pot Meadow

7100'

10,805'

Wood River

River

Little Wood

8100'

118

East Fork

PK Pass
9350'

To Ketchum

0 1 2 3
Miles

19 Pioneer Mountains Traverse

RATINGS (1–10)			MILES	ELEVATION GAIN	DAYS	SHUTTLE MILEAGE
Scenery	Solitude	Difficulty	26*	8200	3-4	50*
9	8	6	(27)*	(8900)	(3-4)	

* The distance may be slightly longer for the hike, and shorter for the car shuttle, depending on how far you can drive on the access road to the south trailhead.

MAPS USGS - Copper Basin SW, Grays Peak, Muldoon Canyon NW, Standhope Peak.

USUALLY OPEN Late June to October.

BEST July.

PERMITS None.

RULES The usual no-trace principles apply.

CONTACT Lost River Ranger District, (208) 588-3400; Ketchum Ranger District, (208) 622-5371.

SPECIAL ATTRACTIONS Solitude; beautiful alpine lakes; fine mountain scenery.

PROBLEMS High altitude hiking; some sketchy trails; poor access road to south trailhead.

HOW TO GET THERE To reach the exit point at the south trailhead, drive 5.8 miles south of downtown Ketchum (or about 6 miles north of Hailey) on State Highway 75, then turn east on paved East Fork Road. The pavement ends after 6.0 miles at an old mining town with the wonderfully optimistic name of Triumph, after which the road turns to badly washboarded gravel. About 1.2 miles past Triumph, bear right at a junction, following signs to Federal Gulch Campground, and, 1.0 mile later, bear left at a junction with Cove Creek Road. Another 3.4 miles take you to Federal Gulch Campground, where the road becomes increasingly rocky and miserable. A passenger car can make it (just barely), but it is very slow and challenging. Most hikers will prefer to park and walk the rest of the way. The road ends at an unsigned trailhead 4.3 miles past Federal Gulch Campground.

To reach the starting point at the north trailhead, return to downtown Ketchum and turn right (northeast) at a traffic light, following signs for Sun Valley. Continue straight through busy Sun Valley, now on the Trail Creek Road. This road narrows and eventually turns from paved to rocky gravel as it makes a very scenic 12-mile climb to a high point at Trail Creek Pass.

> **Warning:** *Trail Creek Road gets a fair amount of traffic during the summer months, often by tourists from Sun Valley who are unfamiliar with driving on mountain roads. This fact, along with dust and excess speed, contributes to numerous accidents. Drive defensively and follow the posted speed limit, so you don't become a statistic.*

Drive 10.5 miles beyond the pass to a prominent junction. Turn right, following signs to Wildhorse and Copper Basin, and drive 2.1 miles to a fork. Bear right, following signs to Wildhorse Guard Station, and drive 3.5 miles to a junction immediately after a bridge over Wildhorse Creek. Turn left and go 0.5 mile on a narrow gravel road to the roadend trailhead, which has an outhouse and a picnic table. The gravel upper parking lot is for dayhikers, so please leave your car in the grassy lower lot.

INTRODUCTION The Pioneer Mountains feature many of the best attributes of other Idaho ranges while avoiding their negative qualities to create the perfect mix for backpackers. The mountains have spectacular, jagged peaks and sparkling cirque lakes that will remind you of the popular Sawtooth Mountains. But unlike in the Sawtooths, the trails here are little traveled, so backpackers can enjoy solitude comparable to the much more remote Lemhi and Lost River ranges. Unlike in those ranges, however, the road access to most trailheads in the Pioneers is fairly reasonable, so you shouldn't have to sacrifice an oil pan or a set of tires to reach your chosen trail. And as in the Lemhis and the mountains of Frank Church-River of No Return Wilderness, wildlife is common, including elk, black bear, mountain goats, and even a few moose. Finally, although none of this magnificent range is protected as wilderness (a situation that should, someday, be corrected), you can still find many trails, including those described here, that are closed to motorbikes by local forest rules, so you can hike blissfully free of the noise, fumes, and badly eroded trails that plague the Bear River and Snake River ranges.

This short, rough, and very scenic traverse is equally good in either direction. It is described from north to south to avoid having to climb up the loose scree slope on the west side of Johnstone Pass.

DESCRIPTION The poorly signed trail starts from the grassy lower parking lot, crosses a bridge over rushing Fall Creek, and comes to a junction with an overgrown jeep road. You turn right on this road, which has been closed to motorized traffic for so long it now has the look and feel of a backcountry trail, and climb fairly steeply across partly forested slopes well above the north bank of Fall Creek. Although there are a couple of waterfalls on the creek, they are so far below the trail you won't be able to see them. The old road ends after 2 miles. Here you level off and cross a couple of sagebrush-covered meadows to a log across Left Fork Fall Creek. Immediately after this crossing is an unsigned junction with the trail up the Left Fork, which is so obscure you probably won't notice it.

You turn south and gradually climb in forests and meadows, never straying very far from Fall Creek. There are some nice views over the meadows to several nearby peaks, which despite reaching to well over 10,000 feet have no names. The trail forks a little less than 1 mile from the Left Fork crossing, where a confusing sign says simply TRAIL and points to the right. This route goes to relatively popular Moose Lake, but it is *not* your trail.

Tip: There is a good campsite about 150 yards down the Moose Lake Trail, a little before it crosses Fall Creek.

Your route bears slightly left at the fork, climbs fairly steeply through attractive forests, and soon passes a good-sized cascading waterfall on Fall Creek. You'll have to go off the trail a short distance to get a good look at this falls, but it's worth it. A little less than 0.5 mile from the Moose Lake turnoff is another junction, this time with a sign saying SURPRISE VALLEY TRAIL and pointing left. You turn onto this trail and soon climb a series of 18 short, steep switchbacks, which gain approximately 750 feet in a little over 0.5 mile, so you'll get a good workout. At the top of the switchbacks, the trail temporarily levels off, then goes around a small meadow. From there, you ascend a dry, rocky gully to another meadow, then climb over a rocky area where the increasingly sketchy route is marked with cairns.

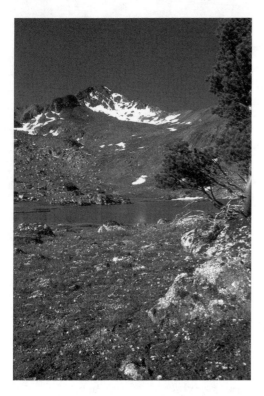

Standhope Peak over Lake 10148

The climbing finally abates as you enter the lower part of Surprise Valley. This beautiful, subalpine valley is bordered by high peaks and cliffs to the east and a lower, jagged ridge to the west. The first surprise here is a large pond, where you'll find a good campsite in the trees above the north shore and enjoy excellent views of the nearby peaks. The second surprise that the creek that drains the valley flows through a narrow and previously hidden low spot in the western ridge and creates a long, sloping waterfall.

The now-very-sketchy trail goes around the west side of the pond, then the tread disappears as you cross a large, wet meadow just above where the valley's creek drops over the waterfall to the west. To relocate the trail, cross the creek and search in the trees to the south, where the trail, here an indistinct path, is easier to find. The path follows the creek upstream for a short distance, then goes up a fairly steep, rocky slope, where a few cairns help to guide you along. You finally enter the meadows in the upper part of Surprise Valley, where a couple of cairns lead you to an easy rock-hop crossing of the creek. The path disappears here, although you may come across its faint tread from time to time if you happen to get lucky.

But who needs a trail? The terrain is open, the hiking is easy, and you'll prefer to wander around a bit anyway to better enjoy the scenery. In July, the meadows come alive with wildflowers, including lots of elephant's head, shooting star, alpine buttercup, bistort, phlox, and aster. In addition, the views of the surrounding peaks and ridges (most of which are unnamed) are excellent. Quiet hikers may even startle a herd of elk, which are not accustomed to seeing people in this high valley. There are few established campsites in this remote area, but there is no shortage of likely flat spots where you can pitch your tent and enjoy the scenery.

At the head of the valley, your trailless course angles up open slopes to the right, as you head for what looks like (and is) a cirque basin that holds a lake. The lake sits at 10,148 feet and has a terrific view across its sparkling waters to snow-streaked Standhope Peak, an 11,878-foot mountain that dominates this area. Unfortunately, the lake does not have any fish and its camps are very exposed. You'll be more comfortable if you spend the night in the valley below.

To exit Surprise Valley, go southeast from the lake and head cross-country through a rocky area with a few scraggly whitebark pines and alpine meadows covered with pink and white heather. Your destination is an obvious low point in the ridge northeast of Standhope Peak. After about 0.2 mile of scrambling, you'll come across a surprisingly well-constructed trail that seems to appear from nowhere. Follow this trail as it ascends a series of switchbacks over a very rocky slope, which often has snow patches well into July. The trail tops out at a windy, 11,000-foot pass, which provides excellent views of Surprise Valley to the north, Broad Canyon to the southeast, and numerous unnamed peaks all around.

Warning: This is the highest elevation of any trail described in this book. Take it slow and breathe deeply if you're not yet acclimated.

The trail goes downhill to the left from the pass and soon gives you a view down of lovely Betty Lake in the basin to the southwest. To reach this lake, the trail completes a fairly long, slightly downhill traverse, then makes six short switchbacks that take you down to the bottom of a rocky slope. From there, you wander gradually downhill, following cairns or faint stretches of tread where available, through an area of alpine vegetation with numerous huge boulders (some as big as houses). After a final switchback, the trail drops past a few stunted whitebark pines to the meadow-rimmed shores of Betty Lake. Camping is poor here due to the exposed nature of the lake, but the fishing for cutthroat trout is excellent, and the view of Standhope Peak is superb. If those qualities aren't enough to warrant at least a short stay, then consider a side trip to spectacular Goat Lake. The obvious bootpath climbs the open slopes southwest of Betty Lake, passes a small upper lake, then goes through a low saddle and drops to Goat Lake. This rock-lined gem

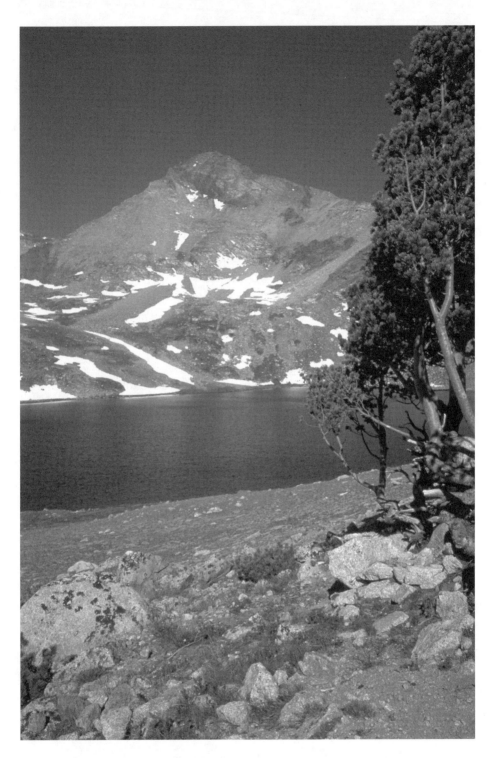

Betty Lake and Standhope Peak

is set in a gorgeous basin beneath a semi-circle of jagged cliffs and mostly unnamed peaks.

The trail down from Betty Lake closely follows the small outlet creek into Broad Canyon. For the most part, this canyon lives up to its name, with a wide bottom and several impressive peaks that rise on either side. About 0.5 mile from Betty Lake, you leave the high meadows, veer away from the creek, and enter pleasantly open forests of Englemann spruce and subalpine fir. You soon pass near a swampy area that is given the generous title of Bench Lake (but which is mostly just a breeding ground for mosquitoes), then rejoin the clear, cascading stream. Several small side creeks join the flow in this area and provide good habitat for wildflowers like bluebells and Lewis' monkeyflowers, which prefer a wet environment.

You make a rock-hop crossing of the creek, then descend steeply through several avalanche chutes, where the trees struggle to reach about 10 feet in height before a new snow slide halts any further upward progress. The avalanches also clear out some lovely, sloping wildflower meadows and bring down large quantities of debris, which makes the path rocky in places. At a particularly attractive meadow, the trail crosses the creek again, this time via a ford or a careful rock-hop.

> **Warning:** *Although the rock-hop looks easy, be sure to use a sturdy stick to test the stability of each rock before you jump. I leaped onto what looked like a large, stable boulder and was rewarded with wet clothes and bruises to my tailbone and ego.*

From this crossing, it's a little less than 1 mile of gentle downhill through lodgepole-pine forests to a junction.

You turn right, following signs for the White Mountains, and immediately cross the creek again, this time on logs. There is plenty of flat ground near this crossing to set up a tent. The trail climbs steeply for the next mile, but the frequent rest stops you'll require are rewarded with nice views through the trees back to Broad Canyon and Standhope Peak. Near the top of the climb, you pass through a small, wet meadow, which usually has a trickle of water through August, then come to a wide, viewless saddle and an unsigned fork. The main trail goes downhill to the left, but you go straight and, 100 yards later, go straight again where another unsigned trail angles in from the left. From here, you briefly lose elevation, cross a tiny creek, then climb to another pass just above an intensely green little meadow with a shallow pond.

Beyond this pass, the trail (shown incorrectly on the Forest Service map) goes southwest beside a tiny creek in a rather steep little gully. You pass a moderate-sized spring, then go through a narrow chasm to where the main branch of Pot Creek joins the flow of your smaller creek. You cross the creek here, then continue downstream to a large, generally flat meadow where you cross the creek again. There are several good campsites in this area.

Now on the north side of Pot Creek, you leave the meadow and descend a moderately steep grade for nearly 1 mile to an easily overlooked and unsigned junction near the edge of Pot Meadow. You go straight, walk another 200 hundred yards to a second junction, then bear right and pass a couple of nice campsites near the lower end of Pot Meadow. Immediately after these campsites is an easy ford of the Little Wood River.

Your next challenge is the long, tough climb up Box Canyon, so take time to rest beside the Little Wood River and stock up on water, because it's a difficult, 2900-foot ascent. The climb is gradual at first, but it soon gets steeper as you make your way up a hillside above a small creek. You cross open slopes with nice views of the high peaks to the southwest, round a small side ridge, then briefly approach the creek before turning back up the canyon and resuming the steady uphill trudge. The climb is relentless and can be tiring, especially on a hot afternoon, but you are rewarded with ever-improving views as you gain elevation.

About two-thirds of the way up from the Little Wood River, you cross a trickling side creek, then turn left and contour briefly before climbing a bit more to the edge of a lovely basin. The ascent gets easier as you slowly curve northwest and follow the creek through rolling meadows in the upper basin of Box Canyon.

A little less than 1 mile after entering these meadows, you come to the headwall of the basin. The trail makes a sharp left turn here and begins the final set of switchbacks to Johnstone Pass. Before climbing these, however, take the time for a short side trip to the north on a sketchy bootpath that climbs over rolling terrain to Upper Box Canyon Lake. This lovely mountain lake, one of the brightest jewels in the Gem State, sits beneath a ring of cliffs and talus slopes and has good fishing. To enjoy this quiet spot in style, spend the night at one of the idyllic campsites amid the wind-sculpted whitebark pines near the lake's south shore.

After returning to the main trail, you make 12 switchbacks up a steep slope of loose talus and scree to 10,000-foot Johnstone Pass. Although only a tiny notch in the ridge, this pass affords extensive views, not only northeast to the canyons and peaks through which you have already traveled, but also west to an entirely new vista – the huge glacial canyon of the East Fork Wood River.

Warning: Nice as the view is, Johnstone Pass is exposed and no place to be when a thunderstorm is approaching.

To reach the East Fork Wood River, you descend a very steep gully of loose sand and small rocks that is easy enough to dig your boot heels into on the way down, but is torture to climb. Fortunately, the steepness of the descent is lessened by two dozen switchbacks and several other twists and turns that could be categorized as switchbacks. Near the bottom, you reach firmer footing and a gentler grade where the trail enters open forests and scenic meadows.

The trail now turns down the canyon and descends through rocky meadows that are swept clear of trees by frequent avalanches. In summer, it isn't snow but waterfalls that streak down the steep walls, adding to the scenic appeal of the area. Also appealing is the view of a tall pinnacle near the head of the canyon. Although this pinnacle didn't look like much when viewed from Johnstone Pass, it is quite impressive from this angle. About 1 mile down the canyon, you cross the creek on a logjam, then continue another mile through sometimes wet meadows and across talus slopes to the roadend trailhead.

Tip: In drier areas near the trailhead look for displays of a particularly striking variety of July-blooming mariposa lily, which has a distinctive purple spot in the middle of each white petal.

POSSIBLE ITINERARY

	Camp	Miles	Elevation Gain
Day 1	Surprise Valley	7	2700
Day 2	Lower Broad Canyon (with side trip to Goat Lake)	7	2000
Day 3	Upper Box Canyon Lake	8	3600
Day 4	Out	5*	600

* This distance may be greater, depending on where you parked.

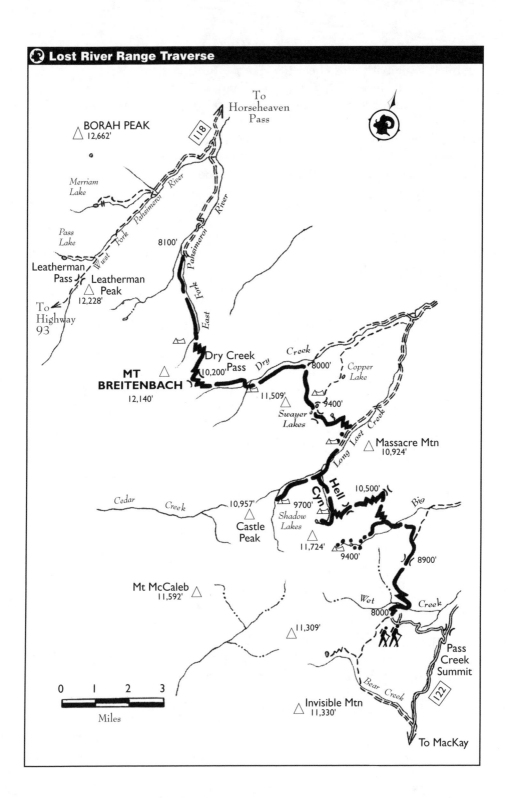

BORAH PEAK
△ 12,662'

To Horseheaven Pass

118

Merriam Lake

Pass Lake

Wust Fork Pahsimeroi River

8100'

East Fork Pahsimeroi River

Leatherman Pass

△ Leatherman Peak
12,228'

To Highway 93

Dry Creek Pass
10,200'

MT BREITENBACH
12,140'

11,509'

Dry Creek

8000'

Copper Lake

9400'

Swayer Lakes

Long Lost Creek

△ Massacre Mtn
10,924'

Cedar Creek

10,957'

△ Castle Peak

9700'

Shadow Lakes

11,724'

Hell Cyn

10,500'

Big

9400'

8900'

Mt McCaleb △
11,592'

11,309'

Wet Creek

8000'

Pass Creek Summit

122

0   1   2   3

Miles

△ Invisible Mtn
11,330'

Bear Creek

To MacKay

20 Lost River Range Traverse

RATINGS (1–10)			MILES	ELEVATION GAIN	DAYS	SHUTTLE MILEAGE
Scenery	Solitude	Difficulty	24*	7300	3-5	67*
10	9	8	(28)*	(8400)	(3-5)	

* The mileage numbers are from the "official" ending point. Since you probably won't be able to drive that far, the actual distance is likely to be somewhat longer for the hike and shorter for the car shuttle.

MAPS USGS - Burnt Creek, Hawley Mountain SW, Leatherman Peak, Massacre Mountain.

USUALLY OPEN Late June to October.

BEST Late June and July.

PERMITS None.

RULES The usual no-trace principles apply. Call ahead about periodic fire restrictions.

CONTACT Lost River Ranger District, (208) 588-3400; Challis Ranger District, (208) 879-4100.

SPECIAL ATTRACTIONS Solitude; outstanding mountain scenery; hiking amid the highest peaks in Idaho.

PROBLEMS Miserable road access; sketchy trail in places; motorbikes on some trails; thin air at high altitudes; in places the route is too dangerous for horses.

HOW TO GET THERE The road access to the ending point at the northwest trailhead is complicated and extremely rough. Drive 23 miles northwest of MacKay on U.S. Highway 93 to a junction with Doublespring Road. Turn right (north) and stay on this good but bumpy gravel road for 10.7 scenic miles, then turn right onto Forest Road 117 at a sign for Horseheaven Pass. This rough dirt road is rather bumpy, but it is passable for almost any car, if you are careful and drive slowly. Exactly 6.3 miles from Doublespring Road is an unsigned junction with Forest Road 118, where you bear right.

Although not, strictly speaking, a jeep road, this is one of those roads that you drive on until sanity finally kicks in and you realize that the potential damage to your car just isn't worth saving a couple of hours of hiking. For the first mile the only problems are that the road is bumpy and has a very high center. Then you come to an ominous sign reading NOT ADVISED FOR TRAILERS AND CARS, which should *really* get you worried. Most passenger cars should pull off the road and park here. This adds about 7 miles to the hike.

Immediately after the sign, the road goes steeply down a very rocky section, then fords shallow Mahogany Creek. On the other side of the creek is an intersection, where you turn left and immediately come to a second junction. The more-heavily-used road to the left is a user-constructed shortcut that goes up a very steep hill, where good ground clearance and four-wheel-drive are just about mandatory. A slightly better choice is to take the bumpy but less steep "official" road that makes a longer loop to the right. These two roads reunite at the top of the hill, after which you bounce along at perhaps 5 miles per hour, a snail's pace that is slowed even further by the need for you to get out from time to time to move some of the more hazardous mini-boulders in your way. About 2.8 miles from Mahogany Creek is a junction just past a small cabin and corral. The West Fork Pahsimeroi Road goes to the right on its way to the Merriam Lake trailhead (a great side trip).

Unless you own a jeep or good SUV, you are almost certainly parked by now. If not, bear left at the junction and, 0.5 mile later, come to a cold, one-foot-deep ford of West Fork Pahsimeroi River. This ford is reasonable on foot, but should definitely *not* to be attempted in most vehicles. After the crossing, the jeep road continues making its bumpy, miserable way along for 2 miles to an unsigned fork. Bear left (downhill) and proceed another 1.5 miles, including a difficult ford of East Fork Pahsimeroi River, to a signed trailhead just before the "road" ends. The reward for this miserable drive is the constant outstanding view of a host of towering, snow-streaked summits.

The starting point at the southeast trailhead has much better road access. To reach it, drive 7.3 miles southeast of MacKay on U.S. Highway 93 to a junction with Pass Creek Road. (Coming from the south, this junction is 19.0 miles north of Arco.) Turn left (north) onto this gravel road and drive 1.2 miles to a junction. Angle slightly right and continue for 7.5 miles on this gravel then good dirt road, which becomes Forest Road 122, to a junction at Pass Creek Summit. Turn left (west), following signs to Loristica Group Campground, and drive 1.9 miles on this reasonably good dirt road to a junction. Keep straight and proceed another 0.3 mile, then park at a gate with a ROAD CLOSED sign.

INTRODUCTION The little-traveled Lost River Range is virtually unknown to hikers outside of Idaho, and even many residents of the Gem State have only a vague concept of where these mountains are. The most popular hike in the range is the route up Borah Peak, which isn't even an established trail. Elsewhere in the range only the occasional intrusion of a noisy motorbike gets in the way of complete solitude for hikers.

The best extended backpacking trip in the range is this rugged traverse that runs northwest from near Pass Creek Pass to the headwaters of the East Fork Pahsimeroi River, where you are smack in the middle of the highest peaks in the state. Along the way are countless open views, lots of wildflowers, and plenty of wildlife.

Although gloriously scenic, significant parts of this trail are so sketchy that much of the walking is effectively cross-country. In addition, junctions are almost never signed and many trails shown on the Forest Service maps either do not exist or are literally miles from where they are indicated. (The USGS maps show no trails at all.) Therefore, this trip is recommended only for experienced hikers who don't mind doing some bushwhacking to follow a poorly signed and rarely traveled route.

Tip: If the winter's snowpack was below or near normal, the best time to take this trip is in mid-to-late June, before the local bovines have been released to "graze" the high meadows.

DESCRIPTION From the southeast trailhead, you walk around the road-closure gate and go 25 yards along a jeep road to an unadorned post marking the start of a trail that angles left. You turn onto this trail and follow it downhill through a selectively logged area to the lush, green meadow holding Wet Creek.

At this point, the USGS map shows no trail at all, while the Challis National Forest map shows the trail going left (southwest) up the canyon of Wet Creek. After hours of difficult bushwhacking, I discovered that this "trail" exists solely in the imagination of some Forest Service cartographer. The actual route goes about 200 yards down Wet Creek, then crosses the creek on an unstable log (or you can make an easy ford). You then go downstream another 100 yards, curve left, and pick up an old jeep road that cuts across the base of a reddish rock outcropping. The trail then climbs the narrow jeep track up a hillside, makes two switchbacks, and heads up a side drainage that goes generally northwest. You turn left off the jeep track where a post has a small but helpful sign stating simply TRAIL.

The trail, which is now easy to follow despite being in the "wrong" place according to the map, climbs at an uneven grade through forests and meadows with fine views of the surrounding mountains. Peak 11,309 to the southwest and another rounded mountain that tops out at over 11,200 feet (there is no specific elevation because it hasn't even been accurately surveyed) dominate the scene. Like most peaks in this remote range, these summits have no names. If you shift your gaze downward to the lower and middle elevations of these peaks, you'll see a wide belt of attractive forests made up of Douglas-firs, Engelmann spruces, and lodgepole and limber pines. The magical scene is completed by the beauty at your feet, where several small meadows and rocky areas come alive in late June and early July with phlox, yarrow, valerian, bistort,

---

▲ Lost River Range: Growing & Changing ▲

Despite being overlooked by the hiking public, the range is both lofty and spectacular. Most of the state's tallest mountains are found in the Lost River Range. In addition to 12,662-foot Borah Peak, the highest summit in Idaho, the range has eight other peaks over 12,000 feet in elevation (most of them unnamed), and a host of summits exceeding 11,000 feet. And there may be more to come, because the Lost River Range is a geologically young range that is still growing. Dramatic evidence of this came on October 28, 1983, with the Borah Peak earthquake, a 7.3 magnitude temblor that raised the mountains – and/or lowered the neighboring Thousand Springs Valley – by as much as 20 feet. The quake also started numerous landslides, left behind an interesting 21-mile-long crack in the ground, and was large enough to disrupt the geysers and hydrothermal activity in Yellowstone National Park 150 miles away.

wallflower, larkspur, lupine, skyrocket gilia, dandelion, alpine buttercup, forget-me-not, and many other wildflowers.

The trail crosses the seasonal flow of a tiny creek, climbs briefly
to an intensely green little meadow, then ascends to a view-packed,
grassy saddle just west of a jagged, reddish rock formation.

*Tip: A side path goes to an excellent viewpoint at the top of this rock
formation.*

The trail disappears briefly here, but you can find it again if you
go directly north through the saddle and descend to the bottom of
an open meadow where the tread becomes more obvious. After losing about 350 feet, you bear left at an unsigned fork, then cross a
small, sagebrush-covered flat and curve to the left.

The trail now makes a downhill traverse across a densely forested hillside and crosses the base of a large rockslide, where pikas
squeak at passing hikers. Shortly after the rockslide, the trail crosses Big Creek, which has reliable water although the name greatly
overstates the creek's size, and climbs very steeply away from the
water up a little gully to the northwest. After quickly gaining about
250 feet, the gully splits and trails follow both branches. As usual in
these mountains, there are no signs to help you determine the correct direction. However, you bear left and continue climbing steeply
for 0.2 mile to another unsigned trail fork.

The main route goes to the right, but for a terrific (and difficult)
side trip, keep straight. This trail soon levels out and gradually
ascends through a low area, where the tread is often obscured by
deadfall and cow paths. Following blazes, you climb left to a low
point in the small spur ridge that separates you from Big Creek,
then go steeply down the other side. The now-quite-faint trail
makes its way back down to Big Creek, where the water disappears
under the porous limestone rocks and the trail stops. Directly ahead
of you is a towering cliff of tilted sedimentary rocks with a crumbly
talus slope at its base.

*Tip: Like many such places in the Lost River Range, this is a good area to
look for fossils of shells, leaves, and other recognizable flora and fauna.*

You follow the rubble-strewn creekbed upstream for about 0.5
mile, go around a rocky knoll, then come to a circular lake near the
head of Big Creek. This small, deep lake is surrounded by spectacular, tan-colored cliffs and rockslides, and is backed by an unnamed

11,724-foot mountain. Unfortunately, lack of flat ground near the lake precludes any comfortable camping. If you want to explore this area further, then scramble up the lake's cascading inlet creek to a stunning upper valley with a spring, flat ground where you can camp, and jaw-dropping views of the towering cliffs and peaks enclosing this little basin.

After this tough but very scenic side trip, return to the unsigned fork above Big Creek and follow the main trail. This path climbs through a rolling, sagebrush-covered meadow, ascends 12 short, steep switchbacks on a partly forested slope, then makes a long uphill traverse to a high saddle just above timberline.

North of this saddle, a gentle slope goes down to an undulating alpine meadow that looks very inviting. But the trail does not go that way. Instead, it turns left and goes up a steep, treeless slope that is covered with lichens, low grasses, and tundra wildflowers. The tread is very faint, but helpful cairns mark almost every turn in a series of switchbacks, which makes the trail easy to follow. You eventually end up just below the top of a nameless 10,535-foot summit. Alpine wildflowers sprinkle this tundra environment and invite you to lie back and enjoy the outstanding views. Rolling Massacre Mountain rises to the north, while the contorted crags of the Lost River Range spread out to the west and south. In the distance to the east is the Lemhi Range, dominated by Bell Mountain and Diamond Peak.

The tread completely disappears on the side of this 10,535-foot mountain. The correct route follows a string of low, strategically placed cairns that lead southwest down to a windy saddle, overlooking the rocky basin that holds the two very stark Shadow Lakes. From the low point at the southwest end of this saddle, the trail descends a talus slope via a series of very steep switchbacks, often across loose scree. The going is quite difficult, because time and lack of maintenance have obliterated many of the switchbacks. It's worth the effort to find them, however, because off the trail it is extremely easy to turn an ankle on the loose rocks. You reach bottom at an unsigned junction in a lovely alpine basin near a wandering creek about 0.2 mile below the Shadow Lakes. The deadend path to the left goes to the lakes, while the trail to the right descends along the outlet creek.

Tip: *The best campsites are in the lower meadow, because those near the lakes are very exposed and rocky. Due to the rocky ground, a free-standing tent is a necessity.*

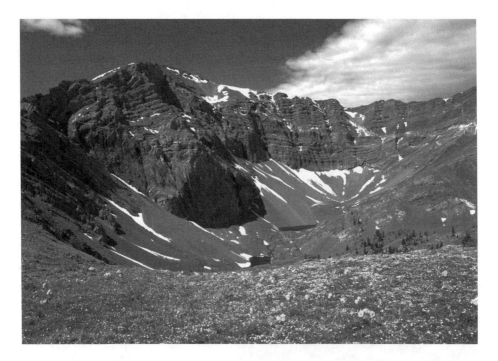

Shadow Lakes from alpine saddle near Massacre Mountain

To continue your trip, follow the sketchy trail along the lake's outlet creek, first through the undulating meadow, then into the forests and down what the map labels as Hell Canyon. If you were coming *up* this increasingly steep trail, that name would probably seem appropriate, but going downhill it's not that bad. The trail can be easy to lose, but it generally stays close to the right side of the creek. After about 1 mile, you make an easy rock-hop crossing of the creek, then drop very steeply through forest to the bottom of Long Lost Creek canyon and an unsigned junction.

The main trail goes right, but if you have an extra hour or two, spend them on a side trip up the trail to the left. This path often has lots of deadfall, but it is easy to follow as it slowly climbs through forests for a little over 1 mile to a lovely meadow in the upper reaches of Long Lost Creek. Wildflowers abound in this rarely visited basin, which is backed by the imposing limestone ramparts of Castle Peak and several unnamed mountains. There are some wonderfully scenic campsites in this area.

From the Hell Canyon junction, the main trail quickly drops to an ankle-deep ford of Long Lost Creek, then follows an undulating,

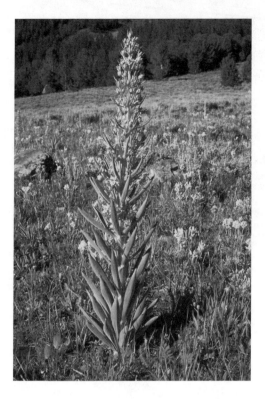

Monument Plant

sometimes rocky course a little above the creek for 0.5 mile to the end of a primitive jeep road. You follow this jeep road across a huge, nearly level meadow that has lots of sagebrush and wildflowers such as phlox, groundsel, owls clover, and the tall spikes of monument plant. The acres of flat ground here make it possible for you to camp almost anywhere here and share an evening with the local coyotes, which hunt for ground squirrels in the daytime and howl during the night. About halfway across the meadow is a junction that, amazingly for these mountains, actually has a sign. The sign tells you that the Swauger Lakes, your next goal, are 2 miles away.

You turn left, leaving the jeep road for a trail that is often used by motorbikes, especially on weekends. One thing you'll immediately notice is that while hiker's trails in this range receive almost no maintenance (and aren't even accurately mapped), this motorbike trail has been very expensively built and is well maintained. The well-constructed route steadily climbs six moderately graded switchbacks over a partly forested hillside to a seasonal trickle of water in a little gully. You then make one more switchback to the base of a rolling, sagebrush-covered meadow and slowly ascend past a little spring to a windswept, 9400-foot high point. From here, the trail curves right and loses about 350 feet of elevation to reach the two small but very scenic Swauger Lakes. There is a fair campsite near the outlet of the upper lake, which gives anglers the chance to spend an evening trying to catch some of the plump cutthroat trout that live here.

A trail built specifically for motorbikes meets your route at Upper Swauger Lake and heads north toward Copper Lake, which is worth a visit if you have the time. Your less-traveled trail goes downhill to the left, passes lower Swauger Lake, then follows a dry creekbed. For the next 2 miles you descend beside this dry creek, crossing its rocky bed several times and sometimes just picking your way along the bottom. A little before the bottom of the canyon, you cross the creekbed a last time and come to a signed junction with the Dry Creek Trail beside a small, marshy pond.

You turn left, walk past the marshy pond, and go up the canyon of misnamed Dry Creek. The trail stays well away from the water for the first 0.5 mile, then gets closer to the clear creek as the canyon gradually curves to the southwest.

Tip: *A waterfall downstream leaves these upper reaches of Dry Creek with no fish, so anglers should not waste their time here.*

Amid the marshes and willow thickets below the trail you can see many beaver dams along the creek. The views across these marshy meadows is stupendous, especially looking toward the head of the canyon, where a massive, snow-streaked wall of mountains is anchored by 12,140-foot Mt. Breitenbach on the right and a string of unnamed 11,000- and 12,000-foot peaks spread out to the left.

The trail crosses a rocky slope, then wanders across a large, gently sloping meadow covered with sagebrush and a sprinkling of wildflowers. After the meadow, you go over a dry creekbed, then splash across a fork of Dry Creek and enter a very green meadow, where the trail disappears. Angle slightly right and pick up the tread again near some good campsites just before an ankle-deep ford of the main branch of Dry Creek.

The sketchy trail turns left after the ford and, about 30 yards later, makes a short but very steep climb to the top of a little ridge bordering the creek. The trail follows the top of this ridge, gradually getting closer to the imposing wall of mountains ahead. The way through that wall is visible on your right at Dry Creek Pass on the northeast shoulder of Mt. Breitenbach.

The way to Dry Creek Pass is indistinct (to say the least), so you will probably lose the trail several times. The pass is usually visible, however, and it's a straightforward scramble to make your way up. Once above timberline, you'll see several paths going up a very steep, rocky slope to the pass. Most of these are game paths, which are indistinguishable from the actual trail. The best advice is to follow whatever route looks to be the easiest.

The views from 10,200-foot Dry Creek Pass make the considerable effort of getting there worthwhile. Tiny alpine wildflowers add color to the scene, but your attention is more likely to be drawn to the splendid views, especially down the U-shaped glacial valley of the East Fork Pahsimeroi River. Equally impressive is the awesome amphitheater created by the semi-circle of 2500-foot-high cliffs on the north wall of Mt. Breitenbach. This is one of the most impressive scenes in all of Idaho.

To descend from Dry Creek Pass, follow the obvious trail to the right (north) as it goes gradually downhill for about 150 yards, then very steeply descends a talus-and-scree slope. More game paths cross your route, but it's usually easy to determine which trail is intended for hikers. Eventually, you enter a whitebark-pine woodland, where frequent blazes help you navigate.

Tip: *The switchbacks through this woodland are easy to miss. The best way to locate a switchback, is to check behind you to see which direction the blazes are cut for uphill hikers to see.*

The last of the steep downhill takes you through the forest just above the bottom of the amphitheater at the head of the East Fork Pahsimeroi River. You can leave the trail here and make an exceptionally scenic camp near the basin floor.

The trail then contours through the trees above the river's rocky gorge and drops to some lovely meadows along the creek. The tread often disappears in these meadows, but a few well-placed cairns help mark the route. About 200 yards after entering the first meadow, you hop over the "river" (just a creek here) and follow the west bank downstream. Although the tread becomes increasingly obvious as you go down the valley, it's still easy to lose the trail, because you will probably be distracted by the excellent scenery.

You pass just above a marshy area with numerous beaver ponds, then hike through a gap in an old, broken-down, wooden fence with a sign that almost laughingly says PLEASE CLOSE THE GATE. Shortly after this fence, you hike past a huge rockslide on the other side of the stream, then go downhill through forest for about 1 mile to a rolling, sagebrush-covered meadow. At the bottom of this meadow you cross a log over the East Fork Pahsimeroi River and immediately come to the northwest trailhead at the end of the jeep road.

If you left a vehicle here, your hike is complete. More than likely, however, you must walk some distance along this very rough road to reach your car. Fortunately, the road walk is not the least bit tedious, because the scenery remains outstanding throughout.

POSSIBLE ITINERARY

	Camp	Miles	Elevation Gain
Day 1	Upper Big Creek Basin	6	2600
Day 2	Swauger Lakes (with side trip up Long Lost Creek)	11	3400
Day 3	Upper East Fork Pahsimeroi River	8	2300
Day 4	Out	3*	100

*This distance will probably be much greater, depending on where you parked.

VARIATIONS This hike presents several options for making rugged but highly worthwhile cross-country side trips. One of the best of these is the scramble over alpine ridges to the top of Massacre Mountain. You should also consider making the bushwhacks up to the high meadows and cirque lakes on the eastern branch of East Fork Pahsimeroi River and up the forks of Dry Creek.

If you have a couple of extra days for hiking and want to avoid the awful road to the northwest trailhead, then you can extend this hike through more wildly scenic terrain to a much-easier-to-reach trailhead. To do this, walk down the jeep road from the northwest trailhead to its junction with the West Fork Pahsimeroi Road. Turn left and hike 3 miles along that road to the trailhead and primitive campground at road's end. From there, follow a signed foot trail that soon crosses two side creeks and comes to the junction with the Merriam Lake Trail, a not-to-be-missed side trip. The main trail goes straight, up the West Fork Pahsimeroi River Canyon, to a junction with the short trail to Pass Lake (another worthwhile side trip), then climbs to the top of windswept Leatherman Pass. From this pass, a steep and often sketchy trail goes down Sawmill Gulch to a trail-head less than 2 miles up a rough spur road directly off U.S. Highway 93.

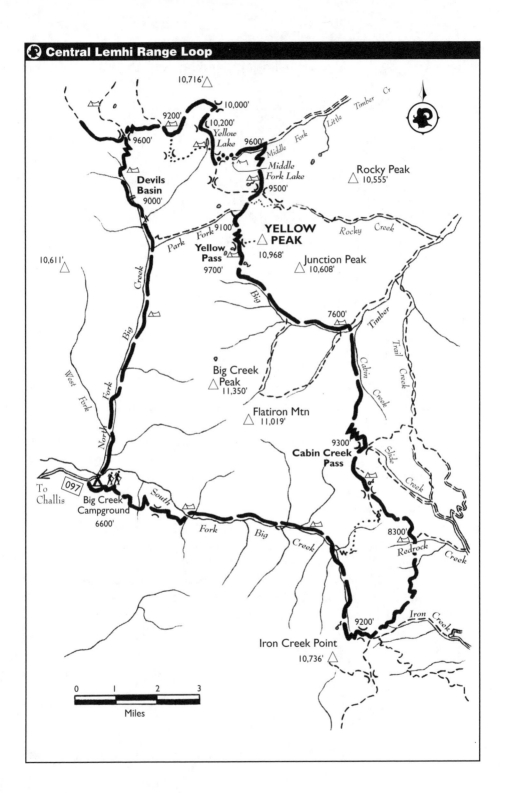

Central Lemhi Range Loop

10,716'

10,000'

9200'

10,200'
Yellow
Lake

9600'

9600'

Middle Fork

Little Timber Cr

Rocky Peak
10,555'

Middle
Fork Lake

Devils
Basin
9000'

9500'

Park Fork 9100'

Yellow
Pass
9700'

YELLOW
PEAK
10,968'

Rocky Creek

Junction Peak
10,608'

10,611'

Big Creek

West Fork

North Fork

Big

7600'

Timber

Cabin Creek

Trail Creek

Big Creek
Peak
11,350'

Flatiron Mtn
11,019'

9300'

Cabin Creek
Pass

Slide Creek

To
Challis

097

Big Creek
Campground
6600'

South

Fork

Big

Creek

8300'

Redrock Creek

9200'

Iron Creek

Iron Creek Point

10,736'

0   1   2   3
Miles

21 Central Lemhi Range Loop

RATINGS (1–10)			MILES	ELEVATION GAIN	DAYS	SHUTTLE MILEAGE
Scenery	Solitude	Difficulty	45	10,300	4-6	N/A
8	9	8	(48)	(10,500)	(4-6)	

MAPS USGS - Donkey Hills NE, Gilmore NW, Patterson SE.

USUALLY OPEN Late June to October.

BEST Late June and July.

PERMITS None.

RULES The usual no-trace principles apply.

CONTACT Challis Ranger District, (208) 879-4321; Lost River Ranger District, (208) 588-3400; Leadore Ranger District, (208) 768-2500.

SPECIAL ATTRACTIONS Solitude; outstanding mountain scenery; abundant wildlife.

PROBLEMS Sketchy trail in places; motorcycles allowed on some trails; potentially difficult stream crossings; new and rerouted trails not shown on the USGS maps.

HOW TO GET THERE From Challis, drive 17.2 miles north on U.S. Highway 93 to a junction at the tiny crossroads community of Ellis. Turn right (southeast) onto a paved county road, following signs for the Pahsimeroi Fish Hatchery, and proceed 30.5 miles to a signed junction with Big Creek Road. (Coming from the south, this turnoff is about 50 miles north of the tiny town of Howe.) Turn left (east) and slowly drive 3.6 miles on this rutted, dirt-and-gravel road to its end at primitive Big Creek Campground. The North Fork Big Creek Trail, which is signed simply trail 075, starts at a T-junction just after a culvert over South Fork Big Creek. Since there is almost no long-term parking at the campground, it is usually better just to park at the signed South Fork Big Creek trailhead at the top of the steep hill 0.2 mile before you reach the campground.

INTRODUCTION To call the Lemhi Range "remote" is a little like saying that the weather in Siberia can get a bit nippy. Hidden behind the already isolated Lost River Range, the Lemhis may be the least known significant mountain range in the lower 48 United States. The nearest city is Idaho Falls, about 100 miles to the southeast, and the outdoor lovers of that town almost always head east to Grand Teton and Yellowstone national parks rather than northwest to the Lemhis. So hikers in the Lemhi Range can expect plenty of solitude, even on holiday weekends. Since few people have even heard of this range, it might be difficult for you to convince potential hiking partners to come along. But persevere in your efforts, because the Lemhis are worth it.

This magnificent loop trip explores a spectacularly scenic part of this range, and does so from a trailhead with reasonably good road access, something of a rarity in these mountains. Wildlife is incredibly abundant in this area. In fact, at times the trail is turned into an obstacle course where it is virtually impossible to avoid stepping in the droppings of elk, deer, mountain goats, moose, and black bears. If you like this trip – and it would be hard not to – then you will probably find yourself joining that small group of devoted individuals who come back to these mountains time and again. You may also want to get involved in the effort to set aside this spectacular part of the Lemhi Range in the proposed Sacagawea Wilderness, a name chosen to honor the extraordinary young Native-American woman who helped guide Lewis and Clark across the continent, and whose branch of the Shoshone tribe lived in the adjacent Lemhi Valley.

> **Tip:** I recommend doing this loop clockwise, especially early in the season, so you can get the most difficult stream crossings done at the start of the trip. This way you still have time to turn around if they look too intimidating.

DESCRIPTION Shortly after the trailhead, you go through a gate, then begin a gradual ascent that always stays close to the lush environment beside North Fork Big Creek. The vegetation is an interesting mix that fills a transition zone between the dry, sagebrush plains of the Pahsimeroi Valley and the wetter, coniferous forests of the Lemhi Mountains. On your left, the stream is crowded with riparian shrubs and trees such as willows and birches, while the open slopes on your right are dominated by grasses and sagebrush. In between are forests of quaking aspen, mountain mahogany, and Douglas-fir. There are also some lodgepole pines in this area, although many of these are dead, having been killed by a bug infestation.

In late June wildflowers are abundant, including the yellow of arnica, the red of paintbrush, the white of yarrow, the blue of lupine, and both red and yellow from columbine.

After about 1 mile, you pass a sign that identifies West Fork Big Creek, which comes down a side canyon on the left. A few yards later, you come to the first ford of North Fork Big Creek. The ford is cold, swift, and well over knee-deep in early summer, but experienced hikers should have little trouble. If the crossing looks too intimidating, you might try scouting around for a log, although the few that span the creek are usually very small and unstable. Now on the west side of the creek, the trail gradually climbs across a series of boulder and talus slopes for a little over 1 mile to the second ford, which is also cold and about knee-deep, but it's a bit easier than the first one.

Having passed these two potential obstacles, you now set out at a carefree pace, gradually gaining altitude through an increasingly dense forest that is dominated by lodgepole pines. The first good campsite comes at about the 4.5-mile point, just before you enter a pretty, creekside meadow. Whether you camp here or not, this is a good spot to rest and try your luck at catching some of the hungry trout that live in North Fork Big Creek. The best fishing is usually in the ponds behind this creek's many beaver dams. Evidence of other wildlife comes in the form of large hoofprints and piles of pelletized droppings in the trail. Although elk are responsible for some of these signs, others are made by moose. On my trip, I was surprised to come face to face with a large, gangly bull moose, who stood for some time just staring at me, perhaps trying to figure out what I was, since so few people hike these trails.

The trail crosses the base of a talus slope, then, at about the 7-mile point, goes across several fairly small branches of Park Fork Big Creek and comes to a junction. If you want a somewhat shorter and easier loop, turn right and climb 3 miles up the valley of Park Fork Big Creek to a junction below Yellow Pass. Hikers who are not accustomed to route finding should take this trail, because the

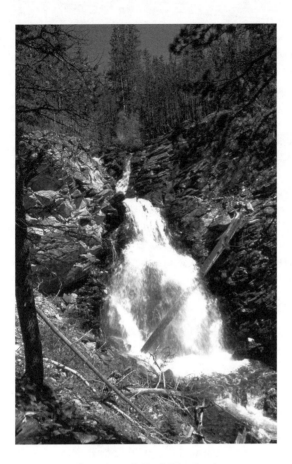
Falls on North Fork Big Creek

recommended route presents some navigation challenges. On the other hand, the trail up Park Fork Big Creek misses both Devils Basin and Yellow Lake, so I recommend that experienced hikers bear left and stick with the main branch of North Fork Big Creek.

Up to now the hike has been fairly easy, but after this junction the grade steepens. Also, the path is sketchy in places (keep an eye out for blazes) and in early summer numerous trickling tributaries cause the tread to be muddy in spots, which makes the going slow and messy. A little less than 1 mile from the Park Fork junction, you ford a tributary creek in the middle of a two-tiered sliding cascade, then cross the main branch of North Fork Big Creek on a log. The forests at this elevation are more interesting than they were below, with some Engelmann spruces and subalpine firs added to the lodgepole pines and Douglas-firs. The scenery has become more interesting as well, because the forests are more open and provide occasional glimpses of the surrounding peaks.

About 1 mile from the last crossing, you pass an impressive waterfall on the main creek, which is worth a short, off-trail detour to fully appreciate. You cross the creek again above the falls, then hop over numerous small creeks that comprise the headwaters of North Fork Big Creek. The last of these crossings comes at the edge of Devils Basin, a gorgeous mountain meadow that must have been named in error, because Satan would never want to be associated with such a heavenly place. The basin is bisected by a clear creek and carpeted with yellow buttercups and white marsh marigolds. The meadow also provides the first complete break in the tree cover, so you can appreciate unobstructed views of the surrounding mountains. There is a very nice campsite on a little rise just after the creek crossing.

The trail disappears shortly after it enters Devils Basin. To relocate it, walk along the right side of the meadow for about 150 yards, then turn onto an obvious path that goes into the trees on the right. This trail is gentle for a short while, then it steeply climbs a rocky slope where your pace is slowed by frequent stops to enjoy the ever-improving views and by the thinner air at this relatively high elevation. The last 0.5 mile of the climb is over a boulder field where the route is marked by occasional cairns.

You top out at a wide, windy, 9600-foot pass, where the harsh environment limits the treelife to only scattered subalpine firs and whitebark pines. Wildflowers are limited as well, to stunted varieties of shooting star and alpine buttercup, mostly in wet areas.

Warning: The trail is easy to lose here, so look carefully for cairns and blazes.

On the left side of this wide pass is a poorly signed junction. The trail that goes sharply left follows a wildly scenic ridgeline and is an excellent side trip, although it may be hard to know when to turn around. Another path, which is not shown on the USGS or Forest Service maps, goes straight, contours for a while, then drops into a scenic basin with a shallow tarn and some decent campsites. This is a good side trip as well, if you don't mind making the steep climb back up to the pass.

Your trail, which is unsigned and the hardest one to locate, goes right and steeply descends a partly forested slope. If you can't find the trail, go downhill to the east over generally open terrain to where the tread becomes a little more obvious in the trees. The trail eventually turns right, levels, and crosses several small snowmelt creeks before intersecting an obvious trail at a junction marked by a cairn.

Tip: The USGS map incorrectly shows this junction about 400 feet lower in elevation.

You turn right on a good trail, then walk gradually uphill for about 350 yards. Here you'll see a sign on a tree 50 yards to the right that points to Big Eightmile Creek in one direction and Timber Creek in the other. There are several good campsites in this area.

The old trail went south from this sign, climbed over a rocky pass, then dropped to Yellow Lake. The somewhat longer new trail, which is not shown on the USGS maps, is much better graded and easier to hike. So, stick with the well-built new trail as it curves up a wide, sub-alpine valley of meadows, rocks, and scattered trees. Directly ahead of you to the northeast is an unnamed, pyramid-shaped peak covered with loose, tan-colored talus and boulders. The path slowly curves to the east around the base of this peak, then climbs to a wide pass. From here, you can see Gunsight Peak to the northeast and look down the scenic valley of North Fork Little Timber Creek.

Instead of going through this pass, the trail turns right and gradually traverses uphill across a rocky slope to a 10,200-foot pass. From this above-timberline location, the trail curves gradually down to the east side of Yellow Lake, a sparkling gem in a grassy cirque surrounded by talus fields and the bare, tan-colored slopes of several nearby ridges and peaks. The beautiful tan color of these mountains is from quartzite, a rock which comprises most of the Lemhi Range. The best campsites are in some clumps of trees near the outlet creek a few hundred yards below the lake.

Tip: *In the evening and morning be sure to check the slopes around Yellow Lake for tiny, misplaced snow patches. If they move, they're mountain goats.*

To exit the Yellow Lake basin, follow the well-maintained trail that gradually climbs the side of the sloping ridge southeast of the lake. After about 0.5 mile, this trail leaves a grove of stunted white-bark pines and presents you with a choice. If you want to stick with the official trail, then continue straight, climb to a high saddle, then descend gradually on a relatively new trail to a junction in the pass above Park Fork Big Creek. For a longer and more scenic alternative, leave the trail where it emerges from the trees and walk a short distance to the left over alpine grasses to an obvious wide pass. Below you to the northeast is the canyon of Middle Fork Little Timber Creek and, in the distance, the Lemhi Valley and the Beaverhead Mountains. Directly below you is enticing Middle Fork Lake, which is your immediate goal.

The way to the lake follows the course of countless thousands of mountain goat hooves on an obvious track that goes down a very

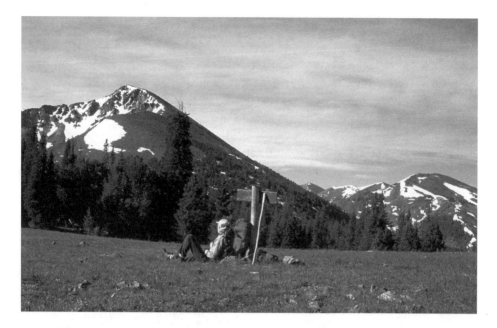

Yellow Peak from 9500-foot pass above Park Fork Big Creek

steep rocky slope. Amazingly, the crafty goats have included a few steep switchbacks. The downhill grade lessens and the track disappears near a grassy spring, but a path is no longer necessary, because it's easy to make your way down from here past a small pond to Middle Fork Lake. On the north side of this scenic lake is a good trail and several excellent campsites.

The trail down from Middle Fork Lake, which is not shown on any map, follows the lake's cascading outlet stream for a little less than 1 mile to an unsigned junction with the Middle Fork Little Timber Creek Trail.

Warning: *This trail is open to motorbikes and ATVs, so it's possible that your peace and quiet will be disturbed by machines.*

You turn right, cross the creek on logs, then steeply climb the wide trail to a pretty little basin with a spring and possible campsites. Black bears and elk both frequent this area, so keep quiet and look for movement in the meadows and near the edge of the forest. The trail goes up a grassy slope above the basin to a 9500-foot pass, where the view to the south is dominated by a striking, orange-yellow peak called, appropriately enough, Yellow Peak. Many other lesser summits are also visible from the pass, but they have no names.

There is a four-way junction at the pass, although the USGS map shows no junction at all. The trail to the right is the trail from Yellow Lake. The trail to the left contours to a wide saddle with a scenic pond, then drops down the canyon of Rocky Creek. Your route bears slightly right, following signs to North Fork Big Creek, and descends through lovely sloping meadows and strips of trees to an unsigned junction with the old trail to Rocky Creek. You go straight and descend a bit more to a junction with the trail down Park Fork Big Creek. This is where the alternate trail that skips Devils Basin and Yellow Lake rejoins your route. You bear left, climb through forest, then skirt a small, rocky basin, and steeply switchback seven times up a talus slope to 9700-foot Yellow Pass.

The view from Yellow Pass presents a whole new panorama of rugged peaks, dominated by Big Creek Peak and Flatiron Mountain to the south. Both of these summits top out above 11,000 feet, which makes them the highest in this part of the Lemhi Range.

Tip: *It is relatively simple for ambitious hikers to make the scramble up open, rocky slopes east of the pass to the top of 10,968-foot Yellow Peak. The commanding views from this summit stretch for hundreds of miles and encompass several nearby mountain ranges and valleys.*

The trail now makes a long descent from Yellow Pass into the curving canyon of Big Timber Creek. Just below the pass is a shallow lakelet with a possible campsite above its northeast shore. The trail then gradually drops past a series of springs in a huge, sloping meadow that is home to a large herd of Rocky Mountain elk throughout the summer months. Observant hikers are almost certain to see some elk, or at least hear their distinctive grunts and high-pitched squeals.

At the bottom of this high meadow, the trail turns left and makes a lovely descent of Big Timber Creek's scenic canyon, generally staying on the slopes above the creek. In the lower canyon, these slopes are open, drier, and covered with sagebrush and a sprinkling of June-blooming wildflowers such as death camas, phlox, lupine, and dandelion. Views are superb from these slopes, especially of Flatiron Mountain and its surrounding ridges. In a particularly large sloping meadow is a signed junction with the upper end of the little-used Flatiron Mountain Trail. You go straight and continue gradually downhill, now mostly in lodgepole-pine forests with a few meadows and aspen glades. Almost 5 miles from Yellow

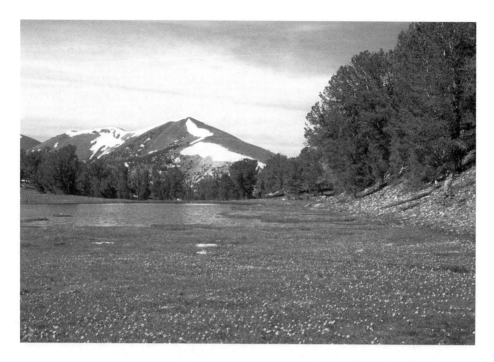

Big Creek Peak over pond below Yellow Pass

Pass, the trail levels and goes through a large meadow to a junction with the lower end of the Flatiron Mountain Trail.

Tip: *There is a comfortable and spacious campsite about 100 yards down the Flatiron Mountain Trail in the trees at the meadow's border.*

Just 200 yards past the Flatiron Mountain Trail is a junction with the Cabin Creek Trail, where you turn right and soon come to a ford of Big Timber Creek. You may be able to find a helpful log in this area, but, if not, the ford is only about 20 feet across and no more than calf-deep.

The Cabin Creek Trail goes upstream beside its namesake creek through attractive forests and small meadows. The ascent is fairly gradual for the first 1.5 miles, then the trail enters a side canyon and starts to climb more seriously. Things ease off again for the next mile as you go through a series of delightful rolling meadows, where the trail has been rerouted to make the grade much more gentle. The trail completes its ascent at a four-way junction in 9300-foot Cabin Creek Pass. An extended rest stop is called for here, not only to recharge your system, but also to enjoy the excellent views looking northwest

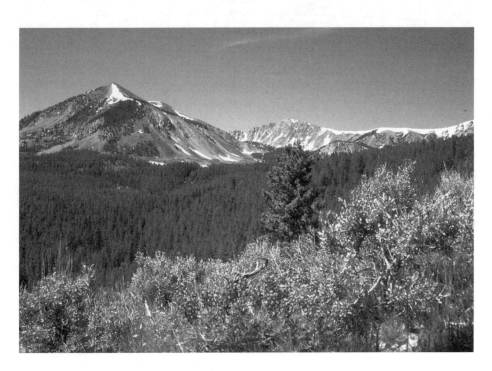

Flatiron Mountain from Big Timber Creek Trail

to Yellow Peak and southeast to an entirely new vista that stretches all the way to towering Bell Mountain.

You turn right at the junction, following signs to Iron Creek, and make a short, steep climb up the shoulder of a hill to an unsigned junction. The trail to the right goes to the top of an unnamed knoll. Your route bears left, traverses the east side of the knoll, then passes through some lovely ridgetop meadows.

Tip: *The trail is easy to lose in these meadows. The correct route crosses the meadow with almost no change in elevation, then picks up again in the woods.*

The trail now gradually descends along the top of a ridge for about 1 mile to an unsigned fork, where you bear right. A few hundred yards past this fork, you travel above a meadow with a small spring and a possible campsite. Unfortunately, cattle often graze in this meadow, which reduces its appeal.

About 0.5 mile past this meadow the trail comes to a saddle and disappears. The only obvious route from here is a game path that angles downhill to the right (west) and goes 0.5 mile to a spring where it deadends. This trail is not shown on any map. The *official* trail, which is very hard to find, goes downhill to the left from the saddle.

Tip: An alternate way to find the official trail is to walk down to the spring, then follow a sketchy game path over a saddle to the east and scramble down the other side until you hit the trail.

For those who don't mind a couple of miles of moderate cross-country travel, there is an alternate route to complete this loop. Take the trail to the spring, then turn right (west) and make your way steeply down through open, creekside meadows and across sagebrush slopes. Whenever possible, try to follow game paths, because experience has taught the animals the best routes. At the bottom of the descent, you enter a steep-sided and heavily wooded canyon where the route gets rugged and quite brushy. Eventually, you hit a switchbacking trail, not shown on the USGS or Forest Service maps, that takes you down to an unsigned junction with the trail along South Fork Big Creek. This cross-country section is all downhill and should only take you a little over 1 hour to complete. Keep in mind, however, that this isolated area is no place to be stranded with a sprained ankle, so never travel alone and do this cross-country section only if you're confident, careful, and experienced.

If you prefer to take the longer, more scenic, official trail (assuming you can find it), then pick up the sketchy route at the saddle and go gradually downhill at an uneven grade across partly forested slopes. One immediately apparent feature of this area is the reddish rock, which here has replaced the tan-colored quartzite and limestone that comprise most of the Lemhi Range. This colorful rock is part of the Challis Volcanic formations and adds greatly to the area's scenic appeal. In honor of this change in geology, the next landmark you come to is Redrock Creek, where there is a junction with a trail that drops to the east. You'll find a possible campsite on the south side of the easy creek crossing.

Having lost about 1300 feet from the knoll above Cabin Creek Pass, the trail now sets about regaining most of that elevation in an irregular ascent that mixes uphill sections with contours and even some downhills. Views are good throughout and keep the hiking interesting. About 0.5 mile beyond Redrock Creek, you hop over an unnamed creek, then go up and down for the next 3.5 miles to a four-way junction below towering Iron Creek Point.

To complete the loop, turn right (west) at the four-way junction below Iron Creek Point and soon cross the trickling headwaters of Iron Creek. The trail then climbs fairly steeply through spacious meadows, gaining a little over 400 feet to a wide saddle. After this, you descend a few switchbacks, pass some springs, then follow an unnamed creek that flows almost directly north on its way to meet South Fork Big Creek. Even though you must cross this creek, or various tributaries, numerous times, it's always easy to keep your feet dry at the crossings. After about 2.5 miles, you intersect an unsigned side trail (the cross-country alternative route) and come to the confluence of your creek with South Fork Big Creek.

Below this junction, the trail travels across a hillside staying just above the creek for 1 mile to a spacious horse camp that is very comfortable but smells badly of equines. If you prefer the aroma of pines and wildflowers, there are many smaller campsites under the trees near the creek.

Beyond the camp, you hop over a side creek, then go around the base of a talus slope of colorful red and tan rocks. Less than 0.5 mile later, you ford or make a slippery rock-hop crossing of an unnamed tributary creek that comes out of a good-sized canyon to the north.

Tip: *You may find a log across this creek hidden in the willows a bit downstream from the trail crossing.*

Almost immediately after this crossing, the trail goes down to a horse ford of South Fork Big Creek. There is no need for hikers to make this ford. Instead, simply scramble a few yards to the right and pick up an obvious trail across a crumbly talus slope. Horses cannot safely negotiate this slope, but hikers should have no problem. After about 200 yards, the horse trail fords the creek again and rejoins your route.

Iron Creek Point Lookout

If you're feeling ambitious, go straight at the junction below Iron Creek Point and hike 1 mile to a second junction. Turn right and climb steadily to the lookout site atop 10,736-foot Iron Creek Point. As with all lookout sites, the views from here are exceptional, including almost the entire southwest side of the Lemhi Range and the broad expanse of the Pahsimeroi Valley to the west. You can even pick out Borah Peak, the highest mountain in Idaho, in the Lost River Range to the southwest.

Below these fords, the trail travels through a grove of willows and aspens, where you'll probably notice that many of the young trees have been chewed through and hauled away by beavers. You then go up and down through a mix of wet meadows and dense riparian shrubbery, and across rocky slopes covered with sagebrush and wildflowers. Although the landscape is very pleasant, it's not as wildly scenic as the high county earlier in the trip. Less than 0.5 mile after leaving the last large sagebrush-covered slope, the trail drops to a nice campsite and a ford of South Fork Big Creek. The easy ford is only calf-deep and the cold water feels great on a hot afternoon.

After the ford, the trail climbs steeply beside a tiny tributary, the banks of which are crowded with 3-foot-tall bluebells, then contours for 0.5 mile and steeply climbs to a sagebrush- and grass-covered saddle with good views.

Tip: For even better views, wander a short distance north to the top of a knoll directly overlooking the steep canyon of South Fork Big Creek.

You descend one long switchback to the bottom of the next side canyon, which contains a trickling creek, then make a final, tough, sun-exposed climb. At the top of a spur ridge, you level off, travel through forest for a few hundred yards, then leave the trees and enjoy a superb view of the Pahsimeroi Valley and the Lost River Range. The last 0.5 mile winds down open, view-packed slopes to the South Fork Big Creek trailhead.

POSSIBLE ITINERARY

	Camp	Miles	Elevation Gain
Day 1	Devils Basin	10	2500
Day 2	Yellow Lake (with side trip out ridge west of the pass above Devils Basin)	8	1900
Day 3	Lower meadow on Big Timber Creek	10	1700
Day 4	South Fork Big Creek Canyon	13	3200
Day 5	Out	7	1200

VARIATIONS As mentioned in the text, you can shorten this loop by about 6 miles, and avoid some of the most sketchy trails, by taking the Park Fork Big Creek Trail directly up from North Fork Big Creek to Yellow Pass.

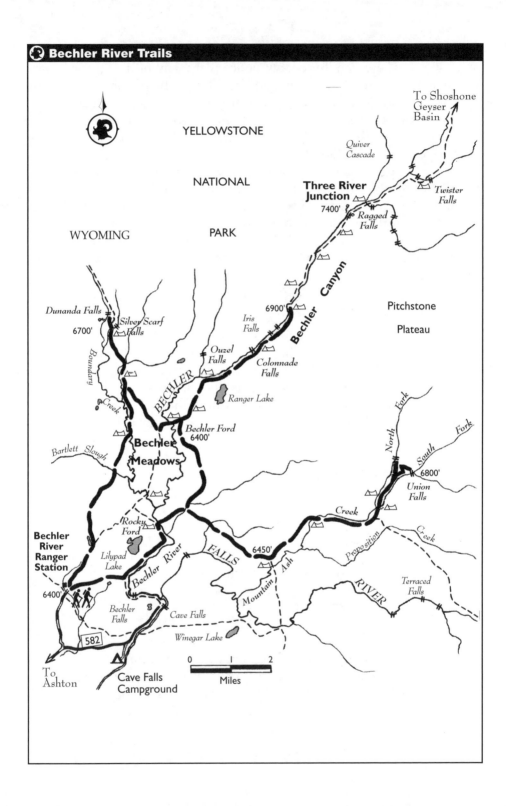

22 Bechler River Trails

RATINGS (1–10)			MILES	ELEVATION GAIN	DAYS	SHUTTLE MILEAGE
Scenery	Solitude	Difficulty	41	1700	3-5	N/A
7	3	3*				

* Except for the fords, which can be very challenging.

MAP Trails Illustrated - Old Faithful and SW Yellowstone National Park.

USUALLY OPEN July 15 to October.

BEST Late August to early October.

PERMITS Yes. Only a limited number of permits are available. The surest way to get the campsites you want is with a reservation. For a fee, you can reserve a permit in advance by writing to: Backcountry Office, Box 168, Yellowstone National Park, WY 82190.

RULES Camping is allowed only at designated sites. Campfires are prohibited except in established fire pits at some campsites. For the safety of yourself, other hikers, and the bears, you are legally required to keep a clean camp; to properly hang all food, garbage, and other odorous items; and to report any aggressive bear activity. Anglers are required to have a special Yellowstone fishing license.

CONTACT Yellowstone National Park, Backcountry Office, (307) 344-2160. (Ask specifically for the informative brochure entitled *Backcountry Trip Planner.*)

SPECIAL ATTRACTIONS Waterfalls; wildlife.

PROBLEMS Bears - both grizzly and black; several difficult stream crossings, especially before August; flooded areas in Bechler Meadows in early summer; clouds of mosquitoes from June through early August.

HOW TO GET THERE From Idaho Falls, drive 53 miles northeast on U.S. Highway 20 to a junction in the town of Ashton. Turn right (east) on State Highway 47, following signs to Mesa Falls Scenic Byway, and drive 1.0 mile to a junction just east of town. Go straight, staying on Highway 47, and drive another 5.2 miles to a junction with Cave Falls Road. Turn right (east) on this paved road, which turns to gravel after 5.8 miles and becomes Forest Road 582. Exactly 16.6 miles from Highway 47 is a junction immediately after the sign marking where you enter Wyoming. Turn left and drive 1.5 miles to the trailhead parking area beside the Bechler River Ranger Station. If you don't already have a reservation, you can pick up a back-country permit at this station, which opens at 8 A.M.

INTRODUCTION If you like the sight and sound of falling water, then you've hit the mother lode, because waterfalls are the prime attraction in this quiet corner of Yellowstone National Park. Sometimes called "Cascade Corner," this compact area contains well over half of the park's waterfalls. The beauty and variety of the dozens of waterfalls here more than compensate for the lack of geysers, mud pots, and roadside bears, which have combined to make other parts of the park so famous. If the many accessible waterfalls aren't enough, adventurous hikers can spend weeks happily bushwhacking to the numerous cascades hidden in side canyons or on isolated sections of the main streams that the trails do not reach.

Although visitors to the Bechler (pronounced Bek-ler) River country may be sorry to miss Yellowstone's famous geysers, they will be glad to be rid of the crowds, for which Yellowstone is also famous. Although the trails here certainly aren't deserted, the number of visitors is only a tiny fraction of what it is in other parts of the park.

> *Warning:* *Both grizzly and black bears are present in this part of Yellowstone National Park. Although grizzly bears are uncommon here, you need to plan for their presence and act accordingly. See page 12 for more information on traveling in grizzly country. Black bears, though not as aggressive as their larger cousins, can be dangerous, and these smaller bruins are quite common in the Bechler River area. Park rangers strictly enforce the rules which require that hikers properly hang their food and other odorous items from the wires provided at all designated campsites any time they are away from camp, even for a few minutes.*

The only road access to this area is from Idaho, so even though these trails are actually in the state of Wyoming, logic dictates that this trip is properly classified as an *Idaho* hike.

This hike is strictly for those who don't mind getting their feet, calves, knees, thighs, and maybe even waist wet. To enhance the area's wild character, the Park Service has removed most of the trail bridges, which forces hikers to make numerous wet and potentially dangerous fords of the Bechler River and its tributaries. Bring a walking stick and wading shoes for improved stability at the crossings, and save this trip for late summer when water levels are lower. Unfortunately, the waterfalls are marginally less impressive at that time, but it beats drowning.

DESCRIPTION The Bechler Meadows Trail, which is marked only with a small metal sign, begins at the northeast end of the complex of historic buildings around the Bechler River Ranger Station. After 100 yards, the trail crosses a trickling creek on a log bridge and reaches a junction. If Union Falls is your first destination, then turn right and walk a nearly level trail through open forests of lodgepole pine with grasses, huckleberries, and various wildflowers on the forest floor. After 1 mile, you pass a large meadow with a shallow, lily-pad-filled lake at its center, then come to a junction beside the slow-moving waters of Bechler River.

You turn left, following signs for Rocky Ford, and closely follow the glassy river upstream. By late summer, which is the best season to take this hike, most of the wildflowers in this area are long past, but there should still be a few yellow goldenrod and blue harebells in bloom. Unlike the flowers, birds are common throughout the hiking season, especially woodpeckers and various small songbirds. As for larger birds, you are likely to see great blue herons, ospreys, and, if you are really lucky, you might even see a goshawk swoop down and catch an unlucky duck off the river.

> *Tip:* In the stream itself are plenty of rainbow and cutthroat trout, but if you want to try to catch any of them, you'll need a special Yellowstone fishing permit and barbless hooks, because the river is managed strictly for catch-and-release fishing.

The trail follows the Bechler River for 2 miles to a junction, where you turn right and immediately face the prospect of going across 100-foot-wide Rocky Ford. In early summer this crossing can be extremely treacherous, but by late summer it's only a little over knee-deep. The water is *always* cold, however, and slippery rocks make the footing difficult, so be careful. The best place to ford is about 30 feet downstream from here.

The trail leaves the river at Rocky Ford and wanders across somewhat drier terrain covered with a nice mix of open forests and grassy meadows. Just under 1 mile from the ford is a junction with the Mountain Ash Creek Trail, where you bear slightly right and walk 0.5 mile to a flat-topped log over a small creek at the edge of a beautiful, grassy meadow. The trail then goes through gently rolling terrain covered with lodgepole-pine forests, a few quaking aspen trees, and dry meadows that are sparsely vegetated with scattered wildflowers and some sagebrush. Eventually, you come to a large meadow and a junction with a dusty, heavily used trail coming from the south.

You bear left, still following signs to Union Falls, and walk 1 mile to a junction with a short side trail to Camp 9U2. About 200 yards past this turnoff is the tricky, knee-deep ford of swift-flowing Mountain Ash Creek. In 2002 there was a rather precarious log over this creek a little upstream from the ford, but its future seemed pretty doubtful, so you should expect to get wet. Right after the crossing is Camp 9U3, a primitive, low-impact site, where fires are prohibited.

To continue on to Union Falls, walk gradually up Mountain Ash Creek through increasingly wet forests and meadows that now include more Engelmann spruces and Douglas-firs as well as wildflowers such as coneflower and monkshood. Although the flora has changed, the terrain remains nearly flat, so you may start to wonder how such a gentle landscape can have so many waterfalls. The answer lies a short distance to the north, where a line of rocky cliffs marks the edge of the Pitchstone Plateau. It is over these cliffs that the falls drop.

About 1.5 miles from the ford of Mountain Ash Creek is a junction. You bear slightly left and walk 0.5 mile to a junction with a side trail to comfortable Camp 9U4 and a ford of South Fork Mountain Ash Creek.

Tip: *To keep your feet dry, simply walk 60 yards up the side trail to the camp, then cross the creek on a flat-topped log.*

After the crossing the trail goes 150 yards up the peninsula of land between the north and south forks of Mountain Ash Creek to

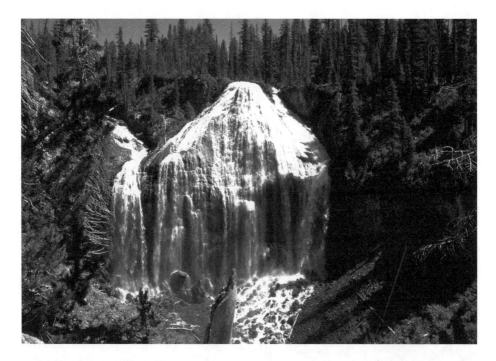

Union Falls

the tiny, A-frame building at the Union Falls Ranger Station. The trail then passes the turnoff to Camp 9U5 and gradually climbs 1 mile on a sometimes-sandy tread to a trail fork.

Both forks of this deadend trail are worth taking. For more subtle scenery, take the left fork, which leads 0.5 mile up North Fork Mountain Ash Creek to a small, cascading waterfall and a nice swimming hole. The more spectacular right fork climbs two switchbacks to an overlook of 260-foot-high Union Falls, a broad veil of water that will take your breath away.

To see more of Yellowstone's waterfalls, return to the junction northeast of Rocky Ford and turn right (north) on the Bechler River Trail. This trail goes a few hundred yards through a meadow to a slow-moving creek, which you cross either on an unstable log or by a simple, knee-deep ford. A short walk through shady forest then takes you to a second creek crossing, this time on a larger, more stable log. After this, the trail climbs 200 feet up a small ridge, then goes up and down on a mostly wooded hillside, where several small, splashing creeks provide water and nice places to rest. After 1 mile on this hillside, you lose a bit of elevation, then walk beside the gently meandering Bechler River to a junction and your next choice of destinations.

To see Bechler Canyon, turn right at the junction and walk through a northeast extension of grassy Bechler Meadows to Camp 9B3. The trail leaves the meadows here and wanders through forests for 0.5 mile back to the banks of Bechler River at very attractive Camp 9B4. If you look north through the trees here you can see impressive, 235-foot-high Ouzel Falls, which drops over a cliff on the other side river. Unfortunately, a tricky river ford and a large marshy area prohibit easy access to the base of this falls.

The trail now follows the river upstream into beautiful, cliff-lined Bechler Canyon, which is a haven for some of Yellowstone's most charismatic wildlife. Don't be surprised to see black bears, which typically take a look at you, give a dismissive huff, then go about their business. Or you could see moose, which are remarkably nonchalant and obligingly allow hikers to take their picture, as long as you don't get too close and make these large and potentially dangerous animals nervous.

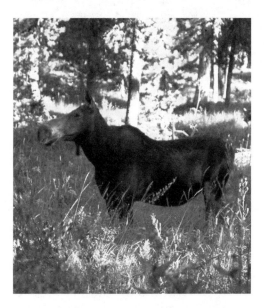

Moose near Bechler Meadows

In addition to wildlife and beautiful scenery, Bechler Canyon features unusually lush vegetation. The Bechler River area is the wettest part of Yellowstone National Park, because winter storms, which normally come from the southwest, dump their precipitation here first. The result of all this moisture is a dense forest of large Douglas-firs and Engelmann spruces with a thick understory of mountain ash, buffaloberry, horsetails, and gooseberry. The fern-lined trail also passes many wildflowers, including birchleaf spiraea, coneflower, monkshood, Queen Anne's lace, grass of parnassus, and a tall, white aster. In the latter half of August you can feast on both thimbleberries and huckleberries, although you'll be in competition with the bears for these tasty treats.

The trail closely follows the clear river upstream, often passing between the river and some large talus slopes where cute little pikas can often be seen and heard. Despite the rugged terrain on both sides of the narrow canyon, the trail manages to remain remarkably gentle as it stays in the shady forest beside the river. Not quite 2 miles from where it started up the canyon, the trail climbs more noticeably and you soon hear the thunderous roar of the canyon's first major cataract, Colonnade Falls. A 100-yard side trail descends to a dramatic overlook of this two-part falls, the lower half of which is a broad sheet of water that drops over a cliff into a basalt amphitheater. A short distance above Colonnade Falls is very inviting Camp 9B5. This is an exceptionally nice place to spend the night, because not only is Colonnade Falls nearby, but just 400 yards upstream from this camp is Iris Falls. On sunny afternoons this wide falls produces a lovely rainbow in its mist.

For the next mile above Iris Falls the river drops over a series of beautiful, gently sloping cascades. The trail provides lots of good views of these cascades as it gradually climbs to Camp 9B6 and, shortly thereafter, a knee-deep river ford over slippery rocks. This is far enough for most hikers, because in addition to this ford, you must make another one about 1 mile upstream, then climb 2 more miles before you reach the next major highlight at Ragged Falls. If you are willing to make the hike, however, the rewards are great, including a series of hot springs, the impressive rock formation of Batchelder Column, and Three River Junction, where the three main forks of Bechler River all converge. If the sight of Ragged Falls inspires you to keep going, then continue fairly steeply uphill for 1.5 miles to the spinning drop of Twister Falls. Above this falls the trail gets more gentle and you leave the lush canyon environment in favor of the drier, lodgepole-pine forests that dominate most of Yellowstone National Park. Really ambitious hikers can keep going another 12 miles to Shoshone Geyser Basin and, from there, on to Old Faithful.

Having explored the wonders of Bechler Canyon, return to the junction at the edge of Bechler Meadows and bear right (west) toward your next major destination, Dunanda Falls. You soon go past a side trail to Camp 9B2 and, immediately thereafter, reach

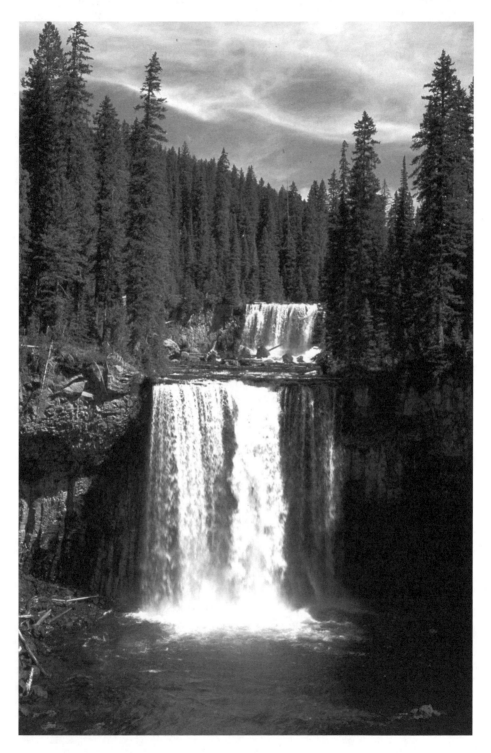

Colonnade Falls

thigh-deep Bechler Ford. This is one of the easiest major fords on this trip, because the water is slow moving and the sandy bottom provides good footing. The meadows near Bechler Ford are a good place to look for moose and sandhill cranes.

The trail immediately leaves the river and crosses part of expansive Bechler Meadows, where you can look south across the waving fields of grass to the jagged spires of the distant Teton Range.

> **Warning:** *In early summer, much of Bechler Meadows is flooded with a foot or more of water, which makes travel difficult and provides a breeding ground for an enormous population of voracious mosquitoes. The flying vampires don't completely disappear until sometime in September, so come prepared with bug repellent, long sleeves, and maybe even a headnet.*

About 0.5 mile from Bechler Ford is a junction, where you turn sharply right and walk 2 miles through meadows and forested terrain to a junction at the edge of a small meadow. Turn right and walk 600 yards through the meadow to a knee-deep ford of a branch of Boundary Creek. Immediately after the ford is the side trail to the designated backpacker area for Camp 9A2.

> **Tip:** *If you want to avoid the ford, walk about 75 yards downstream to a log across the creek, then return on the trail from the backpacker's camping area.*

After the creek crossing, the trail goes gradually uphill for 1 mile through a 1995 burn area that is now covered with fields of bracken fern, sunflowers, and small lodgepole pines. You splash across several small creeks, then reenter unburned forests and take a narrow log over a larger side creek. The trail soon passes a side trail to Camp 9A3, climbs steeply past the tall, flowing cascade of Silver Scarf Falls, then comes to a junction, where the Boundary Creek Trail goes steeply uphill and right.

To see Dunanda Falls, bear left and walk 200 yards to the top of this wide sheet of water, which drops into a scenic canyon of dark-gray rock. A very steep scramble route drops to the base of the falls, where you can soak for hours in an idyllic hot-springs pool looking up at the spectacular, 110-foot falls and the rainbow it creates on sunny days. Life just doesn't get much better than that!

To return to the Bechler River Ranger Station, go back to the junction just south of Camp 9A2 and bear right (south) on the Boundary Creek Trail. This nearly level route travels through forest,

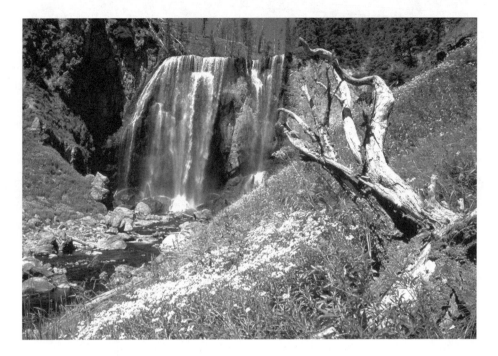

Dunanda Falls

then goes through the grassy, wildlife-rich area between the forest and the willow thickets beside slow-moving Boundary Creek. Moose and beaver are common in this environment. After about 1 mile, you leave this life zone and cross the western part of Bechler Meadows to a calf-deep ford of Boundary Creek. Signs direct you to the best place to ford, which is about 100 yards downstream from here. Right after the ford is scenic Camp 9A1 in a clump of trees near a lazy meander in the creek.

You go south from Camp 9A1 past a series of small tree islands amid the vast expanse of Bechler Meadows. You are likely to see at least a couple of pairs of tall sandhill cranes in this area, either feeding in the meadow or flying overhead and croaking out their loud, guttural call. Less than 1 mile from the Boundary Creek crossing is a ford of Bartlett Slough, a stagnant backwater filled with lily pads. The slough can be up to 4 feet deep in early summer, but is usually only thigh deep by August.

> **Tip:** The bottom of Bartlett Slough is very muddy. Be sure that your wading shoes are securely tied, so they don't get sucked permanently into the goo.

After this crossing, the trail follows a gently rolling course through lodgepole-pine woods, skirts a few small meadows, then passes a lily pond to a junction with the Bechler Meadows Trail. You bear slightly right and wander through open woods on a generally flat trail back to the junction just 100 yards east of the Bechler River Ranger Station.

POSSIBLE ITINERARY

	Camp	Miles	Elevation Gain
Day 1	Camp 9U4 - below Union Falls (with side trip to Union Falls)	13.5	400
Day 2	Camp 9B5 - above Colonnade Falls (with side trip up Bechler Canyon)	12	600
Day 3	Camp 9A3 - below Dunanda Falls	7.5	500
Day 4	Out	8	200

VARIATIONS If you have some extra time and feel that a trip to Yellowstone just isn't complete unless you see a geyser, then continue up the Bechler Canyon Trail all the way to the Shoshone Geyser Basin. Since this area is too far away from the Bechler Canyon campsites for a comfortable dayhike, you will need an overnight permit to stay at a nearby campsite, something that is nearly impossible without advance reservations.

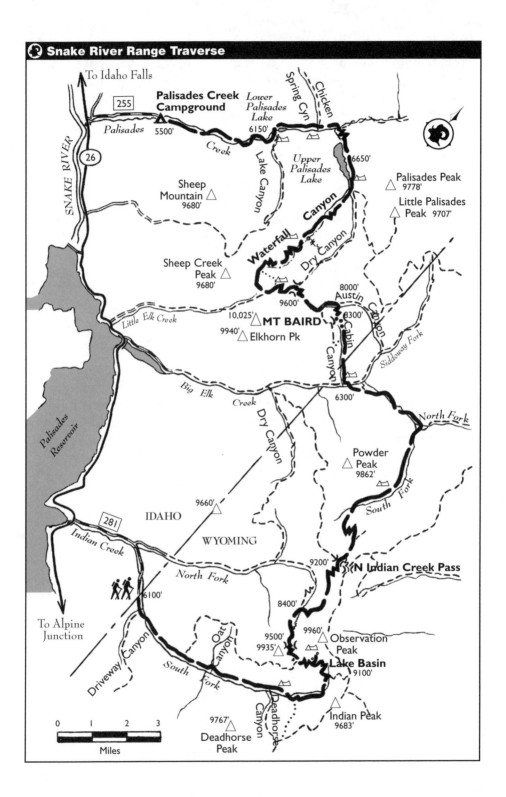

Snake River Range Traverse

To Idaho Falls

255
Palisades Creek Campground 5500'

Palisades Creek

SNAKE RIVER

26

Lower Palisades Lake

Spring Cyn

Chicken

6150'

Upper Palisades Lake

6650'

Lake Canyon

Sheep Mountain 9680'

Palisades Peak 9778'

Little Palisades Peak 9707'

Waterfall Canyon

Dry Canyon

Sheep Creek Peak 9680'

9600'

8000'

Austin Canyon

Little Elk Creek

10,025' MT BAIRD

9940' Elkhorn Pk

8300'

Cabin Canyon

Siddoway Fork

Big Elk Creek

6300'

North Fork

Palisades Reservoir

Dry Canyon

Powder Peak 9862'

South Fork

281

IDAHO

9660'

Indian Creek

WYOMING

North Fork

9200'

N Indian Creek Pass

6100'

To Alpine Junction

8400'

Oat Canyon

9500'

9960'

Observation Peak

9935'

Lake Basin 9100'

Driveway Canyon

South Fork

Deadhorse Canyon

Indian Peak 9683'

9767'
Deadhorse Peak

0   1   2   3
Miles

23 Snake River Range Traverse

RATINGS (1–10)			MILES	ELEVATION GAIN	DAYS	SHUTTLE MILEAGE
Scenery	Solitude	Difficulty	45	9800	3-6	19
8	6	8				

MAPS USGS - Alpine, Ferry Peak, Mt. Baird, Observation Peak, Palisades Peak, Teton Pass, Thompson Peak.

USUALLY OPEN Mid-June to Mid-October.

BEST Mid-July; late September to early October.

PERMITS None.

RULES The usual no-trace principles apply.

CONTACT Palisades Ranger District, (208) 523-1412.

SPECIAL ATTRACTIONS Fall colors; great wildflower displays; wildlife.

PROBLEMS Several moderately difficult stream crossings; mosquitoes in July; motorbikes allowed in the Indian Creek area; sketchy trail in places; several long, dry, steep climbs.

HOW TO GET THERE Start by driving 50 miles southeast of Idaho Falls on U.S. Highway 26 to a signed junction with Palisades Creek Road. To leave a car at the north trailhead, turn left (northeast) on this oiled gravel road, following signs for Palisades Creek Campground, and drive 2.1 miles to the campground and well-developed trailhead. Horse trailers and livestock facilities dominate the trailhead area, so the best parking for hikers is in a gravel lot just before the bridge over Palisades Creek.

To reach the recommended starting point, continue southeast on Highway 26 for 13.7 miles past the Palisades Creek turnoff, then turn left (east) onto Forest Road 281 at the head of a large inlet in Palisades Reservoir. Proceed 1.9 miles on this narrow gravel road to a fork near the confluence of North and South forks Indian Creek.

Go straight, staying on the better road, and drive 1.6 miles to the South Fork Indian Creek trailhead, where a fence line marks the border with Wyoming.

INTRODUCTION The Snake River Range contains the most jagged peaks, the prettiest lakes, and the best fishing streams of any mountains in southeast Idaho. The range is at its scenic best in mid-July, when the meadows are ablaze with colorful wildflowers, and again in late September and early October, when the hillsides are covered with the yellow, orange, and red of aspens, cottonwoods, and maples. Regardless of the season, wildlife is a common sight along the trails, including elk, moose, and black bear. There are even reports of an occasional stray grizzly bear, although they are so rare hikers don't need to take any special precautions.

Although much of this hike is in Wyoming, it is categorized as an Idaho trip, because the road access and both trailheads are in that state.

It is better to start this hike from the south trailhead, especially if you begin on a weekend, because the popular north trailhead is often very busy then. This also allows you to benefit from a net elevation loss of 600 feet. This hike includes several relentless uphills that have no water or shade. Avoid this trip during a spell of hot weather.

DESCRIPTION From the east end of the trailhead parking lot, you cross the fence at the state line, then walk along a jeep road for 100 yards to the start of the trail. This route is open to motorbikes, so the path is wide, dusty, and can be noisy. Apart from the motorbike problems, the hiking is very pleasant, as the trail goes upstream beside lovely South Fork Indian Creek through a lush mix of grasses and tall wildflowers such as coneflower and cow parsnip. The tree cover includes both evergreen and deciduous species, especially Engelmann spruces, Douglas-firs, quaking aspens, and narrowleaf cottonwoods.

About 0.5 mile from the trailhead, you bear left at a junction with the Driveway Canyon Trail and, 200 yards later, come to a crossing of South Fork Indian Creek. On a hot afternoon during the June snowmelt this stream can be a raging torrent, but by mid-July it's no more than ankle deep. There may even be a convenient log over the flow. Now on the north side of the creek, the trail goes

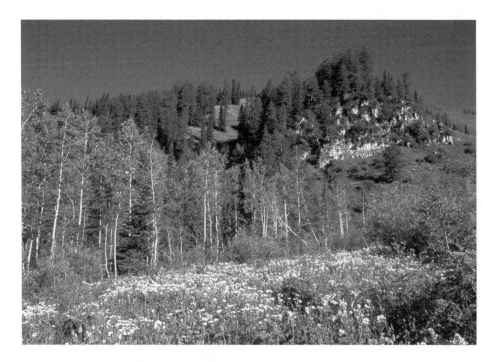

Along South Fork Indian Creek near Oat Canyon

gradually uphill, either traveling close to the creek's bank amid lush, riparian vegetation or crossing rocky slopes a little above the water. These drier slopes feature a different mix of colorful wildflowers, including skyrocket gilia, groundsel, yarrow, aster, pink geranium, birchleaf spiraea, and harebells.

With every added mile the scenery becomes more dramatic, as you pass through increasingly large avalanche meadows that provide ever-improving views of the high peaks on either side of the canyon. In late September, the quaking aspens trees that rim these meadows put on an impressive display of color.

> **Warning:** *The avalanche meadows encountered along this trip are often filled with stinging nettles. Wear long pants and be careful what you brush up against.*

At one of the largest of these meadows, about 3 miles from the trailhead, an easily overlooked sign marks a junction with the Little Oat Canyon Trail, a faint path that angles left. You continue straight and for the next 2 miles climb through brushy avalanche meadows crossed by a series of small side creeks that splash down from the

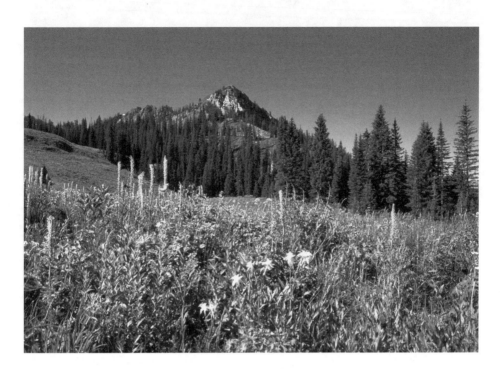

Near Cabin Creek canyon

high ridge to the north. In addition to wildflowers, the meadows are home to many deer and, in early summer, it is common to come across a small, spotted fawn squeaking out an alarm call at your arrival. The meadows are also excellent habitat for black bears, so keep an eye out for them.

About 5 miles from the trailhead the meadows are broken by strips of trees, which give you a chance to rest in the shade. This opportunity is welcome, because the grade of the climb picks up in this area and you'll really start to feel that heavy pack on your back. At the 6.5-mile point is a junction with an unsigned and little-used trail up Deadhorse Canyon, a grassy defile to the south that is worth exploring if you have the time. Just after this junction you enter a small strip of forest with a good campsite. About 200 yards beyond the campsite is the second crossing of South Fork Indian Creek.

Warning: *Although it looks like an easy rock-hop crossing, the rocks here are very slippery; it is much safer to make the ford.*

The trail then makes a short climb away from the crossing and soon comes to a junction with the abandoned Cabin Creek Trail.

This sketchy path ascends a beautiful sloping meadow that provides good views up to several nearby rocky peaks. In July, however, your attention is more likely to be drawn to the meadow's abundant wildflowers. Look for great displays of pink geranium, locoweed, giant hyssop (a member of the mint family), wild carrot, lousewort, and a large, white variety of columbine.

The main trail goes straight at the Cabin Creek junction and continues its moderately steep ascent, mostly through spacious, rolling meadows. Just before South Fork Indian Creek makes a sweeping curve to the north, you cross the now-small stream a final time, then make a single switchback and resume the long, shadeless climb. The trail passes to the right of some low cliffs, then makes an easy ascent to a junction with the Indian Peak Trail. You turn left and climb through a gently rolling meadowland to the delightful Lake Basin. This large, flowery expanse is backed by Observation Peak to the north and features two medium-sized ponds set in grassy basins above the trail. Obvious bootpaths lead to these ponds, and there are good campsites in the trees near each of them. The campsites near the larger pond to the north are better and more scenic.

Tip: From a base camp in this basin you can make a terrific dayhike up the Indian Peak Trail to the high ridgeline of the Snake River Range. From there, you can follow view-packed routes to the tops of both Indian and Observation peaks.

To exit Lake Basin, the trail turns west, switchbacks three times to the top of a small ridge, then makes a gradual downhill traverse to an obscure junction near a small pond in a scenic basin. You bear right and make a short, steep climb to a 9500-foot pass. From this high vantage point you can not only look south to South Fork Indian Creek canyon, but also north to the rugged peaks and valleys that you'll be traversing for the rest of this trip.

The sometimes-obscure trail now makes an uneven descent across lovely, rolling meadows for about 1.5 miles to a bubbling spring next to an elaborate hunter's camp. This camp is reserved for use by a commercial outfitter from late August to November, but at other times you are allowed to camp here.

Warning: The camp has piles of horse manure and lots of flies, so backpackers probably won't want to stay here.

There is a confusion of horse trails around this camp. The correct route stays below the main camp and follows a little creek

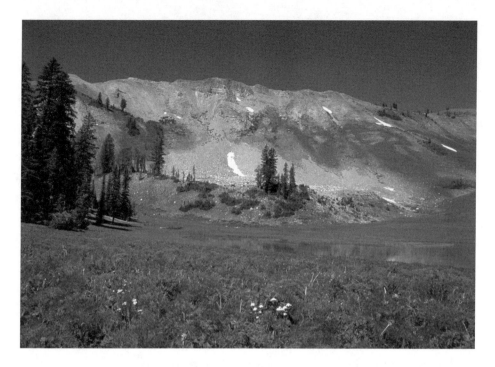

Observation Peak over pond in Lake Basin

through a sloping meadow for 300 yards to a signed junction with a trail to North Indian Creek Pass. If you want to do only a short loop, go straight and hike 7 miles down the North Indian Trail back to the road fork 1.6 miles from your car.

For the full traverse, you turn right, hop over small North Fork Indian Creek, and begin a series of little ups and downs. After climbing over a couple of low ridges, you pass a small spring, then contour across a steeply sloping meadow just below some reddish cliffs. The trail then climbs eight irregularly spaced switchbacks, which steeply gain 600 feet on a sun-exposed slope that can be uncomfortably hot on a summer afternoon. Fortunately, the trail provides great views down the deep canyon of North Fork Indian Creek, so you've got plenty of excuses for rest stops.

The trail tops out at a junction in the wide saddle of North Indian Creek Pass. The trail to the left follows the top of a high, view-packed ridge for several miles before dropping to Big Elk Creek. The first few miles of this trail make a wonderfully scenic side trip. The main trail bears slightly right and winds steeply down into the little basin at the head of South Fork Big Elk Creek. Near the top of this basin is a junction with a trail that switchbacks up to a pass on the ridge to the east. This trail is a worthwhile side trip for those who want a nice view into the vastness of Wyoming.

Your trail goes straight at the junction and traverses the steep slopes above the ever-deepening canyon of South Fork Big Elk Creek. After a little less than 1 mile, you bear left (downhill) at an unsigned fork and soon descend a set of eight well-graded switchbacks. These take you down to the meadows at the bottom of the canyon and an easy rock-hop crossing of the creek. The sketchy trail disappears just after the crossing. The correct route gains a little elevation, then turns and closely follows the west bank of the creek. After a short while the trail enters the forest and the tread becomes more obvious. About 0.5 mile below the crossing is a decent campsite in the trees on the right.

The next 3.5 miles are an easy and very attractive walk that takes you gradually downhill through a series of large meadows beside the cascading waters of South Fork Big Elk Creek.

Tip: Be sure to look behind you from time to time to enjoy excellent views over the meadows to the jagged peaks at the creek's headwaters.

About 6 miles from North Indian Creek Pass is an easy, ankle-deep ford of the creek and a sign marking a junction with an obscure trail up North Fork Big Elk Creek. You bear slightly left on the more obvious trail and soon cross North Fork Big Elk Creek on a log.

The trail now follows Big Elk Creek downstream through meadows and open forests and past willow bogs with lots of beaver activity. Look for moose in these bogs feasting on the tasty wet vegetation. Even if there aren't any moose around, you can usually count on seeing birds, which abound in this varied habitat. Mornings are particularly active, because the forest then is filled with the songs of western tanagers, American robins, white-crowned and chipping sparrows, red-breasted nuthatches, yellow and yellow-rumped warblers, various species of hummingbirds, and numerous others. After a little less than 1 mile, you come to a ford of the good-sized creek. The water is cold and about knee-deep, but it isn't very swift, so the crossing is fairly easy. As I was preparing to make this ford, a large mountain lion came sauntering by on the other side of the

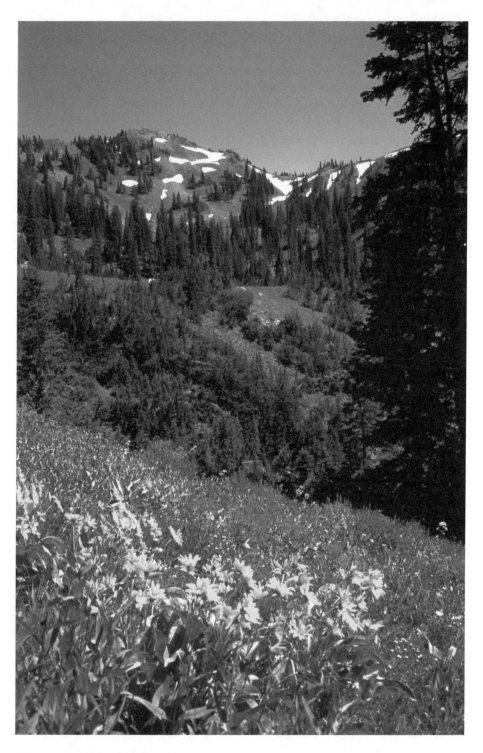

Near North Indian Creek Pass

creek. Once it caught sight of me, the lion slowly walked off into the trees and watched me cross.

Tip: Anglers might want to try their luck in Big Elk Creek, because the stream has lots of good-sized trout.

You may as well leave the wading shoes on for a while, because you'll need them a few hundred yards later, when you have to ford the creek again, and 0.5 mile after that at a third crossing. After the third crossing you can put your boots back on, because the next ford is over 1 mile away.

The trail climbs briefly from the third ford, then makes an up-and-down traverse through the forests above the canyon of Big Elk Creek. You soon come to a small meadow and a junction with a connector to the Siddoway Fork Trail, which angles downhill to the right. You bear slightly left on the more heavily used trail, then descend six switchbacks to the final and most difficult crossing of Big Elk Creek. In early summer this ford is about thigh deep and the water is quite swift, so you might want to scout around for a shallower crossing downstream. Unfortunately, there aren't any logs nearby, so there is no alternative to getting wet.

Once on the other side of the creek, you reach a signed junction with the Siddoway Fork Trail. You go left and almost immediately come to a good campsite on the bench above the creek. Just 150 yards past this campsite is another junction, where you turn right on the very faint Cabin Canyon Trail. The junction is marked only with a small brown sign that faces toward hikers coming from the other direction, so you will have to look carefully for the sign.

Warning: The rugged Cabin Canyon Trail receives little or no maintenance, so be prepared to climb over some deadfall and fight through overgrown areas. In addition to obscuring the trail, these overgrown areas have quite a few blackberries and stinging nettles, so you'll need to wear long pants. The trail's most difficult challenge comes near the head of the canyon, where the route diminishes to little more than a hypothetical dotted line on the map and forces hikers to travel cross-country to relocate the tread.

For a longer, but less challenging, alternate route, try the Austin Canyon Trail. To reach it, turn right on the Siddoway Fork Trail from the junction above the last ford of Big Elk Creek. After 1.5 miles, turn left on the Austin Canyon Trail and climb 4 miles to a junction with the Cabin Canyon Trail. This route is a little over 2 miles longer than the more direct route up Cabin Canyon, but it is easier to follow.

On the Cabin Canyon Trail you face a minor navigation problem almost immediately, as the tread disappears in a narrow, flowery meadow. To relocate the trail, simply walk northwest through the meadow and look for old blazes when you get back to the trees. Once back in the forest, the now-more-obvious tread ascends beside the dry creekbed at the bottom of the canyon past a series of talus slopes that are home to a large population of pikas. Not quite 1 mile into this climb, you cross the unsigned border and reenter Idaho.

For the next 2 miles the fairly steep climb becomes increasingly overgrown. Although the hiking is a bit tedious, you shouldn't lose the tread if you just stick to the right (northeast) side of the dry creekbed. About one third of the way up the canyon an intermittent trickle of water flows at the bottom of the creekbed, which allows you to splash water over your head and cool off on a hot afternoon.

Tip: *Fill up on water here, because this is the last water source for several very tough miles.*

From here on the climbing is almost entirely in meadows, either of tall grasses, which obscure the trail in the lower canyon, or of shorter wildflowers that dominate the upper canyon slopes. In both places shade is nonexistent, so on a hot day you'll pour out gallons of sweat.

About halfway up the canyon the trail pulls its disappearing act. The overgrown tread fades away completely in the grasses and, adding to the confusion, sketchy game paths head up almost every side canyon. The newly rerouted trail shown on the Forest Service map, which is *extremely* difficult to locate on the ground, turns left *somewhere*, goes up one of several side canyons, then climbs around the left (west) side of an unnamed high point to a junction with the Austin Canyon Trail. Since you probably won't be able to find this trail, your best bet is to go cross-country straight through the upper canyon's grassy meadows, then climb the very steep slopes on the canyon's headwall to a low notch in the ridge just to the right of a high, unnamed peak.

Once you reach the pass, the trail becomes obvious as it goes down several extremely steep switchbacks to the meadow at the bottom of Austin Canyon. You cross a small creek in this canyon, with its much needed water, and come to a cairn marking the junction with the Austin Canyon Trail, where you join the alternate route from the Siddoway Fork.

You turn left (west) and climb at a moderately steep grade for 0.5 mile to where the creek goes under a small but interesting stone arch. More climbing takes you through steep, view-packed meadows, then the trail flattens out, goes over the now-dry creekbed, and crosses to the left side of a large meadow. On the south side of the meadow is a waterless camp and a signed junction with the newly rerouted but faint Cabin Canyon Trail.

You turn right at the junction and gradually climb through meadows and past a few groves of subalpine firs toward the impressive, tan-colored cliffs at the head of Austin Canyon. The trail disappears in these upper meadows, but you can find it again if you angle right and look for an obvious trail that goes up the steep slopes on the north headwall. The last 0.5 mile climbs very steeply up a shadeless slope of loose rocks to a junction in a pass with a good view north down Dry Canyon. The trail to the right follows Dry Canyon to Upper Palisades Lake and is a pleasant shortcut, especially if the weather has turned bad. If you take that trail, however, you will miss Waterfall Canyon, one of the highlights of the trip, so I recommend that you turn left.

After the long climb to the pass, you were probably looking forward to some downhill. But you'll have to put those hopes on hold for a little while longer, because first the trail steeply climbs along the top of a ridge. After gaining another 300 feet, the trail finally tops out on a side ridge and makes a long downhill traverse. At the bottom of this traverse are two switchbacks just before you enter a basin directly beneath a unnamed, pyramid-shaped mountain. In early summer a tiny snowmelt creek flows out of this basin, providing water for a scenic campsite.

The faint trail goes several hundred yards across the basin, then steeply ascends the ridge to the south. It is possible, and fairly easy, to avoid this climb by leaving the trail and rambling to the west across rolling meadows for about 1 mile until you hit the Waterfall Canyon Trail. But if you do that, you will miss perhaps the best views of the trip. So take the sketchy trail to the top of the ridge, then drop your pack and gawk. The high peak to the south is 10,025-foot Mt. Baird, the tallest summit in this area. To the southwest you can see a part of large Palisades Reservoir, while to the northwest is

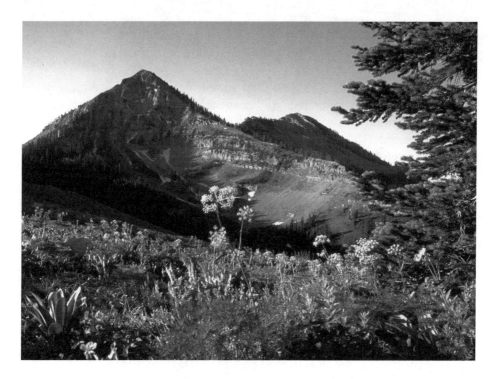

Mt. Baird from the north

a rolling, grassy basin at the head of Waterfall Canyon. On a *really* clear day you can even see the jagged Teton Range in the distance to the northeast. As if the views weren't enough, the flowers on this high ridge are also outstanding. The peak bloom, in mid-July, features a colorful collage of blue larkspur, pink vetch and geranium, white wild carrot, red paintbrush, and yellow balsamroot.

The official trail descends a short distance, then turns right and climbs back up the south side of the ridge. But there's no need for you to lose this elevation, because it's just as easy, and more scenic, to simply turn right and walk along the open, view-packed ridge-line for several hundred yards until you meet the official trail angling up from the left. Shortly after this, you go straight at a signed junction with the Little Elk Trail and make a moderately graded downhill traverse to the rolling basin at the head of Waterfall Canyon.

The trail wanders down through this delightful basin, which has lots of flowers and excellent views of the surrounding peaks and ridges. You soon pass an easily overlooked junction with an abandoned trail, then exit the basin via six gently graded switch-backs through a pleasant mix of forest and small meadows.

Tip: *Quiet hikers stand a good chance of seeing deer and elk in this area.*

After these switchbacks, you follow a dry creekbed (the water flows underground) past a pair of seasonal waterfalls, then make seven more downhill switchbacks. When the trail levels out, you cross the rocky creekbed twice, then enter a large meadow that holds a small lake. The highlight of the scenery here is a tall water-fall that emerges from a cave high on the canyon's east wall and drops several hundred feet in a series of cascades to the lake. It's quite impressive and dramatically demonstrates how Waterfall Canyon got its name. There are some very good campsites at the north end of the lake, although they tend to be quite buggy.

Immediately below the lake, the water goes back underground, so you are left to follow a dry creekbed once again as you gradual-ly descend through meadows and forested areas. Things get steep-er when you come to the edge of an old glacial basin and descend eight well-graded switchbacks past an unseen spring on your left. At the bottom of the switchbacks the trail lazily descends through a forested area with lots of huckleberries to a horse camp and a log over the clear creek that drains misnamed Dry Canyon. About 100 yards later is a junction with the Dry Canyon Trail.

You bear left, walk past some silvery snags in an old burn area, then make your way around the northeast shore of long Upper Palisades Lake. This deep subalpine lake was created when a large landslide blocked the canyon and streams filled the basin behind the slide. The lake is a fairly popular goal for both hikers and eques-trians, in part because it has good fishing for cutthroat trout (although it can be hard to get to the fish without a boat). There are several camps above the lake's inlet and near the outlet, but else-where the lakeside slopes are too steep for camping. Unfortunately, all the best campsites smell badly of horses. When you get to the lake's landslide dam, you will no doubt note that there is no outlet flowing over the dam. Instead, the water emerges from a large spring partway down the ancient landslide.

From Upper Palisades Lake, you lose almost 400 feet in lazy switchbacks, then come to a junction just before an unstable log bridge over Palisades Creek. You turn left, cross the bridge, then climb about 100 feet up the opposite bank and turn to the left (downstream). About 0.5 mile from the bridge is a small log cabin and a junction at the mouth of Chicken Spring Canyon. To reach the spacious designated camping area at Chicken Spring, walk 100 yards downstream from the cabin, then cross Palisades Creek on a log bridge to the camp.

If you are not going to the camping area, continue straight beside the creek. There are several little ups and downs along the way, as the trail follows the lazy stream for 1 mile to willow-lined Lower Palisades Lake, which is a good place to fish and watch for moose. At the southwest end of this lake is a sturdy bridge over the lake's rushing outlet creek and a good-sized camp area near a junction with the Lake Canyon Trail.

You can expect crowds from here on, because the trail from Lower Palisades Lake to Palisades Creek Campground is very popular with dayhikers, weekend backpackers, and equestrians. Although the people are almost always friendly, the horses leave behind smelly souvenirs in the form of an entire orchard's worth of horse apples in the middle of the trail. Surprisingly, despite all the pounding it receives, the trail has very little of the dust and erosion commonly associated with popular horse trails.

From the Lake Canyon junction, you descend a half dozen gentle switchbacks, then make three bridged crossings of cascading Palisades Creek as it snakes through a scenic, steep-walled gorge. After the third bridge the trail stays in the trees above the creek's north bank and travels past a series of scenic cliffs and rock outcroppings in a narrow canyon. Near the bottom of the canyon you enter a noticeably drier vegetation zone, where scattered Douglas-firs, bushy Rocky Mountain maples, and twisted Rocky Mountain junipers are added to the mix of trees. About 1 mile after a final bridged crossing of the creek, the trail skirts the left side of Palisades Creek Campground to the spacious trailhead.

POSSIBLE ITINERARY

	Camp	Miles	Elevation Gain
Day 1	Lake Basin	9	3300
Day 2	Upper Canyon of South Fork Big Elk Creek	9	1900
Day 3	Big Elk Creek (at last ford)	8	400
Day 4	Lake in Waterfall Canyon	10	3900
Day 5	Out	9	300

VARIATIONS There are hundreds of miles of interconnected trails in the Snake River Range, so you can design a trip of almost any length to fit your schedule. The best short option is to make a two- or three-day loop that goes up South Fork Indian Creek and comes back via North Fork Indian Creek. If you have an extra day, add a side trip to the viewpoint atop Observation Peak.

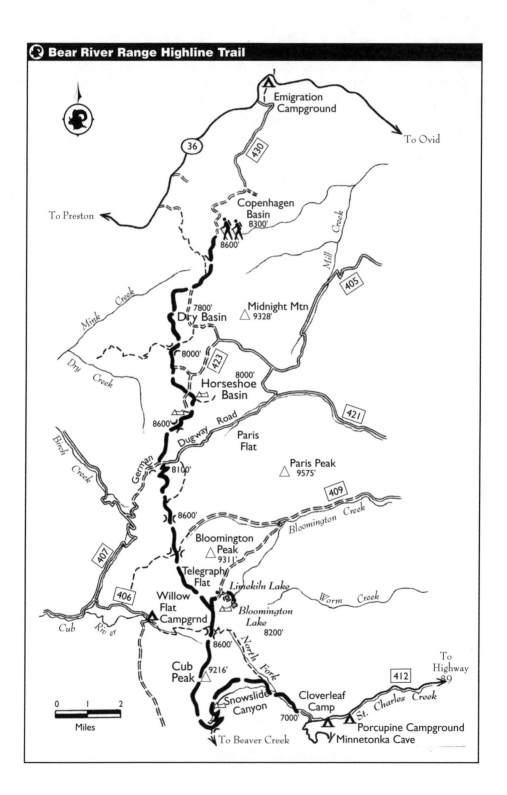

Bear River Range Highline Trail

To Ovid

Emigration Campground

36

430

405

To Preston

Copenhagen Basin
8300'

8600'

Mill Creek

Mink Creek

7800'
Dry Basin

Midnight Mtn
9328'

Dry Creek

8000'

423

8000'
Horseshoe Basin

421

8600'

Dugway Road

Paris Flat

Birch Creek

German

8100'

Paris Peak
9575'

409

8600'

Bloomington Creek

407

Bloomington Peak
9311'

Telegraph Flat

Limekiln Lake

Worm Creek

406

Willow Flat Campgrnd

Bloomington Lake
8200'

Cub River

8600'

North Fork

Cub Peak
9216'

Snowslide Canyon

Cloverleaf Camp

St. Charles Creek

412

To Highway 89

7000'

Porcupine Campground

To Beaver Creek

Minnetonka Cave

0   1   2
Miles

24 Bear River Range Highline Trail

RATINGS (1–10)			MILES	ELEVATION GAIN	DAYS	SHUTTLE MILEAGE
Scenery	Solitude	Difficulty	25*	2800	3-4	37
8	7	5				

* The distance may be slightly longer for the hike, and shorter for the car shuttle, depending on how far you can drive on the access road to the north trailhead.

MAPS USGS - Egan Basin, Midnight Mountain, Paris Peak.

USUALLY OPEN Late June to October.

BEST Late June to mid-July for flowers; late September and early October for fall colors.

PERMITS None.

RULES The usual no-trace principles apply.

CONTACT Montpelier Ranger District, (208) 847-0375.

SPECIAL ATTRACTIONS Fine views; exceptional wildflower displays in from late June to mid-July; fall colors.

PROBLEMS Very limited water and campsites; mosquitoes in July; motorbikes along the entire trail.

HOW TO GET THERE From Montpelier, drive 6 miles southwest on U.S. Highway 89 to the tiny crossroads town of Ovid. To reach the exit point at the south trailhead, continue 11.3 miles south on Highway 89 to a well-signed junction with St. Charles Canyon Road. Turn right (west), following signs for Minnetonka Cave, and drive 8.2 miles on this paved road, which becomes Forest Road 412, to a junction 0.1 mile past Cloverleaf Campground. Turn right onto Forest Road 716 and drive 0.2 mile on this narrow gravel road to the trailhead parking lot.

To reach the recommended starting point, return to Ovid and turn left (west) on State Highway 36. Drive 12.2 miles northwest to an unsigned junction 0.2 mile west of the pass at the summit of the Bear River Range. Turn left (south) on a paved road and proceed 200 yards toward a large snowpark lot, then bear right on a dirt road. This bumpy road steeply climbs for 2 miles, then it levels off and gets increasingly rough. Unless you're driving a jeep or a high-clearance SUV, you should pull off the road and park in this area. About 3.5 miles from Highway 36, you bear right at a fork and go through the huge meadow in Copenhagen Basin, which is covered with countless millions of white bistort blossoms in early July. About 1.5 extremely rough miles from the fork, the road ends at a trailhead sign. There is very limited parking here, but it doesn't really matter, since you probably weren't able to drive this far anyway.

INTRODUCTION The Bear River Range, a northern extension of Utah's famous Wasatch Range, forms the western boundary of popular Bear Lake Basin. Since the lower slopes of these mountains are crowded with lakeside resorts and recreation homes, it is surprising that so few people hike this range's scenic trails. After all, the Bear River Range has plenty of attractions, including view-packed ridges, open forests, and flowered-covered meadows. You'll find plenty of dayhiking options, but for backpackers the best extended trip is the Highline Trail, which samples all of the diverse pleasures this range has to offer.

The most famous attraction in the Bear River Range is Minnetonka Cave. Caves like Minnetonka are typical of areas – the Bear River Range is one – with karst topography. The rock here is mostly limestone, which, unlike granite, allows water to filter down from the surface, slowly dissolving the rock as it goes. Once it gets to the cave, the dripping water deposits dissolved minerals to form stalactites and stalagmites. For hikers, the most important consequence of this geology is that when most of the water filters down from the surface, it leaves very little of that precious commodity above ground. As a result, there are very few lakes and streams to provide water to thirsty hikers. You should carry a minimum of three quarts from the trailhead and a lot more if you plan a dry camp for the first night – which is often a necessity.

> **Tip:** The trail is best done from north to south, because that way you benefit from a net elevation loss of approximately 1600 feet.

DESCRIPTION The Highline Trail starts as a jeep track amid lovely meadows that are framed with stands of lodgepole pine, Engelmann spruce, and white fir. The last species is found almost nowhere else in Idaho. After just 100 yards, you turn onto an obvious trail that leaves the jeep track and veers left into the trees. This trail soon enters a large, sloping meadow, which features a wide variety of colorful, July-blooming wildflowers. Of particular interest is a unique type of white columbine with unusually large blossoms that are both conspicuous and beautiful. This open meadow also has

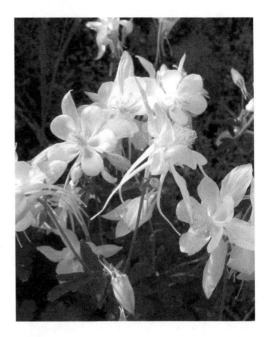

White Columbine

some excellent vistas, both south along the rolling Bear River Range and west to the farmlands around Preston.

> *Warning:* Strangely, even with so little surface water, in early July the mosquitoes can be fierce in these mountains.

Shortly after entering the meadow, you ignore an unsigned motorbike track that angles in from the right, then gradually descend across open slopes to a signed junction with the Snow Hollow Trail. The scenic ridgetop here is carpeted with wildflowers, especially blue lupine and yellow balsamroot, which make colorful foregrounds for some great photographs of the rolling Bear River Range. You go straight at the junction and descend about 400 feet on a wide and often dusty ATV track to the edge of mostly forested Dry Basin and a junction with a jeep road.

You bear right, following a small, brown sign that says simply TRAIL, and travel mostly on the level past a delightful series of rock-garden meadows and a few less appealing logging scars. The trail descends through a sloping meadow ringed by quaking aspens and goes up and down for 2 miles through forests and brushy meadows to a junction with the Dry Basin Trail. You bear slightly right and climb a short distance back to the scenic ridgetop.

At the top of the ridge is an unsigned junction with an obscure trail down Dry Creek. You turn left, gradually climb near the top of the ridge for 0.5 mile, then contour across the west side of the divide on a partly forested slope, which is often covered with thousands of white columbines. At the end of the traverse you come to an open saddle, where your trail is crossed by an old jeep track. Go straight and hike gently up and down for 1 mile to a small, metal-roofed shack on the edge of an expansive meadow called Horseshoe Basin.

The trail crosses a primitive jeep road in this basin, then goes 200 yards up a woodsy side canyon to a stagnant pond. This pond dries up by about late July, but it's the first water on the trip, and it is usually also the *last* water you'll see for another 7 miles. Before drinking the water, I strongly recommend that you treat it *twice*, first by either boiling or iodine, then by filtering it to remove the silt and particulate matter. If you want to play it safe, carry enough water from the trailhead to make a dry camp. There are some decent campsites in the trees near the pond.

About 100 yards past the pond is a junction with a motorbike trail, which is not shown on either the Forest Service or the USGS maps. You veer right, climb over a minor ridge, then go briefly downhill and curve to the left. Shortly after the trail starts to climb again, an unmarked, 100-yard side trail drops to the right to a lovely little meadow with a very pleasant campsite. In early summer there is sometimes a shallow, murky pond on the far side of this meadow (but don't count on it).

 Minnetonka Cave

Minnetonka Cave, a spectacular underground cavern filled with delicate stalactites and stalagmites, is visited by thousands of awestruck tourists every year. Discovered by a grouse hunter in 1907, the cave is now administered by the Forest Service. Since it's only a couple of miles from the south trailhead, interested hikers might want to take the 90-minute, half-mile tour after completing their hike. Guided tours run daily from June to September and they are well worth the relatively modest price. For more information call: (435) 245-4422.

The Highline Trail makes a looping traverse up a forested hillside, then passes two small, grassy basins, which in any other mountain range would almost certainly have water. Here they have only waving grasses and flowers. A short additional climb takes you up to a ridgeline.

The next mile is an especially appealing walk through flower-covered meadows near the top of a ridge with nice vistas to the southeast over the grassy expanse of Paris Flat. Halfway along this section is a saddle, where the trail angles left and makes a long downhill traverse. The descent is steep at first, but then it becomes quite gradual as you cross a sloping meadow liberally covered with picturesque quaking aspens. The trail splits near the bottom of the traverse under a set of powerlines. Bear left and almost immediately come to rough German Dugway Road.

You turn left, walk 20 yards along the road, then turn right onto a dusty trail that is badly churned up by motorbikes. The trail makes one uphill switchback, then gradually winds its way up through open forest and sloping meadows. As usual, there is absolutely no water on this climb, despite the fact that you will probably see a few lingering snowfields on the ridge above the trail in July. A little over 0.5 mile from the road you come to a pretty little basin where an unsigned motorbike trail joins from the left. You go straight, then ascend steeply through forests to a high, grassy saddle just below the crest of the Bear River Range. This is a good spot to rest, have a snack, and enjoy the view southeast to lofty Bloomington Peak.

Tip: For even better views, wander up the open slopes on either side of the pass to the windy summits of two small knolls.

For much of the remainder of the trip the trail goes along a beautiful open ridge, which features flowery meadows, stands of spire-shaped subalpine firs, and great views. The route stays close to the ridgecrest, so you can see not only up and down the Bear River Range, but also west to the relatively dry Bear River Valley and east to the shimmering, turquoise waters of Bear Lake. This easy, beautiful, and inspiring stroll is one of the best ridge walks in Idaho.

About 1.5 miles from the pass is a poorly signed, four-way junction in another saddle with fine views. The large meadow below you to the southeast is Telegraph Flat, but the more interesting view is southeast to the rugged walls encircling the basin of Bloomington Lake. You go straight at the junction and hike 2 very scenic miles to a signed junction with the trail to Bloomington Lake.

Two factors will compel you to make the side trip to Bloomington Lake. The first is the impressive setting of the lake and a natural desire to see it up close. The second is that the lake is a permanent source of water and has good campsites nearby, both of which are extremely rare in these mountains. So turn sharply left, descend about 350 feet to a remote trailhead at the end of a rough dirt road, then walk 400 yards along this road to the signed Bloomington Lake trailhead on your right. This short trail makes a brief climb, splits to form a loop around a shallow, seasonal body of water called Limekiln Lake, then passes a small pond and comes to Bloomington Lake.

Shimmering Bloomington Lake sits beneath a semi-circle of craggy cliffs and is a great place to swim, fish, or just relax and enjoy the view. In recent years beavers have dammed the outlet creek, raising the lake's water level and flooding the angler's path around the shore. The Forest Service recently prohibited camping in the area immediately around the lake. Instead, they recommend that people camp southwest of the Bloomington Lake trailhead.

After returning to the Highline Trail, you continue south and resume the spectacular ridge walk along the crest of the Bear River Range. The trail traverses the west side of a high point, then drops to a saddle where a large cairn marks a four-way junction. If you want to shorten the trip, turn left and descend 4 miles on the pleasant North St. Charles Trail to the south trailhead.

For the longer and more scenic route, go straight at the four-way junction and resume the gorgeous, up-and-down ridge hike. The remaining ridge walk is about 3 miles long, but the excellent scenery will make it seem like a lot less. The route never strays very far from the top of the divide, so the views in all directions are superb. The beauty at your feet is a match for the distant views, with an abundance of colorful early summer wildflowers. The most common varieties are cinquefoil, wild carrot, lupine, pink geranium, skyrocket gilia, and sulfurflower. Distracted by all this fine scenery, you will barely notice as the trail climbs high on the slopes of Cub Peak, then gradually descends to a low saddle and a signed junction with the Snowslide Trail.

Tip: Quiet hikers may see both deer and elk in this area.

You turn left and descend four switchbacks to a partly forested basin at the head of Snowslide Canyon. Surprisingly, you'll find a creek in Snowslide Canyon, the first reliable running water on this entire trip. Just downstream from where you cross this trickling creek is a comfortable campsite at the edge of a small meadow choked with bluebells and false hellebore.

You briefly follow the tiny creek, then contour across a partly forested hillside through thickets of quaking aspen trees and ceonothus bushes. After splashing across the second of two spring-fed creeks, you make a gradual, 1-mile descent to a junction with the North St. Charles Trail. You bear slightly right and follow this wide, gently graded, and dusty trail to a bridge over Snowslide Creek and, shortly thereafter, a bridge across North Fork St. Charles Creek. You pass through a gate, and then, about 1 mile after the first crossing, come to a second bridge over North Fork St. Charles Creek. Just 300 yards later is the south trailhead and your car.

Tip: North Fork St. Charles Creek has good trout fishing.

POSSIBLE ITINERARY

	Camp	Miles	Elevation Gain
Day 1	Upper Horseshoe Basin	8	500
Day 2	Bloomington Lake	8.5	1400
Day 3	Out	8.5	900

VARIATIONS If you don't mind doing a fair amount of road walking, consider hiking all 55 miles of the Highline Trail from Beaver Creek, near the Utah border, to Soda Point, at the north end of the range. Unfortunately, the road access to these remote trailheads is long, rough, and complicated.

For a shorter version of the trip, start at the south trailhead, climb Snowslide Canyon, then turn north and walk along the ridge to Bloomington Lake. On day two, make a dayhike along the very scenic ridge that goes north from Bloomington Lake, turning back whenever you feel you've seen enough. You can then return to your car via the shorter trail down North Fork St. Charles Creek.

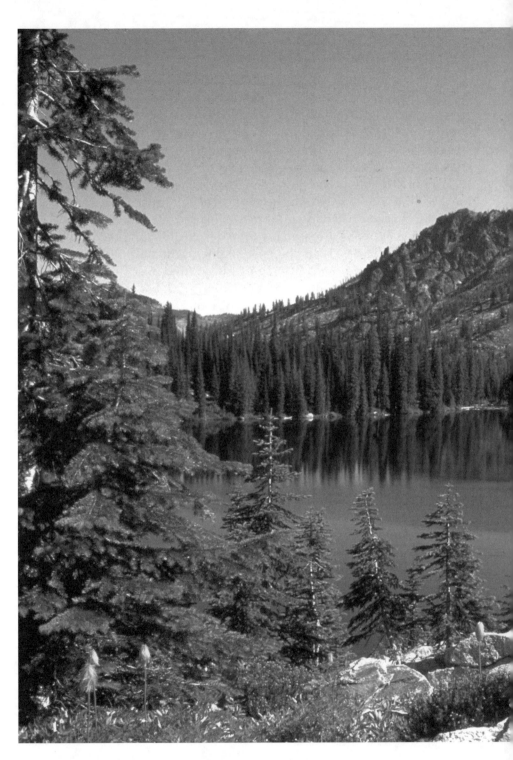

296   *Lloyd Lake, Selway Crags Trip 26*

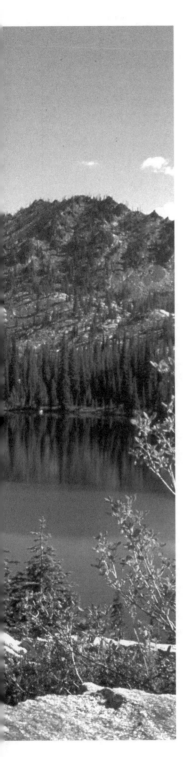

Other Backpacking Trips

Although this book highlights my choices for the best long backpacking trips in Idaho, there are many other options for the adventurous backpacker. With some creativity and a good set of topographic maps, a backpacker could spend a lifetime exploring the mountains, canyons, and deserts of this state.

What follows is an overview of some additional recommended trips, with just enough description to whet the appetite.

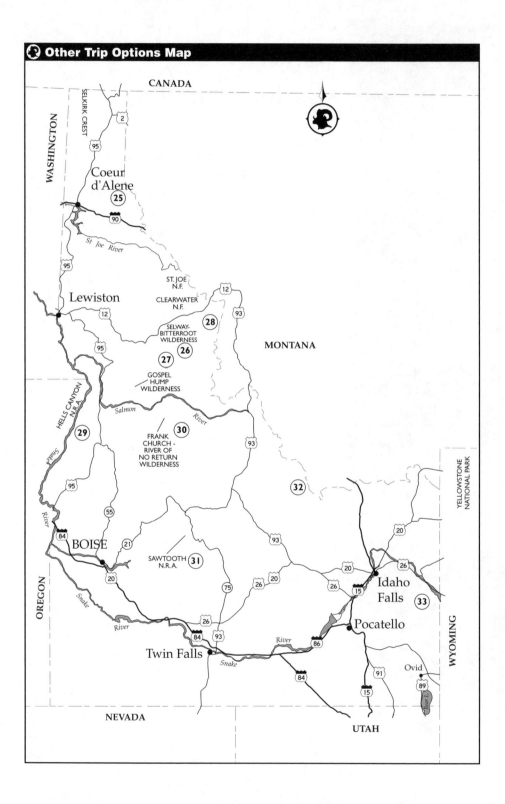

25 Coeur-d'Alene River Trail

RATINGS (1–10)			MILES	DAYS
Scenery	Solitude	Difficulty	14	2-3
6	5	3		

MAPS USGS - Cathedral Peak, Jordon Creek.

USUALLY OPEN May to October.

BEST Mid-May to October.

SPECIAL ATTRACTIONS Good fishing; early-season hiking.

PROBLEMS The trail generally stays well above the river, so hikers must bushwhack to get to the water.

For most of its length, the Coeur-d'Alene River is a tame stream that flows lazily through bottomlands where it is closely followed by roads. Near its headwaters, however, the river runs swift and wild through a scenic, forested canyon. A pleasant, 14-mile trail parallels this section of the river, with only one brief interruption by a logging road. The trail gives backpackers a wonderful introduction to one of the state's best fly-fishing streams, without the crowds found elsewhere on the river. But even if you aren't an angler, this relatively easy trail is worth hiking for the excellent canyon scenery. The stream is managed as a catch-and-release fishery; barbless hooks are required.

26 Selway Crags

RATINGS (1–10)			MILES	DAYS
Scenery	Solitude	Difficulty	Var	Var
8	5	4		

MAP USFS - Selway-Bitterroot Wilderness - North Half.

USUALLY OPEN July to October.

BEST Mid-to-late July.

SPECIAL ATTRACTIONS High, craggy, granite peaks; cirque lakes.

PROBLEMS Mosquitoes in July.

This is a relatively popular hike into one of the most scenic parts of Selway-Bitterroot Wilderness. The Selway Crags feature classic mountain scenery with dozens of beautiful lakes tucked into glacial cirques amid a small group of granite peaks. There are two possible approaches to the area. The shorter and easier trail starts from Big Fog Saddle, at the end of a rugged, narrow, and steep dirt road that climbs from the Selway River Road near the Selway Falls Guard Station. The other trail is longer and much more tiring, but it starts from a good paved road, U.S. Highway 12 along the Lochsa River. Whichever route you choose, once you reach the Selway Crags, the best plan is to set up a base camp and spend several days exploring the area's many lakes and viewpoints. The Cove Lakes are the most popular choice for a base camp, but other nearby lakes, some off-trail, provide better scenery and more solitude.

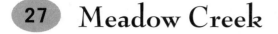

27 Meadow Creek

RATINGS (1–10)			MILES	DAYS
Scenery	Solitude	Difficulty	Var	Var
5	8	5		

MAP USFS - Selway-Bitterroot Wilderness - South Half.

USUALLY OPEN Late June to October.

BEST Late June to October.

SPECIAL ATTRACTIONS Good fishing; wildlife.

PROBLEMS Long car shuttle if done as a one-way hike.

Meadow Creek flows out of an unprotected roadless area west of Selway-Bitterroot Wilderness. The scenery is relatively subdued, with forested ridges on either side of the creek providing pleasant if not spectacular views. The main attractions are fishing, which is excellent, and abundant wildlife. A good trail starts near the Selway River and parallels Meadow Creek for about half the stream's length. Once the trail leaves the creek, you can either loop back to Indian Hill Lookout on view-packed ridge trails to the north and east, or make a one-way trip by going south to Red River Hot Springs. The latter exit gives you the chance to soak in the soothing hot water before making the dusty drive back to civilization.

28 Big Sand Creek – Hidden Peak Loop

RATINGS (1–10)			MILES	DAYS
Scenery	Solitude	Difficulty	30	3-5
7	7	6		

MAP USFS - Selway-Bitterroot Wilderness - North Half.

USUALLY OPEN Mid-July to October.

BEST Late July.

SPECIAL ATTRACTIONS Good fishing; wildlife.

PROBLEMS Mosquitoes in July; bumpy access road.

This scenic loop explores the remote northeast corner of Selway-Bitterroot Wilderness and includes an excellent sampling of the wilderness's best attributes – lovely forests, quiet lakes, and clear streams. Not-to-be-missed side trips lead to glorious viewpoints atop Diablo Mountain and Hidden Peak, each of which sports a fire lookout. The trail starts from bumpy Forest Road 360 south of Powell and makes a long loop via Horse Heaven Meadows, Big Sand Creek, and Hidden Creek.

29 Southern Seven Devils Mountains

RATINGS (1–10)			MILES	DAYS
Scenery	Solitude	Difficulty	24	3-5
7	7	6		

MAP USFS - Hells Canyon National Recreation Area.

USUALLY OPEN July to October.

BEST July.

SPECIAL ATTRACTIONS High, craggy, peaks; cirque lakes; solitude.

PROBLEMS Mosquitoes in July; rough road access.

Although not as well known as the loop through the northern Seven Devils Mountains (Trip 8), the southern Seven Devils have a wonderful loop trail of their own with similarly grand scenery. This trip starts at remote Black Lake Campground, at the end of a long, rough dirt road from the town of Council. From here, most hikers head west to Six Lake Basin, but to do the loop, you go north past beautiful Emerald Lake, then circle east around the craggy towers of Monument Peak and Black Imp. Excellent side trips lead to spectacular Ruth Lake and well-named Crystal Lake, the latter requiring a cross-county scramble.

30 Big Creek

RATINGS (1–10)			MILES	DAYS
Scenery	Solitude	Difficulty	26	3-5
6	5	3	(one way)	

MAP USFS - Frank Church-River of No Return Wilderness - North.

USUALLY OPEN April to October.

BEST Late June to October.

SPECIAL ATTRACTIONS Excellent fishing; good canyon scenery.

PROBLEMS Hot weather in midsummer; difficult transportation logistics.

Beginning from the alternate trailhead for Trip 10, this is an easy, extended walk along the entire length of Big Creek, a first-class fishing stream that knifes through the heart of Frank Church-River of No Return Wilderness. In addition to fishing, hikers can gawk at the canyon scenery and watch the abundant wildlife. Snow usually blocks the road to the upper trailhead until late June or early July, so even though the lower parts of this trail are open as early as April, accessing the trail at that time requires either taking a long float trip down the Middle Fork Salmon River or hiring a bush plane to fly you into a remote airstrip.

After hiking downstream to the mouth of Big Creek, you face the prospect of either going back the way you came or finding another way out. Some people elect to make the long hike out on the relatively easy Middle Fork Salmon River Trail (see Trip 13). Others opt for the shorter but much more difficult Waterfall Trail, which makes a tortuous climb out of the canyon and exits through the Bighorn Crags to the east (see Trip 11). For a change of pace, you can also arrange to be picked up by a bush plane or float back to civilization on a raft. Both options are fun but rather expensive.

31　Smoky Mountains Loop

RATINGS (1–10)			MILES	DAYS
Scenery	Solitude	Difficulty	Var	4-6
7	8	6		

MAPS USGS - Baker Peak, Frenchman Creek, Galena, Paradise Peak.

USUALLY OPEN Late June to October.

BEST July.

SPECIAL ATTRACTIONS Solitude; wildflowers.

PROBLEMS Motorcycles are allowed on some trails.

Although they are located relatively close to Idaho's largest population centers, the Smoky Mountains remain unknown to most Idaho outdoor lovers. In almost every way, these rolling, forested mountains are overshadowed by the neighboring Sawtooth Range. Unlike the Sawtooths, the Smokys have almost no lakes and few spectacular peaks. But even though they fall short in these important qualities, that doesn't mean they deserve to be ignored. Open forests, extensive views, colorful wildflowers, and solitude are more than enough to make a trip here worthwhile. For proof, try any of several possible loops that start from the Big Smoky Guard Station north of Fairfield. Probably the best trip goes up Smoky and Big Peak creeks all the way to scenic Baker Lake, which is about the only location in these mountains that sees many hikers. From there, you circle back to the north and west via Royal Gorge, West Fork Big Smoky Creek, and Skillern Creek to your starting point.

Tip: A side trip from Skillern Creek to tiny Paradise Lake is well worth your time.

32　Continental Divide Trail

RATINGS (1–10)			MILES	DAYS
Scenery	Solitude	Difficulty	57-85	5-9
7	6	7		

MAPS USGS - Bannock Pass, Deadman Lake, Deadman Pass, Eighteenmile Peak, Morrison Lake, Tepee Mountain. (Unfortunately, the recently completed trail sections are not shown on these USGS maps.)

USUALLY OPEN Late June to October.

BEST Late June (to avoid the cows).

SPECIAL ATTRACTIONS Great views; lovely mountain scenery.

PROBLEMS Some walking on primitive roads and incomplete trails; cows are allowed to graze in the high meadows in July.

Once complete, the Continental Divide Trail will go 3200 miles through America's Rocky Mountains from Mexico to Canada. Only a small section of this classic trail is in Idaho, where it travels through the Centennial and Bitterroot mountains along the border with Montana. Some of the trail is still under construction, so hikers occasionally have to walk on primitive roads or travel cross-country. Construction is complete, however, on one particularly attractive section, where you can enjoy some great scenery.

Start at Bannack Pass, northwest of Dubois, and travel north through the Beaverhead Mountains to the recommended exit point at Bannock Pass (it's pronounced the same, but spelled differently). If you want more exercise, continue north from Bannock Pass to Lemhi Pass, where Lewis and Clark first crossed the Continental Divide. Don't miss the side trip into the ruggedly beautiful Italian Peaks, not far from the starting point.

33 Caribou Mountains

RATINGS (1–10)			MILES	DAYS
Scenery	Solitude	Difficulty	Var	Var
6	7	6		

MAPS USGS - Commissary Ridge, Palisades Dam, Red Ridge.

USUALLY OPEN Late June to October.

BEST July; late September.

SPECIAL ATTRACTIONS Excellent fall colors; solitude.

PROBLEMS Lots of hunters in October; many trails are open to motor-bikes.

There are many miles of interconnected trails in the Caribou Mountains southeast of Idaho Falls, and a hiker could spend several weeks happily traveling all of them. Those efforts would be especially rewarding in the fall, when the maples, willows, cottonwoods, and quaking aspens turn the hillsides into a colorful palette of yellow, red, and orange. The scenery is more subdued than in the nearby Snake River Range to the east, but wildlife is more abundant here and, except for hunters, people are few. No one trail is better than another, but most hikers start at the Bear Creek trailhead near Palisades Dam and select from any of several possible loops to viewpoints atop Red Peak and Deadhorse Ridge.

THE WILDERNESS SOCIETY

The Idaho office of The Wilderness Society works to protect wilderness and wildlife through public education, scientific analysis and advocacy. Its goal is to ensure that future generations will enjoy the clean air and water, wildlife, beauty, and opportunities for recreation and renewal that pristine forests, rivers, deserts and mountains provide.

The Idaho office is working with local conservation groups and citizens to include additional Idaho areas in the National Wilderness system so they will be protected forever. For more information on how you can help, or to make a donation contact:

The Wilderness Society
2600 Rose Hill, Ste. 201
Boise, ID 83705
208/343-8153
208/343-8184 (Fax)
id_office@tws.org

Index

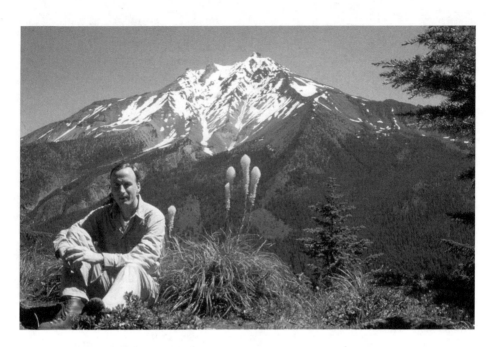

ABOUT THE AUTHOR

Doug Lorain claims that as a youngster he was frequently told to "take a hike" and that eventually he decided to take this advice to heart. Much of the more than 35 years he has lived in the Northwest has been spent hiking the trails and backcountry of Oregon, Washington, and Idaho. Spurred by an unquenchable thirst for new trails to explore and a great enthusiasm for backpacking, he has now hiked over 25,000 miles through every corner of the American Northwest and many thousands more in other western states and Canadian provinces. Despite a history that includes being charged by a grizzly bear, bitten by a rattlesnake, shot at by a hunter, and donating gallons of blood to mosquitoes, Doug claims that he wouldn't trade one moment of it, because he has also been blessed to see some of the most beautiful scenery on Earth.

His earlier books for Wilderness Press include *Afoot & Afield Portland/Vancouver* and *Backpacking Oregon* and *Backpacking Washington*. His photos have appeared in numerous magazines, calendars, and scenic books and have been used to illustrate all five of his guidebooks.

Backpacking Books from Wilderness Press

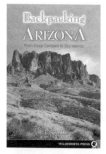

Backpacking Arizona
32 of the best backpacking trips in Arizona, from easy overnighters to 10-day challenges. Trips in the Colorado Plateau (including Grand Canyon), Rim Country (Mogollon Rim, Mazatzal, and Superstition mountains) and Sky Islands (Galiuro, Chiricahua, and Santa Rita mountain ranges), plus more.
ISBN 0-89997-324-8

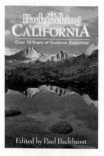

Backpacking California
Compendium of the best California backpacking adventures with 62 trips by 17 Wilderness Press authors. Trips range from one night to two weeks in the Coast Ranges, Sierra Nevada, Cascades, and Warner Mountains.
ISBN 0-89997-286-1

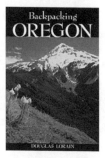

Backpacking Oregon
The most intriguing backpacking trips along the Oregon Coast, through the Columbia gorge, atop the High Cascades, Klamath, Siskiyou, Blue and Wallowa mountains, and into Hells Canyon. Adventures range from a weekend to over a week in length
ISBN 0-89997-252-7

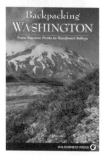

Backpacking Washington
Top backpack trips sample the diversity of Washington's finest natural areas on the Olympic Coast, Mt. Rainier, Mt. St. Helens, Pasayten and Salmo Priest wildernesses, and North Cascades.
ISBN 0-89997-272-1

For ordering information, contact your local bookseller or Wilderness Press, www.wildernesspress.com